Mental Hospitali

MENTAL HOSPITALIZATION
Myths and Facts
about a National Crisis

CHARLES A. KIESLER
AMY E. SIBULKIN

To Kevin and Eric Kiesler
—CAK

To my parents
—AES

For information address:

SAGE Publications, Inc.
2111 West Hillcrest Drive
Newbury Park, California 91320

SAGE Publications Inc. SAGE Publications Ltd.
275 South Beverly Drive 28 Banner Street
Beverly Hills London EC1Y 8QE
California 90212 England

SAGE PUBLICATIONS India Pvt. Ltd.
M-32 Market
Greater Kailash I
New Delhi 110 048 India

Printed in the United States of America

Library of Congress Cataloging-in-Publication Data

Kiesler, Charles A., 1934-
  Mental hospitalization.
  Bibliography: p.
  1. Psychiatric hospitals—United States—Utilization. 2. Psychiatric hospitals—United States—Length of stay. 3. Psychiatric hospital care—Economic aspects—United States. 4. Mental health policy—United States. I. Sibulkin, Amy E. II. Title. [DNLM: 1. Deinstitutionalization—trends—United States. 2. Health Policy—trends—United States. 3. Hospitalization—trends—United States. 4. Hospitals, Psychiatric—trends—United States. 5. Mental Disorders—therapy. WM 35 K47m]
  RC443.K54 1987   362.2'1'0973   86-15571
  ISBN 0-8039-2878-5

Table of Contents

Acknowledgments 7

SECTION I 9

Chapter 1. The Problem 11
Chapter 2. The History of Mental Hospitalization 27

SECTION II Trends in Hospitalization for Mental Disorders: A Reanalysis of National Data 41

Chapter 3. Current Trends in the Annual Number of Inpatient
         Psychiatric Episodes 46
Chapter 4. Episodic Rate of Mental Hospitalization 70
Chapter 5. Trends in Length of Stay per Psychiatric Episode 83
Chapter 6. Trends in the Proportion of Total Hospital Days That Are
         for Mental Health Care 104
Chapter 7. Nursing Homes and Deinstitutionalization 114
Chapter 8. Readmissions 131

SECTION III Attempts to Treat the Hospitalized and Hospitalizable 147

Chapter 9. Alternative Treatment: Noninstitutionalization 152
Chapter 10. Deinstitutionalization and the Problems of Subsequent
         Treatment, Chronicity, and the Homeless 181

SECTION IV Problems with the Overall System 203

Chapter 11. National Expenditures for Mental Hospitalization 205
Chapter 12. Needs for New Knowledge 238
Chapter 13. Barriers to Effective Knowledge Acquisition and Use 260
Chapter 14. Summary and Conclusions 271

References 278
Indexes 299
About the Authors 311

Acknowledgments

All of the national data and descriptions of government programs presented in this book result from careful study of government documents prepared by staff members at various agencies. Numerous people at these organizations spent a great deal of time giving us detailed explanations of methodology, providing us with unpublished data, and reviewing manuscripts that used their data. Without their assistance over an extended period of time, our presentations would not be as accurate.

We name the people with whom we communicated the most, while realizing that many people with whom we never spoke provided our contacts with information to answer our questions.

The staff of the National Institute of Mental Health provided data and clarified various aspects of the several NIMH surveys. We particularly thank Rosalyn Bass, Helen Bethel, Paul Henderson, Ronald Manderscheid, Laura Millazzo-Sayre, Marilyn Rosenstein, Carl Taube, and Michael Witkin for giving us much information on many occasions. David Larson was an excellent liaison between us and various NIMH branches. Grants from NIMH facilitated some of this work.

At the National Center for Health Statistics, Barbara Haupt, Eileen McCarthy, and Mary Moien clarified many points about the National Hospital Discharge Survey, and Willberta Swann located unpublished statistics. Esther Hing and Alvin Sirrocco provided National Master Facility Inventory data and explained the differences between the American Hospital Association and National Master Facility Inventory Survey. They also clarified many aspects of the National Nursing Home Survey.

Gary Davis and Peter Kralovec of the American Hospital Association assisted in interpreting *Hospital Statistics* tables and describing the Annual Survey.

Nelda Alkadhimi and William Page of the Veterans Administration assisted in interpreting VA hospital utilization surveys and explicating their methodologies. John Gaegler located data from the cost surveys.

Several staff members at the Health Care Financing Administration were very helpful in clarifying the facts on which the discussions of Medicare and Medicaid are based. Gail Toff at the Intergovernmental Health Policy Project and Mary Uyeda at the American Psychological Association were also instrumental in writing about these health care programs.

Army, Navy, and Air Force personnel provided information and data from their hospital utilization surveys. Aaron Handler and Steven Kaufman of the Indian Health Service gave us similar data for hospitals operated by the IHS.

William Shadish extensively reviewed Chapter 7 and Richard Frank and Mark Kamlet provided background information for Chapter 11.

We were fortunate to have superb secretarial help. Regina Perry and Cheryl Troetshel did excellent word processing, and Dorothea Boemer was exceptional at preparing the tables.

SECTION I

CHAPTER 1

THE PROBLEM

Ask average educated citizens what they have read or heard recently about mental hospitalization, and they will probably mention bag ladies or street people, whom they believe result from deinstitutionalization. Deinstitutionalization refers to a decline in mental hospitalization, a movement begun about 30 years ago, in part the result of economic and social forces.

In our experience, the information readily available to the informed public has focused on three themes regarding mental hospitalization. These themes dominate discussion on radio and television, in newspapers and magazines, and even in professional journals. They are: the problems of the homeless, with the implicit assumption that most have been or should be in a mental hospital; the pros and cons of deinstitutionalization, a public debate that has smoldered, and occasionally raged, for over 30 years; and the fact that the number of residents in public mental hospitals has declined sharply in recent years.

These three themes are indeed issues of major importance for the nation. However, they do not represent the whole picture for public policy regarding mental hospitalization. Further, when discussion is limited to those three themes, the total picture is distorted in serious ways that are critical for responsible public policy and planning.

Consider, for example, the following statements. Answer honestly; is each true or false?

(1) The number of episodes of mental hospitalization has declined in recent years. True or false?
(2) In most places where people are hospitalized for mental disorders, the length of stay has declined. True or false?
(3) Only a very small percentage of total days people spend in hospitals in the United States is for mental disorders. True or false?
(4) For the small number of people with serious mental disorders, they can be treated in mental hospitals more effectively than any place else. True or false?
(5) More money is spent for psychotherapy than for treatment in mental hospitals. True or false?

If you answered true to any of these questions, you are a good candidate to read this book. In our view, the correct answer for each is FALSE. The number of episodes of mental hospitalization has not declined. In fact, it has risen quite sharply over the past 10 to 15 years (see Chapter 4). In two places where people are hospitalized for mental disorders, the length of stay has declined recently. However, in most places, the length of stay for mental hospitalization has remained quite stable in recent years (see Chapter 5). Mental hospitalization is in fact quite a substantial national problem: Currently about one-quarter of all days spent in hospitals in the United States for all health problems are for mental disorders (see Chapter 6). Further, the data suggest that the vast majority of cases of mental disorders now being hospitalized could be more effectively treated outside of a hospital (see Chapter 9). Last, the cost is substantial. Between 70%–75% of total direct mental health expenditures in the United States are specifically for mental hospitalization (see Chapter 11).

This book is really a research monograph. It represents a description of our research program over the past several years in which we have been investigating various aspects of the national de facto system of mental hospitalization. Our intent is to present the most thorough and integrated analysis of data on hospitalization for mental disorders yet attempted.

We emphasize that our approach to hospitalization is not clinical in nature. We are neither clinical psychologists nor psychiatrists. We will not take a close clinical look at any given patient. We do not assume nor assert that we know the best treatment, or that we have intuitive insight into the intricacies of psychiatric diagnosis.

Our approach emphasizes social psychology, epidemiology, economics, and related disciplines. We look at data regarding mental hospitalization for the nation as a whole; we inspect national policies regarding mental health treatment in general and mental hospitalization in particular; we reanalyze the national data base; we determine whether what we do as a nation is in fact what we planned to do; we look at the overall system of mental hospitalization (whether planned or not) and the changing patterns of utilization and care.

There has also been a debate over the last two or three decades about whether mental hospitalization is an effective form of clinical treatment for valid diagnoses or a severe form of institutionalization of social deviants, with greater similarity to confinement in a prison than a hospital. This debate will be described more completely in Chapter 2. However, we say now that we have tried to avoid taking either side. Our intent has been to keep an open mind and, to the extent possible, let the data speak for themselves. We will return to these issues at various points in the book.

Although we look closely at the process and outcome of a national system of mental hospitalization, we do not claim the expertise to second guess the clinical judgment of the committing physician in any given case. However, in certain sections of this book, we will make judgments about the number of people hospitalized, the clinical outcomes of those hospitalizations, and the relative efficacy of mental hospitalization compared to other forms of treatment. We make these judgments as research scientists on the basis of the existing scientific evidence. One does not have to be a trained clinician to evaluate the scientific evidence. Indeed, it is sometimes an advantage to be "only" a researcher, since we have no preformed opinion or judgment as to how the evidence should look clinically.

We sometimes take the clinician's word very literally. When we refer to someone being hospitalized for a mental disorder, we mean the person was labeled with one of the mental disorders in the *Diagnostic and Statistical Manual* (American Psychiatric Association, 1968, 1980a) or the *International Classification of Diseases* (National Center for Health Statistics, 1962, 1967, 1980). In any given case, it is a fact that the diagnostic code was applied to a specific patient; it may not necessarily be a fact that the diagnosis was accurate. Yet the fact of the diagnosis is the only information we have, so we go with that.

The general plan is to stick with the data as closely as possible and not our own preconceptions (at minimum we attempt to label the two as clearly quite different). For example, we are rather certain that many more people are hospitalized for mental disorders than reflected in the national diagnostic data. The evidence suggests that nonpsychiatric physicians are not very accurate in recognizing mental disorders (e.g., Eastwood, 1975; Hoeper, 1980; Marks, Goldberg, & Hillier, 1979; Nielson & Williams, 1980). Except when the most serious symptoms are present, such as hallucinations, nonpsychiatric physicians tend not to recognize mental disorders. This leads to an underestimate in national statistics regarding mental disorders. This could be an issue for public concern if, say, public funds (e.g., Medicaid, Medicare) are used for ineffective and expensive treatment when more effective and appropriate treatment would result from an accurate diagnosis.

Another source of error in the national count of hospitalizations for mental disorders is the intentional mislabeling of diagnoses. We suspect that many attending physicians, particularly nonpsychiatrists, may eschew diagnoses of mental disorder in order to protect the client from an embarrassing label or to obtain reimbursement from insurance, since many plans limit coverage for mental health (e.g., Muszynski, Brady, & Sharfstein, 1983). We are not aware of direct evidence of mislabeling on medical records, but studies comparing insurance claim forms to medical record abstracts or physician records provide evidence that fewer mental disorders will be claimed than actually occurred, for both inpatients and outpatients (e.g., Doyle, 1966; Tenney, 1968).

The data presented in this book are of inpatient medical records or abstracts and not of insurance claim forms. However, we infer that the same underreporting of mental disorders occurs at the level of the original record for similar reasons.[1] Consequently, we are certain that more people are hospitalized for mental disorders than are reflected in national data. However, we do not know how many are in which categories, and so we set that notion aside when analyzing the data.

Mental Health Policy: The Current Context of Mental Hospitalization

Mental health policy is essentially a nonfield; it is at best undeveloped (see Kiesler, 1980). We do have national policies related to housing, urban development, defense, and health, and a good deal of time and money is spent in studying those policies and developing national alternatives. In some sense mental health policy is quite different from other national policies, in that it does not receive national discussion in the public media. That is, some of the specific problems are widely discussed but well-articulated alternative policies are not.

Further, we have not had an adequate data base on which to discuss policy alternatives precisely. For example, we know how many housing starts there are in the country each year, and we know the average price of new houses across the country and by regions. These data play an important role in our housing and economic policies of the country. We know how many hospital beds we have in the country, and how many are occupied in any given week. These data play an essential role in discussions of national health policy and in the need for new physical plants in health.

In mental health, the situation is quite different. We do not know precisely how many people are hospitalized each year for mental health reasons. We do not know how many people are treated as outpatients for mental health problems in the United States each year. We do not even know precisely how many people have mental health problems; estimates vary widely. Within our physical health resources nationally, we are not certain how many people general practitioners treat for mental-health problems.

The Task Panel on the Nature and Scope of the Problem of the President's Commission on Mental Health (Mechanic, 1978) summarized the epidemiological evidence on the incidence and prevalence of mental disorders in the United States. Dohrenwend, Dohrenwend, Gould, Link, Neugebauer, and Wunsch-Hitzig (1980) give a more detailed summary of the studies done between 1951 and 1972. Given the important differences in methodology across the studies, Dohrenwend et al. concluded one could not tell what the national prevalence rate for mental disorders was. They suggested the *hypothesis* that the correct prevalence rate was somewhere between 16% and 25% among adults under 60 years old.

Counting the number of people with mental disorders is a formidable task. First, samples from the entire population must be surveyed, not just those in treatment, because the majority of people with mental health problems are not seen by those who specialize in the provision of mental health services (Dohrenwend et al., 1980; Regier, Goldberg, & Taube, 1978; Shapiro, Skinner, Kessler, Von Korff, German, Tischler, Leaf, Benham, Cottler, & Regier, 1984). The majority is either seen by general health care providers or not at all. Second, what constitutes a mental-disorder "case" must be operationally defined in order to be counted in a replicable way.

The NIMH Epidemiologic Catchment Area (ECA) study addressed these issues by surveying people both in and out of institutions and by using a standardized instrument for eliciting recall of symptoms in face-to-face interviews. The symptoms were then translated into standard diagnostic categories (DSM-III) via computer algorithms.

The results available at this time for three of the five study sites (New Haven, Baltimore, and St. Louis) show six-month prevalence rates[2] of 15% to 20% for noninstitutionalized adults, depending on the city. These rates do not include all mental disorders, only the most common ones. Also, these percentages reflect number of diagnoses, rather than people, since each person could have more than one disorder (Myers, Weissman, Tischler, Holzer, Leaf, Orvaschel, Anthony, Boyd, Burke, Kramer, & Stoltzman, 1984).[3]

Although the individuals selected to be interviewed were carefully sampled to be representative of their respective sites, they do not constitute a national probability sample. The ECA design allows for replication across sites of the relationships among rates of specific diagnoses, age, and gender (e.g., more men than women experience alcohol dependence in all three sites). However, we do not know how representative these sites are of the country; the weights given to the frequencies of diagnoses are designed to reflect the population of the sites and not of the country. The Dohrenwend et al. "hypothesis" of 16%–25% is still probably the best national estimate.

Even when we are reasonably certain about a given datum, the implications of it for national mental health policy may be obscure. For example, we could know that a particular person received psychotherapy from a psychiatrist who was reimbursed from a specific insurance plan. That is, we know that the patient was treated and is no longer receiving treatment. We may not know specifically what the treatment was (so that we might compare that treatment with others at a national level). Nor are we likely to know whether the patients are significantly better now, whether they are working now when not before, whether they are receiving other public funds (such as welfare), whether they are in school or have dropped out, whether they have become married or divorced, and the like.[4]

The lack of precise data has seriously interfered with discussions of national alternatives for mental health policy. Sometimes discussions and challenges to current policy are mounted, but the need for the development of a national data base in mental health is not well understood.

DEFINITION OF MENTAL HEALTH POLICY

Kiesler (1980, p. 1066) has defined national mental health policy as

the de facto or de jure aggregate of laws, practices, social structures, or actions occurring within our society, the intent of which is improved mental health of individuals or groups. The study of such policy includes the descriptive parameters of the aggregate, the comparative assessment of particular techniques, the evaluation of the system and its subparts, human resources available and needed, cost-benefit analysis of practices or actions, and the cause and effect relationships of one set of policies, such as mental health, to others, such as welfare and health, as well as the study of institutions or groups seeking to affect such policy.

Our approach is to attempt to grasp the totality of what is done in the name of mental health. The view here will be very pragmatic and empirically oriented: We assume that our mental health policy consists, de facto, of all the practices that occur in the name of mental health. Thus we can inquire about what is done to handle mental health problems, to whom, with what effect, and at what cost. We will look at both the de facto and de jure national mental health policies, as defined below, and show how they tend to conflict with one another, through the main cornerstones of each—the Medicaid program and the Community Mental Health Centers (CMHC) system, respectively.

DE FACTO AND DE JURE PUBLIC POLICY

We use the terms "de jure" and "de facto" in the same way they were used in discussions of school desegregation. De jure policy is intentional in nature and usually legislated into law. The de facto policy is the net outcome of overall practices, whether the outcome is intended or not. The terms are very useful in mental health policy since, like school desegregation and other practices, the de facto system has certain unintended negative consequences. For example, much social legislation has been oriented toward integrating schools and facilitating the professional advancement of women and minorities. Nonetheless, our de facto systems often work at odds with the intent of our legislative practices, and our social practices often subtly and unintentionally create barriers that exclude minorities and women. In the mental health area, we also have a de facto system that often undercuts and is inconsistent with our formal de jure system of treatment. Let us move to a discussion of how that happens.

DEFINITION OF MENTAL HOSPITALIZATION

We define mental hospitalization as the inpatient treatment of a diagnosed mental disorder. Typically this would involve diagnosis of a mental disorder and admission to and discharge from an institution that is designed to handle overnight stays, whether for general health care or specifically for the treatment of mental disorders. These institutions can be any type of public or private hospital, nursing home, residential treatment center, or the inpatient services of community mental health centers. (We discuss all of these in more detail in Chapter 3.) Halfway houses and other community residences are designed to be less restrictive settings than traditional hospital institutions, and are not included in this analysis.

THE DE JURE MENTAL-HEALTH POLICY

For the last 20 years or more, our national de jure mental health policy has had two main thrusts: outpatient care, largely through community mental health centers; and deinstitutionalization—getting current patients out of mental hospitals and reducing the average length of stay for mental institutionalization. Let's look at each of these in turn.

CMHCs and Outpatient Care. The Community Mental Health Centers Systems Act was originally signed by President Kennedy in 1963. It promoted federal funding of community mental health centers (CMHCs) in specific geographical areas (1500 of them, called catchment areas).[5] As of 1981 there were 691 functioning community mental health centers initiated under this act. The federal program was to provide substantial funding in the beginning stages of a community mental health center. The funding was then decreased over the course of an eight-year period, when the center should theoretically have been able to fund itself from state, county, and city sources as well as fee-for-service and other service provision (such as consulting with school systems). In fact, few of the centers were able to survive that well, and an emergency funding program saved many from having to close their doors at the end of the eight-year period. Although only approximately half of the catchment areas were successful in beginning community mental health centers, these areas tended to be high-population ones and they include well over 75% of the country's population (Edelman, 1978).

The Reagan Administration changed all this dramatically. Under the Omnibus Budget Reconciliation Act of 1981 (PL 97-35), federal funds for mental health services were cut 25% and removed from the control of the National Institute of Mental Health. Although the resulting block grant program to the states does mandate some continuation of mental-health services, the precise impact of PL 97-35 is still difficult to assess (see Kiesler, McGuire, Mechanic, Mosher, Nelson, Newman, Rich, & Schulberg, 1983). However, we still discuss CMHCs because data on their utilization are an important part of national trends as we will see in Chapter 3.

It was originally hoped that the CMHC system would provide a sufficient source of alternative care for less affluent citizens so that state and county mental hospitals could be phased out. As the task force on community mental health centers of the President's Commission on Mental Health says in its report, "it was asserted that the centers would be ultimately financed by increased state and local funds made available through the phasing out of state hospitals and, it was hoped, by the private sector through voluntary insurance" (Edelman, 1978, p. 316).

The movement to promote outpatient care in general and community mental health centers in particular has been claimed as a great success and in many respects this claim is valid. For example, NIMH estimates that in 1955 there were 379,000 episodes of outpatient care in the United

States. By 1975, this figure had grown to 4.6 million, a twelvefold increase over a 20-year period (Witkin, 1980).

The thrust toward outpatient care has been successful not only in numbers but in proportion of episodes nationally. In 1955 inpatient care was the mode of treatment in 77% of the clinical episodes; in 1975 this percentage had decreased to 27%, according to NIMH figures (Witkin, 1980).

CMHCs have also been successful in other ways. In 1975–1976, 11.5% of staff in all mental health facilities were employed by community mental health centers, but those centers provided 29% of the total episodes of care in the United States, an index of efficiency of care. The care was also less expensive than other places: The 29% of total episodes of care were provided at a cost of only 4.2% of the total bill for mental health in the United States. Further, CMHCs were successful in offering care to people who might not otherwise afford it. In 1975, 54% of the new patients served in community mental health centers reported weekly family incomes of less than $100 (all of these statistics are from Edelman, 1978).

This section serves only to introduce the topic of CMHCs. In Chapter 3 we provide a detailed description of the numbers of episodes occurring in various types of hospitals. In Chapter 11, we will also break down the national costs of mental hospitalization in the United States in some detail.

Deinstitutionalization. As a policy, deinstitutionalization encompasses the discharges of patients from psychiatric hospitals and the subsequent care of discharged patients in the community (Bachrach, 1976). Expected outcomes of a successful deinstitutionalization policy include fewer people hospitalized and each for a shorter period of time.

In some respects the move toward deinstitutionalization has been less successful than expected. As mentioned, the proportion of clinical episodes that involve inpatient care has dropped enormously over a 20-year period. However, outpatient care increased so dramatically during that same period that we are in essence talking about a percentage of a much larger base. It is revealing to look at inpatient care independently of outpatient care, as we will in Chapters 3 through 6.

If someone says that the national priority of deinstitutionalization has been successfully implemented, they usually mean one of two things. A typical statement in newspapers and magazines encompasses both aspects: "The number of residents in public mental hospitals and their average length of stay have dropped dramatically over the last 20 years."[6] Both assertions are technically correct, but misleading. The average stay in a public mental hospital has decreased in recent years.

That is accurate. However, the phrase "public mental hospital" refers specifically and only to state and county mental hospitals, the snake pits of the past. The average length of stay in Veterans Administration hospitals has also dropped, but taken together these two sites of hospitalization handle only about 20% of the total national inpatient episodes. All other sites of hospitalization have remained rather constant in length of stay (see Chapter 5). Further, even though the length of stay has remained relatively constant within type of hospital, there is still considerable variation in the length of stay among types of hospital.

It is also true that the number of residents has dropped in state and county mental hospitals as well. Again, the term "residents" is a technical one and refers to the number of patients in a hospital on a given day (usually the first or last day of the calendar year in NIMH data). In fact, over a number of years, the number of *residents* was dropping, while *admissions* were increasing (see Chapter 3).

In summary, it is true that "the number of residents in public mental hospitals and their average lengths of stay have dropped dramatically over the last twenty years." However, we assert now and describe more completely in chapters to follow, that each of these statistical facts is misleading when taken in isolation. The gap between the de jure and de facto policies becomes clearer when trends in all types of inpatient facilities are considered simultaneously.

THE DE FACTO MENTAL HEALTH POLICY

As mentioned, the de jure national mental health policy involves two major elements: (1) deinstitutionalization, including aftercare (described in Chapter 10) and (2) the development of a public system of effective outpatient care. The major impediment to successful implementation of this policy is the design of insurance programs, both public (e.g., Medicaid and Medicare) and private (e.g., Blue Cross/Blue Shield). These insurance programs, quite unintentionally, so dominate the national scene that they in effect have become the national de facto mental health policy.

How could that be? The major aspect of insurance planning for mental health that affects policy is financial disincentives for outpatient and community care. The assumption by insurance executives is that if they fully insured psychotherapy and other community care (such as programmatic alternatives to mental hospitalization), so many people would take advantage of this alternative that the insurance plan would go bankrupt.

Consequently, the tendency is to insure hospitalization at full cost and outpatient care at part cost. The net effect on the patients, particularly if they do not have much money, is clear. The same psychiatric services that might not be fully insured for an outpatient become completely insured for an inpatient. For financial reasons, patients who might otherwise be treated as outpatients are admitted as inpatients (see Chapter 11).

The promotion of inpatient, as opposed to outpatient, care can result from various mechanisms. Private health insurance plans typically limit outpatient reimbursement by imposing deductibles, coinsurance, a maximum dollar limit, and a limit on the number of visits, while a hospital stay is completely covered (although the number of days may be limited). See Muszynski et al. (1983) for a summary of 300 private insurance plans.

Medicare. The federally funded health insurance program for the aged and disabled spent $995 million on mental health care in 1981, and over 80% of it was for inpatient care (Table 1.1). Differences in expenditures for inpatient and outpatient care cannot be directly translated into services delivered, given that a unit of inpatient service will cost more than a unit of outpatient service. Therefore, we would expect beneficiaries of inpatient care to incur expenses disproportionate to their number. However, part of this difference in expenditures between inpatient and outpatient care is likely attributable to the annual $500 limit and 50% coinsurance on physician services provided for mental-health in an outpatient setting. This means that Medicare will pay up to $250 per year for physician office visits for mental health care (half of $500).[7] We will more fully describe the Medicare program and the various coverage limits in Chapter 11 and Appendix 11-A.

Medicaid. This state and federally funded program was designed to provide medical services for the poor. It specifically emphasizes the "categorically" poor: the aged, the blind, the disabled, and members of families with dependent children but with only one parent capable of providing support (HCFA, 1983; SSA, 1984). It thereby excludes a good many of the poor in the United States including intact families, the working poor, single people, and childless couples. In fact, the majority of people between the ages of 21 and 65 are ineligible for medical assistance from Medicaid (Newman, 1978). This is a program designed to serve a narrow segment of the country's population.

Medicaid is intended to be primarily a medical program. However, quite unintentionally Medicaid is also the largest single mental health program in the country. As Table 1.2 shows, in fiscal year 1977, the Medicaid program spent a total of 558 million dollars for care of patients in state, county, and private mental institutions and psychiatric hospitals (see Newman, 1978).[8] Coincidentally this figure exceeds the

TABLE 1.1
Estimated Medicare Program Payments for Identifiable
Treatment of Mental Conditions by Type of Service, 1981[a]

Type of Service	Payments (in millions)	Percentage of Total
Inpatient		
Short-stay hospital	$630	63%
Psychiatric hospital	$190	19%
Outpatient hospital	$ 45	5%
Other institutional	$ 15	2%
Physician	$115	12%
Total	$995	100%

SOURCE: Unpublished data from Health Care Financing Administration.

[a] Identified by type of provider/supplier (i.e., psychiatric hospital, psychiatrist, or psychologist billing independently) or by the principal diagnosis recorded on institutional billings for samples of Medicare enrollees.

total federal cost for the whole community mental health centers system for that year of $240 million (NIMH, 1980). The total dollars that Medicaid spent on mental institutionalization is even much greater. For example, another category listed in their budget is general hospital inpatient, outpatient, and emergency care related to mental health, a category in which 185 million dollars was spent during that same period. Based on other national data, the majority of these funds probably was for inpatient care.[9]

Further, the total Medicaid reimbursement to community mental health centers came to $100 million. Eighty-two million went to physicians and other practitioners in private practice and $110 million was spent on drugs related to mental health. Residential treatment facilities, rehabilitation, and children's programs came to an additional $110 million. These various totals come to an additional $587 million. If we assume that 70%[10] of $587 million was directly related to inpatient care, then an additional $411 million was spent on mental hospitalization. Adding this to the $558 million directly paid to state, county, and private psychiatric hospitals, a total figure of approximately $1 billion was spent in FY 77 on mental hospitalization through Medicaid.

That's not the end of the Medicaid story. In addition to this $1 billion another $2.2 billion was reimbursed directly to nursing homes for mental health services, presumably all inpatient care. This $2.2 billion was

TABLE 1.2
Medicaid Expenditures for Mental Health Services FY 1977[a]

Type of Care or Service	Estimated Expenditures[h] (in millions)
State, county, and private mental institutions and psychiatric hospitals[b]	$558
General hospital, inpatient, outpatient and emergency care, related to mental health[c]	$185
Community mental health centers[d]	$100
Private free-standing clinics	$25
Physicians and other practitioners[e]	$82
Nursing homes[f]	$2,189
ICF/MRs	$702
Residential treatment facilities, rehabilitation and children's programs	$110
Drugs[g]	$110
Total	$4,091

SOURCE: Reprinted from The President's Commission on Mental Health, Report of the Task Panel on Cost and Financing (Newman, 1978), based on data from the Health Care Financing Administration.

[a] Estimates include direct costs to Medicaid for mental illness and retardation.

[b] FY 1977 Budget Estimates, MMB/DOB.

[c] General hospital expenditures are estimated at four percent of Medicaid's projected inpatient general hospital expenditures in FY 1977.

[d] Estimate based on the Medicaid reimbursement to CMHCs as reported by NIMH for FY 1975.

[e] Mental health related expenditures for physicians and other practitioners were estimated at 4% and 1%, respectively, of total projected expenditures to those providers under Title XIX in FY 1977 (DOB).

[f] Nursing home expenditures (SNF, ICF) related to mental health services are estimated at 40% of the projected nursing home expenditures for FY 1977.

[g] Drug expenditures related to mental health under Medicaid are estimated at 11% of projected drug expenditures for FY 1977.

[h] Technique based on methods used by Levine and Levine (1971).

derived from the estimate that payments to nursing homes for mental health services represent 40% of the total Medicaid payments to nursing homes (Levine & Levine, 1975). If the estimate for nursing homes is correct, then the total Medicaid contribution to inpatient mental health care in 1977 was over $3 billion, twelve times as much as the $240 million the federal government spent on the community mental health center system that year.

Medicaid and Medicare are the major underwriters of institutional mental health care in the United States. As we discuss in Chapter 11, the Medicaid and Medicare programs make it easier to be hospitalized than to receive alternative treatment. While it is true these patients receive care that they might not otherwise receive (Newman, 1978), unnecessary hospitalization is probably encouraged for patients who cannot afford other care, either through copayments in the case of Medicare or through lack of coverage of needed community services. Less coverage for outpatient care is typical of most insurance programs, but mental health outpatient coverage is usually less than for general health (Muszynski et al., 1983). This is discriminatory treatment of mental health care, and induces hospitalization in cases where it is not only unnecessary but would not otherwise occur.

The federal government apparently spends about twelve times as much for mental institutionalization through Medicaid as it does to implement its overt de jure policy of outpatient care (through CMHCs). The national policy of outpatient care and deinstitutionalization may get the policy publicity, but inpatient care gets the dollars. It is quite clear that our de jure policy of deinstitutionalization and outpatient care is being seriously undercut by a de facto policy of institutionalization through Medicaid and Medicare. The patient in essence is caught in an unintended policy clash between federal agencies.

Plan of the Book

In the next chapter, we describe some of the history of mental hospitalization to help the reader keep the present and the possible alternative futures in perspective. The first four chapters in Section II describe in detail the trends in basic epidemiological data on mental hospitalization for all types of places in which people are hospitalized: the number of such episodes occurring over time (Chapter 3); the rate of mental hospitalization and its change over time (Chapter 4); the average length of stay over time (Chapter 5); and changes in the proportion of total hospital days that are due to mental disorders (Chapter 6).

Chapter 7 describes trends in nursing home residents and compares these data with state hospital trends. Chapter 8 describes data on hospital readmissions and their role in planning services.

The two chapters in Section III describe research on noninstitutionalization (Chapter 9) and deinstitutionalization (Chapter 10). Noninstitutionalization refers to treatment instead of mental hospitalization, and deinstitutionalization encompasses issues and problems of treating patients after they have been discharged from a mental hospital.

Section IV places these data in some perspective by looking closely at the national system of mental health care. Chapter 11 describes the total expenditures for inpatient care for mental disorders and where that money goes. Chapter 12 describes the need for new knowledge: What sorts of things should we be investigating in order to design an intelligent and effective national mental health policy? Chapter 13 discusses the barriers to effective knowledge use: Why aren't we making better use of what we already know? Chapter 14 tries to sum up some of these recurring themes and lay out some reasonable policy plans for the future.

As we have mentioned, our intent here is to provide the most thorough and complete presentation and analysis of the national data on mental hospitalization yet attempted. At times, the reader may find the wealth and detail of the data almost overwhelming, and perhaps tedious. We both apologize and beg the reader's indulgence.

In almost every detailed investigation we have attempted in this area, we have been surprised by what the data actually show and what is commonly thought to be true, even by sophisticated professionals. Several of our studies, therefore, have been considered to be quite controversial. Given the level of the controversy and the national importance and complexity of the problem, we feel it critical that we be very detailed. We have tried to adopt a style that allows the curious to get through the book without drowning in detail. The counterarguing critic, however, will have to deal with all the data at once, not just the typical sliver or subset.

Notes

1. Within the category of "mental disorders," insurance claim forms for *outpatients* have been shown to record both more and less serious diagnoses than reported on their medical records (Schwartz, Perlman, Paris, Schmidt, & Thornton, 1980; Sharfstein, Towery, & Milowe, 1980). Pressures to minimize the seriousness of mental health problems may result from fear of breached con-

fidentiality (Chodoff, 1978), and pressure to exaggerate the seriousness may result from the need to prove that the case warrants reimbursement.

2. This is the number of people affected during the six months prior to the interview.

3. See the original article for percentage distributions of individual diagnoses.

4. Although we also do not know these outcomes for people treated for physical health problems either, we expect that mental health problems relate more closely to these variables than do physical health problems, on average.

5. Both spellings, "catchment" and "cachement," are used in the literature.

6. The following discussion only relates to the number of patients who become institutionalized. The problems of the deinstitutionalized in receiving care and the problems of coordinating among programs for the deinstitutionalized are a very important but separate issue, which will be taken up in Chapter 10.

7. There is, however, a hefty deductible for hospital stays—$400 in 1985.

8. Data on mental health expenditures under Medicaid are indirectly derived and are quite crude. They are presented to show relative magnitudes of expenditures and not absolute amounts.

9. For example, the American Hospital Association reported inpatient care in general hospitals to be 87% of total expenditures in 1977 (AHA, 1978).

10. A number partly chosen because 70% of the total mental health dollar is projected to be spent on hospitalization (see Chapter 11). This percentage has also been independently estimated by the Health Care Finance Administration (see Newman, 1978).

CHAPTER 2

THE HISTORY OF
MENTAL HOSPITALIZATION

As we discussed in Chapter 1, the delivery of mental health services has changed dramatically in the United States in the last 20 to 30 years. Partly as a result of the Community Mental Health Center System, the number of outpatient episodes in the United States has increased geometrically until today almost 80% of total episodes in mental health are outpatient (Witkin, 1980). However, this increase in number of outpatient episodes should not obscure the picture for inpatient episodes. Chapter 3 documents an overall substantial increase in hospital admissions for mental disorders.

The state and county hospital system used to be the core of mental health services in the United States. It clearly is not anymore. It delivers only a small fraction of the total mental health episodes in the United States (both inpatient and outpatient). For decades, until 1979, there were more inpatient episodes in the state hospitals than anywhere else, at least for the institutions surveyed by NIMH.[1] In that year, general hospitals with psychiatric units treated a slightly larger number of inpatient episodes than did the state and county mental hospital system. However, general hospitals without psychiatric units, facilities not typically surveyed regarding mental disorders, record the most inpatient episodes in mental health. More mental disorder episodes have occurred there than in state and county mental hospitals since 1973.

It is startling for many to learn that the rate of hospitalizing people for mental disorders has continued to increase, both in terms of the absolute number of inpatient episodes and in terms of the rate per 100,000 population (see Chapter 4). We seem to have become so pleased as a nation with a drastic decrease in the number of residents in state and county mental hospitals that we accept that as a summary statement of our overall national system. It is not.

Why do we hospitalize people more frequently than ever before? There are a number of possible reasons. One, we never seem to question whether mental hospitalization is effective, even in its best representations. We will present evidence on the effectiveness of alternative care in Chapter 9. Two, insurance incentives, both public and private, often favor hospitalization for particular patients, and we will discuss how more completely in Chapter 11. A third reason is the subject of this chapter. Hospitalization follows 150 years of traditional professional practice in the field of mental health.

Mental hospitalization has been the treatment of choice for cases of serious mental disorder for over 150 years. Indeed, the history of mental-health policy was the history of mental hospitalization until fairly recently. Thus a short history of the policies and actions related to mental hospitalization seems very appropriate.[2]

Early History

Eaton (1980) provides some interesting early background. Concern with madness occurs throughout recorded history. Depression, for example, was studied quite systematically in 5th century B.C. Greece, and one of the 12 tables of Roman law in 5th century B.C. Rome regards the disposition of a man's goods if he is found "raving mad."

Eaton argues that prior to the Age of Reason (15th–16th century) the treatment of madness mostly consisted of benign neglect—the acceptance of bizarre behavior as culturally deviant, but not requiring confinement. True, there was an asylum in Baghdad in the 8th century and in Damascus in the 9th. Granada, in Arab Spain, also established an asylum in 1365.

However, Foucault (1973) argues that madness represented a special threat of chaos to the rational economic order of the of Age of Reason—a threat that precipitated a need for control and repudiation. He argues that the publication of *Malleus Malificarum* (Witches' Hammer), which equated madness with control by the devil and which led to the inquisition, crystalized a major change in the Western view of the mad. Eaton agrees, "There appears to have been a period in our civilization sometime before the end of the fifteenth century when madness was an 'undifferentiated experience.' If it existed, it was not remarkable and did not require departure from every day life. It is difficult to find references to persons who engaged in bizarre behaviors, and when we do find them, the references are allegorical or only by implication" (1980, p. 22).

For Foucault, the culminating event was what he refers to as the Great Confinement of 1656, in which beggars, lunatics, and vagrants were rounded up and confined in the Hospital General formed for that purpose. Foucault claims that 1% of the population of Paris was locked up at one time.

Colonial United States

By the days of Colonial America, the active treatment for the insane was punishment. The insane members of wealthy families were kept at home and, if violent, were likely to spend their lives locked in a specially constructed room in the attic or cellar. They were considered to be a disgrace to the family and not publicly acknowledged. The less wealthy were considered felons if they were violent, and paupers if they were not.

> Thus, while the violently insane went to the whipping post and into prison dungeons or, as sometimes happened, burned at the stake or hanged, the pauper insane often roamed the countryside as wild men and from time to time were pilloried, whipped, and jailed. . . . If capable of work, a man might be auctioned off as free labor to the farmer who would accept the smallest payment from the town. This was a form of slavery. Eventually, houses of correction, work houses, and alms houses assumed custody of the insane [*Action for Mental Health*, 1961, p. 26].

The Pennsylvania Hospital in the eighteenth century was the first hospital in the United States to admit mental patients. However, punishment was an integral aspect of the approach to treatment. Deutsch (1949, p. 80) quotes Dr. Benjamin Rush, the first director of the hospital, as saying, "Terror acts powerfully on the body through the medium of the mind, and should be employed in the care of madness."

The Joint Commission on Mental Illness and Health, in their volume *Action for Mental Health* (1961), suggests that fear and punishment as a treatment of mental illness was related to Old Testament beliefs that diseases of any kind, whether mental or physical, represented punishment for sin. In the Pennsylvania Hospital, the insane patients were chained to the wall in bolted prison cells in the cellar, and the cell keeper regularly carried a whip and used it freely. It was not until the latter part of the eighteenth century that such practices began to change.

Colonial United States is a reasonable starting point for an introduction to the United States history of mental hospitalization. However, the treatment of the insane has fluctuated throughout the ages. In Belgium, for example, the town of Gheel has served as a center for community care of the insane and retarded for 600 years without resorting to mental hospitals. In medieval times various monasteries were said to house and treat the insane quite humanely. As noted, Foucault argues that the Age of Reason signaled a dramatic change in perception and treatment of the mentally disordered. Whether one agrees with that or not, it is certainly neither the case that treatment during colonial times reflected the accumulated wisdom of the ages nor that such treatment was constant across centuries. However, punitive treatment was typical in the United States in the late eighteenth century.

Two major figures had a dramatic impact on treatment in the last part of the eighteenth century. As one outcome of the French Revolution, Dr. Philippe Pinel was put in charge of two insane asylums in Paris. One of his first acts was to unchain the patients in the asylums much to the shock of his colleagues who thought the patients extremely dangerous (Bockoven, 1956). It is generally accepted that the violence of the patients decreased dramatically once they were able to move about. Pinel had a humanitarian and accepting approach to the treatment of the insane, which he called "moral treatment." Patients were treated sympathetically in a supportive environment. In a startling statement almost 200 years later, the Joint Commission said, "to Pinel's principles for the treatment of psychotics, twentieth century psychiatry can add little, except to convert them into modern terminological dress" (1961, p. 29).

About the same time, the second major figure, William Tuke, started the York Retreat in England, an institution with treatment principles based on permissiveness and kindness as reflected by the Quaker faith. The word "retreat" was to suggest the need for seclusion from the stresses of the increasingly urban society (and is still used in the titles of a number of private mental hospitals).

The 19th Century

In the first third of the nineteenth century, the concepts behind moral treatment and the York Retreat spread to hospitals in the United States, but not very quickly and typically to hospitals to which only the very rich had access. Dorthea Dix has been given major credit for changing this situation. She was very impressed with the effects of moral treatment, particularly in the few state hospitals where it was adopted. She was angry about the treatment of the insane poor, still mostly placed in alms houses and jails. She set about systematically to advocate for the establishment of state hospitals. She would tour an entire state, assessing the treatment of the insane and subsequently make recommendations to the state legislature. Eventually she was given credit for starting state hospitals in over 30 different states, quite an incredible activist effort.

At the same time, a philosophy of public welfare was receiving attention and debate. In 1828, Horace Mann first described the principle that the insane should be considered wards of the state (Eaton, 1980). The developing activist climate of public welfare both supported and probably instigated the efforts of Dix.

The middle third of the nineteenth century was a period of very rapid building of mental hospitals. By 1880 there were almost 140 public and private mental hospitals with over 40,000 patients out of the total of 92,000 insane found in the 1880 census (Grob, 1983). Between 1850 and 1890, 94 state mental hospitals were built. Unfortunately, for what was to follow, those built after 1870 tended to be much larger.

The future of progressive treatment in mental hospitals seemed assured. Yet the movement for the humane treatment of the mentally ill failed and fairly quickly. In the last 100 years there has been a series of cycles in the treatment of the mentally ill that many regard as periods of progressions and retrogressions with no clear accumulation of knowledge regarding treatment. Let us try to look at this issue in a little more detail, because there are several complicated threads that seem to come together.

First, the state mental hospitals rapidly became very large. When the state took over the costs of treating the mentally ill, the local units were glad to empty their jails and alms houses to save on expense. The Joint Commission attributes some of the rapid increase in the size of the state hospitals to the waves of immigration to the new world. This could only partly be true. In 1880, 62% of the inpatients were native born (Grob, 1983). The Joint Commission says, "Our state hospital system never has recovered from this original overcrowding and its facilities have never kept abreast of continued population growth" (1961, p. 63). As Mechanic (1980) notes, it is ironic that the reform movement led to the development of very large custodial institutions. The very size of the institutions led to increased need to regularize the patients' activities to increase efficiency of care. By 1880, the average size of a mental hospital was over 500 patients and many had over 1,000 patients (Grob, 1983). In the process of becoming a bureaucracy, the state hospital also depersonalized and regulated the environment for patients, interfering with the basic premises of moral treatment.

In the early part of the nineteenth century, reformers and hospital superintendents were generally optimistic about the care of the insane. Indeed, many patients did get better, but equally as many never did. Grob reports a 30-year review published in 1877 that estimated that 34% of admissions would recover by the end of the first year, 36% would remain stationary, and 29% would die.

Custodial care became an increasing requirement of the mental hospital. Restraint became a controversial issue. Some states reported success of nonrestraint laws. Other reformers felt restraint violated the rights of patients. Critics of mental hospitals felt mechanical restraints represented evidence of the failure of the whole system of mental hospitals.

Even in the nineteenth century the use of drugs with mental patients was popular. Such drugs as opium, morphine, and chloral hydrate were regularly used. Critics referred to them as "chemical restraints," and noted that hospitals using mechanical restraints tended also to use chemical restraints as well. A report to the Massachusetts legislature in 1875 stressed the importance of such drugs in the treatment of the insane but described puzzlement regarding the variations in use, with some hospitals reporting the use of six times as much drugs as the state average (Grob, 1983).

At the same time, significant changes were occurring in psychiatry and the place of psychiatrists in medicine. The Association of Medical Superintendents of American Institutions for the Insane (AMSAII) was founded in 1844. This organization became the American Medico-Psychological Association in 1892 and ultimately the American Psychiatric Association in 1921. American medicine was becoming more scientific with important pathogenic and bacteriological discoveries. Moral treatment, of course, was environmentally based and behavioral, not medically based and somatic. An argument over the causes of mental disorders ensued.

For example, the Joint Commission (1961) attributed a specific blow to the practice of moral treatment when Dr. John Gray became the implicit spokesman for American psychiatry as editor for the *American Journal for Insanity*. Gray rejected the whole concept behind moral treatment and argued strongly that mental patients were really physically ill with a brain disease. Eventually this became an accepted point of view. When the National Association for the Protection of the Insane and the Prevention of Insanity was organized in 1880 and attacked Dr. Gray and insane asylums, they in turn received public rebuke from the AMSAII. Gray's perception of mental illness as a physical disease, and the generally pessimistic attitudes toward cure, became an accepted point of view in psychiatry. "Mental hospital superintendents who saw patients accumulate and continue to live their lives out in locked wards became steeped in this negative outlook. Far from feeling they had failed in a social or in a medical responsibility, these first psychiatrists apparently were satisfied that they were fulfilling the mission that the state had assigned them. This was to take custody of all persons committed to their institutions by the courts and thenceforth guard the public and patients against the latter's irrational acts. The superintendent's primary responsibility ended, under state laws, with keeping the mentally ill alive, the emphasis being on physical rather than mental well-being. For example, if the patient would not eat, he was force fed; but if he would not talk it was not considered important to encourage him to do so" (Action for Mental Health, 1961, p. 65). This pessimistic view of the mentally ill fit generally with what were regarded as progressive views of Darwinism being expounded at the time (Dain, 1980).

At the same time, the view that mental illness was a physical disease also led to the belief that ultimately a cure for the disease would be found. This belief had a negative effect on the conduct of mental hospitals (Grob, 1966). Grob argues that the belief in ultimate cure led to a feeling that there was little one could do in the interim except custodial care. This attitude undermined both alternative approaches to potential care and the potential of discovering other methods of treating mental patients. Grob further argues that the increasing professionalization of psychiatry inhibited the development of alternative approaches to mental health care. The desire of psychiatrists to professionalize their field led to social distance from other factions and groups interested in the treatment of the mentally ill, and cut off their active involvement in treatment. Mental hospitals were geographically and socially isolated from the rest of society and did not encourage active involvement by community spirited individuals—the same sort of person who provided the impetus behind moral treatment. A good deal of the impetus behind moral treatment was nonprofessional in nature. In fact, those hospitals that followed the example of the York Retreat did not even include physicians in their treatment "plan."

Historically then, several factors destroyed the humanitarian approach to "moral" and humane treatment of the mentally ill. The size of the hospitals was a major factor, because it necessitated bureaucratic developments that led to an impersonal and dehumanizing environment. The notion that mental illness was a physical illness that could be handled by a solely medical approach became a dominant point of view, and was further fed by a general public acceptance of social Darwinism. The expectation that a specific medical cure could be ultimately found for mental illness also inhibited effective treatment because it implied that one had to wait until such a cure was found (without attempting to improve treatment in the interim). All of these factors interfered with actual treatment and the development of alternative treatment strategies, and ultimately led to the acceptance of simple custodial care as the treatment of choice.

Although the data are sparse, there is some evidence that the effectiveness of treatment declined with the move away from the methods of Pinel and Tuke. In studies of early records, moral treatment seems quite effective. A review of 244 case histories of the York retreat prior to

1845 reported a hospital discharge rate of about 50% and a permanent recovery rate of 20% (Bockoven, 1956). A review of Worcester State Hospital records, 1833–1852, reports a discharge rate of 71% (66% recovered; 5% improved) for those ill less than one year prior to admission and 59% (45% recovered; 14% improved) for others. Bockoven also reports an earlier unpublished study of the same hospital, which found a 54% recovery rate, following up patients for 28 years! Modern hospitals today would be quite pleased with those rates.

These studies were not without their critics, even at that time. Pliny Earle, one of the founders of the AMSAII, charged that the recovery rates were grossly exaggerated and that the data were confounded in several respects.

There are not many studies of recovery rates following the move away from moral treatment. Since the emphasis was not active treatment, one can understand why. However, Bond (1954) compared recovery rates for schizophrenic patients in a Pennsylvania hospital for the periods 1925–1934 and 1940–1946. He found recovery rates of 9% in the former period and 22% in the latter.

However flawed, the early research is still surprisingly sophisticated evaluation research carried out over a century ago. It suggests moral treatment did have a positive effect. However, one should not make too much of any specific statistic or comparative statistics. There is not much detail in the studies reported. Certainly, the people judging the recovery of a patient were also those philosophically committed to the form of treatment. Further, whether one is hospitalized or not depends partly on both the tolerance of the culture for deviance at the time, the public's perception of whether the mentally ill are dangerous, and inadvertent effects of a system of care. For example, the definition of insanity varied. When states began to assume responsibility for the care of mental patients, city and county officials began to regard the senile and the aged as insane. This allowed them to remove such people from the local alms houses and shift the financial responsibility to the state. In spite of these variations it seems a good guess that moral treatment was reasonably effective and that the subsequent new medical approach was less effective, particularly since the latter did not emphasize treatment but rather custodial care.

Over the years, the practice of hospitalizing mental patients continued to increase, although there is no real evidence that the incidence of mental illness increased during that time (Goldhamer & Marshall, 1953). There was some fluctuation in the rate of hospitalization. Brenner (1973) found in a review of over 100 years of institutional practices that institutionalization especially increased following periods of economic hardship.

There was considerable variation in state practices over the ensuing years. The State of Nevada, for example, at one time subcontracted the care of all its psychiatric inpatients to California. Wisconsin was regarded the most innovative. It maintained a central facility for the most chronic cases and decentralized responsibility for the remainder to counties. The acute cases tended to be cared for on small farms, emphasizing freedom and occupational opportunities. By 1930 only about 20% of the insane were cared for in the state mental hospital in Wisconsin. (To this day, the episodic rate of mental hospitalization is lowest in Wisconsin.)

Various nonprofessional individuals played important roles in the treatment of the mentally ill. One of the first, Robert Fuller, attacked the McLean Asylum in 1833 as a result of his experience there as a patient. E.P.W. Packard was involuntarily committed to the Illinois State Hospital in 1860 by her husband. At that time public law allowed the institutionalization of married females and children without the procedural safeguards afforded adult males. As a result of her efforts, Illinois passed a law in 1867 providing for jury trials in sanity hearings, with other states subsequently following suit (laws to which hospital superintendents objected).

The 20th Century

Perhaps the most famous individual affecting mental health policy was Clifford Beers, who ultimately founded the National Committee for Mental Hygiene in 1909 (now the Mental Health Association). Beers had spent over three years in public and private mental hospitals. His classic book, *A Mind that Found Itself* (1908), as well as his own activities and efforts, stimulated citizen involvement in mental hygiene, prevention of hospitalization, aftercare, and other modern concepts; activities that the Mental Health Association continues to this day. The National Committee conducted a number of state surveys of mental hygiene and mental hospital facilities over the ensuing years.

In 1930, Beers organized the First International Congress on Mental Hygiene. Ironically, Beers died in a mental hospital in 1943, having spent the last four years of his life there.[3]

In the twentieth century, mental hospitals increasingly became domiciles of the aged. For example, in 1885 the admission rates (per 100,000 population) to state mental hospitals in Massachusetts were 70.4

and 65.5 for males and females over 65, respectively. In 1939–1941, rates were 280 and 223 for the same age group, a fourfold increase.

Treatment outcomes did not improve. Grob (1983) describes a study by Fuller and Johnston in 1931 of patients confined in 1909–1911 and studied for 16 years. Of every 100 patients, 35 were discharged as improved or better, 7 discharged but unimproved, 42 died in the hospital and 16 continued in the hospital throughout the period. For example, of the 2,481 schizophrenics in the study, 722 remained in the hospital for the full 16 years covered by the study. These statistics are, if anything, worse than those alluded to earlier in the middle of the nineteenth century.

As Grob describes, "Between World Wars I and II, the commitment to institutional care of the mentally ill remained unchanged." Indeed, during the depression, perhaps the mentally disturbed fared better in institutions than they could have outside.

Various "innovations" became popular. In the 1920s fever therapy peaked. In the 1930s insulin and metrazol shock therapy and prefrontal lobotomy were popular. Various drugs used 50 years before continued to be popular.

State hospitals continued to grow in size. In 1939 the average sized state hospital had between 1500 and 3000 patients, and state hospitals in general accounted for 83% of all institutionalized patients.

During World War II the financial blight continued, but the war effort required many of the professional staff engaged in treatment in mental hospitals to leave. As the Joint Commission says, ". . . it brought them [state hospitals] to their lowest state, as houses of horror, in the last fifty years" (1961, 12). As late as 1947, Albert Deutsch (1949, p. 449) says, regarding his visits to a number of institutions, "the writer heard state hospital doctors frankly admit that the animals of nearby piggeries were better fed, housed and treated than many of the patients in their wards. He saw hundreds of sick people shackled, strapped, strait-jacketed and bound to their beds; he saw mental patients . . . crawl into beds jammed close together, in dormitories filled to twice or three times their normal capacity."

The National Institute of Mental Health was formed in 1949. In 1955 the Mental Health Study Act was passed and led to the Joint Commission on Mental Illness and Health. A report of that commission argued for community mental health centers and decreased size of mental hospitals. The report was generally well received and eventually led to the establishment of the Community Mental Health Centers Act of 1963. Although it does not seem to be commonly known these days, the Commission generally made very progressive recommendations regarding mental hospitalization. For example, one recommendation was that "no community general hospital should be regarded as rendering a complete service unless it accepts mental patients for short term hospitalization and therefore provides a psychiatric unit or psychiatric beds" (p. 265). The effect would be to decentralize treatment into smaller units and partially segregate acute cases from chronic ones.

Many state mental hospitals at the time had 10,000 to 15,000 patients, but the commission recommended "no further state hospitals of more than one thousand beds should be built, and not one patient should be added to an existing mental hospital already housing a thousand or more patients . . . special techniques are available for the care of the chronically ill and these techniques of socialization, relearning, group living, and gradual rehabilitation or social improvement should be expanded and extended to more people . . ." (p. 268). This argues to reverse the trend toward large hospitals and for the administrative use of known effective techniques for rehabilitation.

"Smaller state hospitals of a thousand beds or less and suitably located for regional service, should be converted as rapidly as possible into intensive treatment centers for those patients with major mental illness in the acute stages, or in the case of a more prolonged illness, those with a good prospect for improvement or recovery" (p. 266). This represents a clear, implicit argument for the treatability of mental disorders.

"The objective of modern treatment of persons with major mental illness is to enable the patient to maintain himself [sic] in the community in a normal manner. To do so, it is necessary (1) to save the patient from the debilitating aspects of institutionalization as much as possible, (2) if the patient requires hospitalization, to return him to home and community life as soon as possible, and (3) thereafter to maintain him in the community as long as possible" (p. 270). This recommendation argues for more treatment, noninstitutionalization if possible, and aftercare.

The commission also argued for prevention; "persons who are emotionally disturbed—that is to say, under psychological stress they cannot tolerate—should have skilled attention and helpful counseling available to them in their community if the development of more serious mental breakdowns is to be prevented. This is known as secondary prevention, and is concerned with the detection of beginning signs and symptoms of mental illness and their relief; in other words, the earliest possible treatment" (p. 256).[4]

These excerpts are provided to give the reader a flavor of the rather far-reaching recommendations of the Joint Commission on Mental Illness and Health in the 1950s. One outcome of that commission, the Community Mental Health Centers Systems Act of 1963, is surely the most progressive piece of legislation in the history of mental health treatment. It also had significant effects on the rates of deinstitutionalization, and on the general acceptance of deinstitutionalization as a national priority.

Deinstitutionalization had begun before the Joint Commission was formed. There is some contention in the literature about who should get credit for deinstitutionalization. Among psychiatrists and many other mental health professionals, the commonly accepted basis for the deinstitutionalization movement was the discovery of tranquilizing drugs, first experimentally used in the treatment of the mentally ill in 1953 and in general use in state hospitals by 1955. Indeed, the Joint Commission says that "estimates from various states indicate that as many as one third of all public mental hospital patients now receive these drugs, the general rule being to tranquilize patients who are hyperactive, unmanageable, excited, highly disturbed or highly disturbing" (1961, p. 39).

They go on (p. 39) to say, "these drugs have revolutionized the management of psychotic patients in American mental hospitals, and probably deserve primary credit for the reversal of the upward spiral of the state hospital inpatient load in the last four years."[5] Of course, we have noted, "chemical restraints" had been in common use in mental hospitals for over a century.

The problem of historical validity in that quote is that there was also a general move afoot toward an open hospital system and removing the restraints formerly imposed on patients; in short, returning to the basic practices of moral treatment. Indeed, the first systematic study of the use of the drugs (Brill & Patton, 1957, 1959) took place in the New York State system with essentially both variables occurring at roughly the same time (drug use and changes in other treatment practices).

In 1955 the Department of Mental Hygiene in New York introduced chlorpromazine and reserpine for general use in the state's 18 mental hospitals. In the first year of the program beginning in 1955, 30,000 patients received treatment with it. Brill and Patton studied the effects of this on the system from 1955 to 1959. However, as they note, in 1956 the Department of Mental Hygiene also began a new program for intensified treatment of newly admitted patients and began converting to an open hospital system. One of the substantial effects noted for these drugs is the reduction of the noise level in the wards and the increased ease of managing the patients. One effect noted in this study and others is that the staff were very enthusiastic about the use of the drugs and staff morale increased after introduction of them. The morale itself and the changing pattern of interacting with patients led to increased discharges of both tranquilized and nontranquilized patients. The drug in essence may have affected the staffs' relationships to all patients and thereby produced better treatment. However, in the Brill and Patton studies, the discharge rate among patients who were on the drugs was twice that of the patients who were not, even prior to the introduction of the open hospital system.

On the basis of such evidence some people argue that drugs have revolutionized psychiatric care. Others disagree. They suggest that the changes in administrative practices toward the more open hospital or social contracts with patients produced the larger effects and drugs only supported this changing philosophical approach to inpatient care (cf. Mechanic, 1980). By looking at the effects in English hospitals following such administrative changes but prior to the introduction of psychotropic drugs, some authors contend that the variance accounted for is largely through administrative changes, not psychotropic drugs (Bockoven, 1972; Scull, 1977). Zusman (1967) says that in those hospitals that adopted intensive treatment methods developed in WWII, treatment was much improved prior to the introduction of drugs. Whatever the separate contributions of drugs and changed social treatment, the march toward deinstitutionalization had begun. Deinstitutionalization, as a movement, has become a national controversy. These issues are discussed more completely in Chapter 10.

In the 1970s, deinstitutionalization was hurried along by a series of court cases. In *Wyatt v. Stickney* in 1972, an Alabama federal court outlined three basic requirements for mental treatment: the right to a humane environment; the right to adequate treatment personnel; and the right to individual treatment. In 1974 the United States Court of Appeals, Fifth Circuit, upheld that decision.

In *O'Connor v. Donaldson* (1975), the Supreme Court ruled that mental illness alone was not constitutionally sufficient for involuntary hospitalization. The concept of the right to the least restrictive treatment alternative became frequently asserted. The full impact of these and several other court cases is yet to be felt by the system of mental hospitalization. Rubin's fine book, *Economics, Mental Health, and the Law* (1978) outlines the potential legal and economic implications of these various cases.

In 1977, President Carter formed a President's Commission on Mental Health (PCMH), which made a set of recommendations in 1978. The three-volume set of task panel reports are of special note to anyone interested in mental health policy. The PCMH urged increased funding for personnel, research, and CMHCs, and increased emphasis on groups in special need, such as women, children, minorities, and the elderly. The major legislation coming out of this effort, the Mental Health

Systems Act, was an attempt to integrate better the system of delivery of services. Unfortunately, this legislation was repealed as a part of the Omnibus Budget Reconciliation Act of 1981.

In some sense perhaps we have come full circle since the days of Pinel. We are committed to discharging people from hospitals and to maintaining them in the community. Yet we are putting them in faster than ever. In the next section we will see there were three million inpatient episodes in the United States in 1981, reflecting a continuing increase over the previous 10-15 years. The site of hospitalization has changed away from state mental hospitals to general hospitals, particularly those without psychiatric units. Yet we have no systematic evidence on the outcomes of this change. That is to say, we do not know how the recovery rate has changed as a function of site of hospitalization.

In the next chapter we take up the issue of the number of inpatient episodes nationally and how it has changed across different types of hospitals.

Notes

1. General hospitals without psychiatric units were not included.

2. For a more complete treatment see Grob, 1966, 1983; Levine, 1981; Deutsch, 1949 or Bockoven, 1972.

3. Dain's (1980) biography of Beers is recommended to the reader.

4. We note that some (e.g., Levine, 1981) criticized the Commission for being too oriented towards hospitals and hospital treatment and too little toward prevention.

5. According to Eaton (1980), eight months after the introduction of chlorpromazine in the United States in 1954, over two million patients had been treated with it. Eaton attributes much of this dramatic increase in use to the intensive marketing of the drug manufacturers, directed at both psychiatrists and legislatures, which had to increase budgets for drug therapy.

SECTION II

TRENDS IN HOSPITALIZATION FOR MENTAL DISORDERS: A REANALYSIS OF NATIONAL DATA

Based on the de jure mental health policy of community mental health centers and deinstitutionalization, one might expect statistics to show fewer people are being hospitalized now and for shorter periods of time than 25 years ago. The chapters in this section will review utilization statistics bearing on these questions. Statistics will show admissions, discharges, residents, and episodes for various types of institutions treating psychiatric inpatients. By reviewing the best available evidence from a variety of sources we can assess what has actually occurred in terms of hospitalizing people.

All of the evidence presented here rests on national surveys of inpatient treatment of mental disorders. Redick, Manderscheid, Witkin, and Rosenstein (1983) provide a history of such surveys. Although modern epidemiological studies of mental disorders in noninstitutionalized populations began at least 30 years ago, culminating in the Epidemiological Catchment Area Study (described in Chapter 1), the United States actually began counting the "insane and idiotic," as well as paupers and convicts, in 1840, under the direction of the secretary of state. The decennial census from 1840 to 1870 was unencumbered by any definitions of "insane" or "idiotic." The census takers, who interviewed each head of household, were simply instructed to ask the respondent whether any members of the household were insane or idiotic. The other categories were deaf and dumb, blind, pauper, or convict. (The pauper and convict categories were omitted from the 1870 census).[1]

The 1880 and 1890 censuses were the first to enumerate the "defectives" in institutions, as well as at home. Institutions included jails and alms houses in addition to institutions for the retarded and those with mental disorders.

Beginning in 1904, an enumeration of the insane and feeble-minded (formerly the idiotic) was limited to those in institutions, because Congress decided it did not want to count what it could not adequately define. (Being in an institution was apparently adequate evidence for having a mental disorder.) The Bureau of the Census did the institutional censuses from 1923 through 1946. Beginning in 1923, the survey was rather detailed in that separate forms were filled out for each resident, first admission, discharge, etc., and characteristics of the institution. Specific diagnoses of mental disorders were first requested in 1923, after the American Psychiatric Association and the National Committee for Mental Hygiene introduced a classification.

The National Institute of Mental Health (NIMH) was formally established in 1949 and took over the census of patients in mental institutions. The organizational unit that became the Biometry Branch actually began its first census in 1948, collecting data for 1947. Rather than collecting detailed information on a separate form for each person, data were consolidated into tables showing the total number of admissions or discharges categorized by sex, age, and/or diagnosis. These "patient movement" data continued to be collected, and these forms have many features in common with the forms used through 1980.

During the 1950s and 1960s, NIMH began collecting data from newly established facilities, such as outpatient clinics, residential treatment centers, and community mental health centers. The Inventories of Mental Health Facilities were designed in 1968 to be a set of uniform survey forms covering all types of mental health facilities. At this time, coverage of institutions for the mentally retarded was shifted out of NIMH to a different division in the Public Health Service. Rather than collecting data on patient characteristics, the Inventory forms collected aggregate data on total admissions, discharges, etc. Separate surveys of probability samples of patient records began in order to obtain patient level data more efficiently.

NIMH periodically compiles trend data from their various surveys and presents them in one source. Their most recent compilations, *Mental Health United States, 1983* and *Mental Health United States, 1985* (Taube & Barrett, 1983, 1985), not only present data on utilization of mental health facilities but also include statistics on service providers and expenditures. Surveys conducted by several other agencies and professional organizations were used as sources of the data on human resources and utilization of facilities in the general health care sector.

Chapters 3 through 6 in this section deal with inpatient data: trends in the number of episodes, admissions, discharges, and residents in all types of institutions housing people with mental disorders. Our data presentations differ from Taube and Barrett's in that we present data from several surveys designed to count the same things, in order to see the extent to which various sources agree. The NIMH data we present will be the same as in their publications,[2] but we consider the NIMH data as only one source to be compared with other sources.

Given the tedious nature of the following data presentations, the reader may wonder why we are going to such great lengths to present data that often result in the same conclusions. The answer is validity. We have more confidence in a trend if independent sources show the same pattern.

The use of independent sources also provides more information about the total universe of institutions than would be apparent from using one source alone. As will be further explained, some surveys cover subsets of institutions or report certain statistics that others do not. Given that a full understanding of the trends in mental hospitalization at the national level requires the simultaneous consideration of several different statistics across the range of facilities, we have compiled the most complete presentation that exists to date.

Chapter 3 compares utilization data from various surveys to show changes in the absolute volume of inpatient service in the last 25 years. Chapter 4 describes these changes in terms of episodes per 100,000 population; that is, the change in rate of episodes. Data on the average length of stay in these institutions are provided in Chapter 5. Another approach to assessing the impact of these policies is to determine the proportion of total hospital days for all health care that are for mental health care. Chapter 6 will show trends in these proportions across the same types of facilities surveyed in Chapters 3, 4, and 5. Chapter 7 will discuss trend data on nursing home residents and their relation to the declining state mental hospital population. Chapter 8 discusses data on readmissions and their role in planning services.

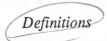

Definitions

In Chapter 1 "mental hospitalization" was defined as the hospitalization of a person for the treatment of mental disorder, regardless of the type of institution in which he or she stays. (We will describe these institutions as we present data for them.) A diagnosis of mental disorder is inferred based on the diagnosis at the time of discharge or because the type of facility is designed to treat primarily mental disorders.

Much of our epidemiological data are expressed in terms of "episodes," because NIMH reports utilization data in terms of episodes, and we conform to their reporting practices when possible. *Episode* refers to the total clinical occurrence of a mental disorder. An inpatient episode begins when a patient is hospitalized and ends when the patient is discharged. In national epidemiological data, episodes typically refer to resident patients at the beginning of a reporting year, plus all admissions during the year.[3]

The term *residents* refers to the number of people in a hospital at a given time. It does not indicate the number of people hospitalized within a year. Unless otherwise noted, *admissions* include first admissions and readmissions. Since an individual may account for more than one episode during the year (by being discharged and subsequently readmitted), most national data include some duplication of people. The problem of duplicated episodes will be further discussed in Chapter 3. Also, other relevant terms will be defined as they arise.

Sources of Data

Our analyses are based on survey data collected by various public and private organizations. Although the National Institute of Mental Health is the most widely cited source of data on utilization of mental health facilities, the Veterans Administration, the National Center for Health Statistics, and the American Hospital Association also regularly conduct surveys that are national in scope. The results of these surveys are intended to represent all facilities in the United States. This representativeness is achieved in one of two ways. Either the whole universe is surveyed, with estimates made for nonresponses, or a probability sample of individual facilities or records is selected, and the estimates are multiplied by the appropriate fraction to reflect the whole universe. Another major distinction among surveys is their unit of analysis, i.e., whether they collect aggregate data at each particular site, e.g., state mental hospital, or whether individual patient records are surveyed. Whereas the first type can provide aggregate numbers of residents, admissions, and the like, only the second type can provide data on patient characteristics. Some data gathering organizations conduct both types of surveys.

The purpose of comparing figures from different surveys, supposedly measuring the same thing, is to establish the reliability of the findings. If two independently conducted surveys report similar figures, then confidence in the conclusions is raised. Another advantage of this "multiple-source" method is that parts of the universe covered sometimes by only one survey are not missed.

Brief descriptions of the surveys we have used are given as the data are introduced in each chapter. For detailed descriptions of the surveys, the reader is referred to the *Guide to National Data on Inpatient Care for Mental Disorders* (Sibulkin & Kiesler, 1982). All the variables on inpatient utilization collected by the surveys are described, and tables show how to obtain the statistics from published and unpublished sources.

Notes

1. The 1850 and 1860 forms indicate they are to be used for "free inhabitants," while the 1870 form only specifies "inhabitants."

2. We also include data from earlier years, taken from other NIMH publications.

3. Epidemiologists typically refer to this statistic as "period prevalence," consisting of the point prevalence at the beginning of a specified period plus all new cases that occur during the period (see Palinkas & Hoiberg, 1982).

CHAPTER 3

CURRENT TRENDS
IN THE ANNUAL NUMBER
OF INPATIENT PSYCHIATRIC EPISODES

At the end of this chapter,[1] we will show the current best estimates of the number of episodes occurring nationally in each type of inpatient facility. To set the stage properly, we need to focus on and review the trends leading up to this current picture in each site of hospitalization. The trends vary for each type of facility, and so we consider them separately.

State Mental Hospitals [2]

These hospitals receive the most publicity regarding deinstitutionalization efforts, although it is important to regard them as only one part of the total mental health inpatient system. Table 3.1 shows the number of these facilities and figures on utilization as reported by NIMH and the American Hospital Association (AHA) from 1948 to 1983.

A first step in searching for consistency among different estimates of the utilization of any type of facility is to determine whether different sources are including the same number of facilities in their data bases. We see that these two independent agencies agree fairly closely that state mental hospitals have not disappeared; the number of them has fluctuated around 300 for the last 35 years.[3] While the number of state mental hospitals has remained fairly stable, they have been "emptying out." According to NIMH, the number of residents has dramatically decreased from the peak of about 559,000 in 1955 to 125,000 in 1981, or 78%. The AHA trend agrees: The average daily census (the average number of residents present per day, rather than the residents on a given day) shows a decrease in census of 77% between 1955 and 1981. However, this sharp decrease in residents is often emphasized to the exclusion of the less- publicized increase in admissions. Both NIMH and AHA show that admissions of 150 to 200 thousand in 1950 had doubled by the mid-1960s. Admissions continued to rise until the early 1970s and have gradually declined to about 300 to 350 thousand, similar to the early 1960s.

Now we can see what happens when residents and admissions are combined to form "episodes," the statistic used most frequently by NIMH to compare the number of contacts across different types of facilities and years. Episodes equal the number of patients in residence at the beginning of the twelve-month reporting period, plus the number admitted during the reporting period.[4]

The NIMH data in Table 3.1 show a 39% decline in episodes from 819,000 in 1955 to 499,000 in 1981. We see that as a summary statistic, the number of episodes can be fairly misleading when the two contributing variables (residents and admissions) have opposite trends over the years. Since the number of residents decreased at a slightly faster rate than the number of admissions increased, the net result of a 39% decrease in episodes masked the important rise in admissions during this time.

Another element critical to understanding the flow of people in and out of state mental hospitals is deaths of the patients. In 1950, 41,000 deaths occurred, and the number of deaths climbed to 50,000 in 1960 before starting to decline. By 1980, only 7,000 deaths occurred (Goldman, Adams, & Taube, 1983). If deaths are added to "net releases"[5] to represent the total number of people exiting state mental hospitals, deaths accounted for 29% of those ultimately leaving these hospitals in 1950 but only 3% in 1975.[6]

SUMMARY

The number of residents in state mental hospitals has decreased by almost 80% (the sharpest decline was in the period 1965–1975). While this decrease was occurring, admissions continued to increase for a long time. Since 1972, admissions have fallen. The number of inpatient episodes, which includes both residents and admissions, did not begin to drop until the late 1960s. But today still about 60% as many inpatient episodes occur in state mental hospitals as did in 1955.

It is interesting that despite widespread use of chlorpromazines in 1954–1955, episodes in state mental hospitals did not begin to decrease until 1965.[7]

TABLE 3.1
Number of Institutions, Inpatient Episodes, Admissions, Residents, and Average Daily Census in State and County Mental Hospitals, According to NIMH and AHA Surveys, 1948-1983

	NIMH					AHA		
Year	No. of Inst.[a]	Inpatient Episodes	Admissions	Additions[b]	Residents (End/Yr.)	No. of Inst.	Admissions	Avg. Daily Census
1948						306	202,162	580,502
1949						302	199,604	581,920
1950	322		152,286		512,501	310	205,665	592,853
1951	322		152,079		520,326	319	187,738	619,905
1952	329		162,908		531,981	322	310,098	633,578
1953	332		170,621		545,045	326	206,834	646,464
1954	352		171,682		553,979	321	204,455	652,328
1955	275	818,832	178,003		558,922	320	217,716	661,743
1956	278		185,597		551,390	301	239,374	643,425
1957	277		194,497		548,626	260	216,614	594,869
1958	278		209,823		545,182	290	272,308	590,583
1959	279		222,791		541,883	296	272,023	627,900
1960	280		234,791		535,540	313	276,121	657,718
1961	285		252,742		527,456	313	294,178	640,141
1962	285		269,854		515,640	320	324,119	634,140
1963	284	799,401	283,591		504,604	328	342,483	639,612
1964	289		299,561		490,449	326	357,282	618,592
1965	290	804,926	316,664		475,202	318	394,215	590,988
1966	298	802,216	328,564		452,089	314	366,319	567,117

Year								
1967	307	801,354	345,673		426,309	312	394,424	526,750
1968	312	791,819	367,461		399,152	333	426,974	517,385
1969	310	767,115	374,771	486,661	369,969	341	449,034	474,777
1970	315		384,511	459,523	337,619	351	483,553	432,520
1971	321	745,259	402,472	474,923	308,983	339	488,324	379,678
1972	327		390,455	460,433	274,837	348	470,653	365,539
1973	334	651,857	377,020	442,530	248,518	343	456,805	329,835
1974	320		374,554	434,345	215,586	340	447,933	293,708
1975	303	598,993	376,156	433,529	191,395	326	443,513	251,167
1976	300			413,559	170,619	313	435,780	216,083
1977	297	574,226		414,703	159,405	309	424,414	195,981
1978	284			406,407	153,544	293	406,944	173,914
1979	280	526,690		383,323	140,355	287	385,185	169,459
1980	276			370,344	132,164	276	356,596	162,093
1981	277	499,169		370,693	125,246	272	338,822	151,434
1982						266	328,889	144,584
1983						275	330,727	138,911

SOURCES: NIMH data: 1950-1968: President's Commission on Mental Health, Vol. 2; Kramer, 1977; Statistical Notes 23, 146, 60. 1969-1981: *Mental Health United States 1983* and *1985*. AHA data: Data from 1948-1970 appear in the journal *Hospitals* published in the following year. Data for 1971-1983 appear in the *Hospital Statistics* editions for each year.

NOTE: See Kiesler and Sibulkin (1983a) for further details on data collection and sources. Some statistics reported here differ slightly from the original article due to NIMH's revisions of their data.

[a] From 1969 to 1981 NIMH reports the number of facilities as of January of the following year. They correspond to the utilization statistics for the years shown here.

[b] NIMH defines *additions* to include new admissions, readmissions, and returns from long-term leave (Taube & Barrett, 1985).

Veterans Administration Medical Centers

The VA conducts detailed surveys of all health care in its medical centers, collecting both aggregate and patient level data. Results are reported in the VA's *Annual Reports*. The National Institute of Mental Health[8] collects data from the VA, as part of their broader surveys. We will start with comparing the number of facilities reported by the two sources and then describe admissions, residents, and episodes.

VA data are complex in that two different kinds of facilities were operated until 1979. With the extensive amount of data collected, VA statistics can be analyzed in a variety of ways. Table 3.2 compares the number of VA hospital facilities and various admission figures according to the VA and NIMH. Hospitals were categorized as "general medical and surgical" or as "psychiatric," indicating the predominant but not exclusive type of care provided. Beginning in 1979, this distinction was no longer made and all hospitals were designated "medical centers." The number of VA psychiatric hospitals has decreased since the 1950s. The number of general hospitals has been fairly constant for years, but recently has been increasing.

NIMH data show a similar trend of a decrease in psychiatric hospitals and an increase in general hospitals that provide psychiatric care.[9] The reason for discrepancies between the two sources is not clear—it should be easy to determine if a hospital exists—but changes in classification of hospitals between the times the two surveys were conducted may have had an effect. It does illustrate the difficulties in obtaining precise national data in this field.

A description of admissions, residents, and episodes is complicated by the VA's classification of "bed sections" as either medical, surgical, or psychiatric. Both psychiatric and general hospitals could have psychiatric as well as medical or surgical bed sections. Bed sections consist of beds classified "according to their intended use; patients are classified according to the classification of the beds they occupy, rather than on a diagnostic basis" (VA *Annual Reports*). Therefore, admissions to a psychiatric bed section do not directly correspond to diagnoses of mental disorder; they are counts of all admissions to the psychiatric bed sections regardless of the diagnosis at admission or discharge.

According to the VA's own data, the trends in general hospital versus psychiatric hospital utilization differ (see Table 3.2). Psychiatric admissions to general hospitals rose from 16,264 in 1954 to 121,186 in 1978, the last year of the general/psychiatric hospital distinction. Admissions to the psychiatric hospitals increased fourfold between 1954 and 1971, but have declined since. Regarding residents in psychiatric hospitals, the VA reports a dramatic decrease in the average daily census in psychiatric hospitals of about 70% between 1954 and 1978. This decrease is almost identical to that reported for residents of state mental hospitals.

Now we combine admissions and residents to create episodes for comparison with NIMH's episodes. Table 3.3 shows VA episodes in all psychiatric bed sections, broken down by type of hospital. We calculated VA episodes in a way that would be equivalent to NIMH episodes.[10]

From 1969 to 1980, total episodes reported by NIMH are in fairly close agreement with episodes derived from VA data. Episodes peaked at 215,000 in 1976 and declined somewhat to 198,000 in 1983. We also see that the decline in episodes beginning in 1976 (according to the VA source) is due to the decline in psychiatric hospital episodes offsetting the rise in general hospital episodes. Although the distinction between general and psychiatric hospitals ceased after 1978, former psychiatric hospitals still have relatively large psychiatric bed sections and probably continue to function in a similar way. Therefore, the continuing decrease in total episodes is likely driven by decreasing episodes in former psychiatric hospitals.

Let us consider the trends in the two components of episodes: numbers of residents and admissions (not shown in Table 3.3). The resident population rose to 69,000 in 1967 and decreased to 21,000 in 1983. Admissions rose to 189,000 in 1976 before a steady downturn. Therefore, the decline in total episodes, beginning in 1976 is due to the decrease in admissions added to the already decreasing residents. Unlike state mental hospital episodes, the net VA episodes are driven more by admissions rather than residents.

We might note a final VA statistic, number of discharges with a principal diagnosis of mental disorder as reported by the VA (Table 3.2). There are two reasons why these figures are higher than admissions to psychiatric bed sections. The discharge records from all bed sections are examined and the principal diagnosis is recorded. Second, the VA defines the principal diagnosis after the fact, as that responsible for the major portion of the hospital stay (rather than the problem causing the admission). If the mental health problem is perceived to be responsible for the majority of the length of stay, it is presumably recorded as principal, regardless of the seriousness of the medical problem. Therefore, people can be discharged from the medical and surgical bed sections with a principal diagnosis of mental disorder. The longer-than-average length of stay for mental disorders would also contribute to a higher count of mental disorders based on principal diagnoses than on treatment in a bed section. Table 3.2 shows discharges with a primary diagnosis of

TABLE 3.2
Number of Institutions, Inpatient Episodes, Admissions, Discharges, Average Daily Census in VA Hospitals, According to Surveys by VA and NIMH, 1954-1983

Year	No. of VA Hosp Providing Psych Care		Admissions to Psych Bed Sections		Average Daily Census in Psych Hosp	Discharges with Primary Diagnosis of Mental Disorder All Hosp[d]	No of[f] VA Hosp		Inpatient[h] Episodes
	Gen[a]	Psy[a]	Gen	Psych			Gen	Psy	
1954	75	38	16,264	12,926	49,528	50,800[e]			88,355
1955	100	40	19,160	14,189	51,328	54,812[e]			
1956	103	40	21,310	17,135	52,624	52,840			
1957	103	41	20,057	17,112	54,518	53,350			
1958	100	41	21,330	16,303	52,674	53,450			
1959	85	39	38,958[c]		52,424	55,230			
1960	74	39	41,452[c]		52,427	59,080			
1961	72	40	45,433[c]		52,773	65,126			
1962	74	41	49,279[c]		52,986	69,413			
1963	72	42	22,073	29,231	54,006	83,208			109,973
1964	75	42	23,505	32,573	54,335	89,413			
1965	75	41	24,238	33,480	52,906	91,078			115,843
1966	76	41	26,385	38,640	52,081	102,865			122,979
1967	75	41	28,917	42,159	50,059	118,731		40	128,196
1968	77	41	34,192	46,216	46,365	130,438			133,503
1969	79	38	39,529	47,621	40,327	144,607	76	34	186,913
1970	70	37	42,775	54,500	34,960	151,323[c]	80	34	176,800
1971	80	33	54,921	54,301	29,851	166,274	110[g]		
1972	89	28	79,291	49,289	24,620	178,654			

1973	92	28	90,612	50,682	24,558	194,465	86	27	208,416
1974	92	27	101,017	47,783	22,955	207,812	89	24	214,264
1975	96	24	110,774	43,661	19,476	218,039			
1976	101	23	117,253	44,716	17,647	219,802	100	22	217,507
1977	103	22	117,977	41,876	16,356	215,132			
1978	105	21	121,186	37,974	15,097	214,084			
1979	127		159,771			212,556			
1980	129		160,417			211,867	127 [g]		205,580
1981	128		157,933			208,390			
1982	128		154,304			205,777			
1983	129 [b]		150,896 [b]			202,772			

SOURCES: VA data: Veterans Administration Annual Report for that year, published by the Government Printing Office in the following year. Discharge figures from 1954 to 1969 appear in the ANNUAL REPORT of the following year. 1955, 1965-1968: Statistical Note Nos. 5, 23; 1963: Kramer, 1977; 1970: Mental Health Statistics. Series A, No. 12; 1969-1980: *Mental Health United States, 1983, 1985.*

NOTE: See Kiesler and Sibulkin (1983a) for further details on data collection and sources. Some statistics reported here differ slightly from the original article due to NIMH's revisions of their data.

[a] These are the number operating during the year. Figures may differ from those reported for the end of the year due to openings, closings, and redesignations of hospitals.

[b] Beginning in 1979, all VA hospitals were called "medical centers" and types of hospitals were no longer distinguished. There were 129 VA medical centers with psychiatric bed sections in 1983 and 150,896 admissions to them.

[c] From 1959 to 1962 the admission figures are for all psychiatric bed sections. Separate figures by type of hospital are not published.

[d] The VA defines "principal diagnosis" as the diagnosis "responsible for the major portion of the patient's length of stay as judged by the attending physician." This is different from the National Center for Health Statistics' criterion of the condition resulting in the admission. These are discharges from all VA medical centers, whether or not they have a psychiatric bed section.

[e] These figures include discharges of veterans from VA and non-VA hospitals.

[f] NIMH reports the number of facilities for 1969 to 1977 as of January of the following year. They correspond to the utilization statistics for the years shown here. The most recent publications (*Mental Health United States*) show only the combined number of psychiatric hospitals and general hospitals with separate psychiatric services. We show the breakdowns by type of hospital as reported in older publications, although they sum to slightly different totals than the currently reported totals.

[g] Includes general hospitals with separate psychiatric units and psychiatric hospitals.

[h] Total episodes in general hospitals with separate psychiatric units and psychiatric hospitals.

TABLE 3.3
Psychiatric Inpatient Episodes in All VA Hospitals as Reported by NIMH and Constructed from VA Data, 1955-1983

| Year | Veterans Administration | | | NIMH | | |
| | Psychiatric Bed Section | | | | | |
	Gen. Hosp.	Psych. Hosp.	Total	Gen. Hosp.	Psychiatric Hospital	Total
1955						88,355
1956						
1957						
1958						
1959			145,552			
1960			150,257			
1961			160,152			
1962			172,982			
1963			193,337			109,973
1964			191,981			
1965			187,890			115,843
1966			195,496			122,979
1967			162,900			128,196

Year						
1968			170,068			133,503
1969			190,503			186,913
1970			185,884			176,800
1971	79,277	114,153	193,430			
1972	107,739	90,290	195,319			
1973	117,703	82,572	200,276	117,000	91,000	208,000
1974	129,697	78,555	208,248			
1975	143,268	68,988	212,259	131,003	83,261	214,264
1976	150,660	67,222	214,775			
1977	150,631	61,961	212,592	140,166	77,341	217,507
1978	155,179	56,790	211,969			
1979			210,593			
1980			209,314			205,580
1981			206,062			
1982			205,030			
1983			198,054			

SOURCES: VA data: The total number of episodes were derived by adding the total on the rolls in all psychiatric bed sections plus gains. Total on rolls equals residents and absent bed occupants. Gains equal admissions plus intra- and interhospital transfers. Totals are from the VA Annual Reports. The breakdowns by type of hospital are unpublished figures from the VA. NIMH data: 1955, 1965-1968: Statistical Note No. 23; 1963: Kramer, 1977; 1969-1980: *Mental Health United States, 1983* and *1985*.

NOTES: The sum of the episodes for years 1972 through 1976 do not exactly match the total reported in the Annual Reports, due to editing at the VA.

mental disorder peaked at 220,000 in 1976 and decreased to 203,000 in 1983, thus following the same trend as episodes.

SUMMARY

There were 198,000 episodes for mental disorders in VA medical centers in 1983. Episodes began to decline in 1976 and were the result of a decline in admissions added to an already declining resident population.

Private Mental Hospitals

Table 3.4 shows NIMH statistics on the number of private mental hospitals, episodes, admissions, and residents from 1955 to 1981. These are combined figures for both profit (investor-owned) and nonprofit facilities.[11]

Episodes in private mental hospitals fluctuated in earlier years but clearly began to increase in the 1970s. NIMH reported an 80% increase in episodes between 1971 and 1981.

In state mental hospitals, a decline in residents was ultimately joined by a decline in admissions. In contrast, for the private sector, both admissions and residents have been increasing since the 1970s. The growth of for-profit psychiatric hospitals, particularly multihospital chains, may account for this rise in private psychiatric hospital use. AHA data show that in 1969 private mental hospitals were equally divided among those run for-profit and not-for-profit. In 1984, 64% were for-profit (Levenson, 1982, 1983).

Community Mental Health Centers

Table 3.5 shows NIMH data for inpatient care in CMHCs. One can see that CMHCs—the flagship of outpatient care—accounted for over a quarter of a million inpatient episodes in 1980, creating a total of nearly 4 million inpatient days. CMHCs did not exist until 1967. At that time there were about 100, and nearly 700 existed in 1980. Almost 10 times the number of inpatient episodes occurred in 1980 as in 1967. It was hoped that CMHCs would provide community care alternatives to state mental hospitalization, but we will see in Chapter 10 that the evidence that CMHCs played this role is unconvincing.

We caution the reader that there is the potential for some CMHC data being counted twice in some national data (specifically, general hos-

TABLE 3.4
Number of Institutions, Inpatient Episodes, Admissions,
Residents, and Average Daily Census in Private Psychiatric
Hospitals, According to NIMH, 1955-1981

		NIMH		
Year	No. of Inst.	Inpatient Episodes	Additions	Residents
1955		123,231		
1956				
1957				
1958				
1959				
1960				
1961				
1962				
1963		127,921		9,998
1964				
1965		125,428 [b]		
1966		103,973		
1967	174	124,258 [a]		
1968	151	118,126 [a]	89,138	10,454
1969	150	102,510	92,056	10,963
1970				10,677
1971	156	97,963	87,106	10,207
1972	177		101,198	11,193
1973	180	123,000	109,516	10,977
1974	180		119,071	11,496
1975	182	137,025	125,529	11,576
1976				
1977	188	150,685	138,151	12,078
1978				
1979	184	150,535	140,831	12,921
1981	211	176,513	162,034	15,123

SOURCES: 1955-1968: Statistical Notes Nos. 5, 23; Report Series on Mental Health Statistics, Series A, No. 18 and B, No. 5; Kramer, 1977; 1969-1981: *Mental Health United States, 1983* and *1985.*

NOTES: See Kiesler and Sibulkin (1983a) for comparisons with American Hospital Association data and details on data collection. Some figures do not agree with the original article, due to NIMH'S revisions of their data. Private psychiatric hospitals include profit, nonprofit, short- and long-term ones. From 1969 to 1981 NIMH reports the number of hospitals as of January of the following year. They correspond to the utilization statistics of the year shown here.

[a] Includes residential treatment centers for children, which began reporting nationally in 1967 (Statistical Note No. 23).
[b] Based on 238 hospitals; 64 were later found ineligible and removed from this category. This reclassification accounts for the drop in episodes between 1965 and 1966 (Statistical Note No. 23).

TABLE 3.5
Number of Federally Funded Community Mental Health Centers,
Inpatient Episodes, Inpatient Days, and Average Daily Census
from NIMH Surveys, 1967-1980

Year	Inpatient Episodes	Number of Inpatient Days	Average Daily Census
1967	27,070		
1968			
1969	65,000	1,924,000 [a]	5,271
1970	110,622		
1971	130,088	2,225,000	6,096
1972	144,601	2,562,000	7,019
1973	192,000	3,276,000	8,975
1974	211,027	3,836,000	10,510
1975	246,891	3,718,000	10,186
1976	270,944	3,951,000	10,825
1977	268,966	3,818,000	10,460
1978	298,897	4,063,000	11,132
1980	254,288	3,609,000	9,888

SOURCES: 1967: Statistical Notes Nos. 5, 127; 1969, 1971, 1973, 1975, 1977, 1980: *Mental Health United States, 1983* and *1985*; other years: Provisional data on federally funded community mental health centers, 1978-1979.

NOTE: Some of the statistics reported here differ slightly from those reported in Kiesler and Sibulkin (1983a) due to NIMH's revisions of their data. Beginning in 1976 the data are based on a random sample of CMHCs rather than the universe, and the figures are estimates inflated from sample counts.

[a] There is some ambiguity in the data sources as to whether these days occurred in 1969 or 1970. The most recent publications show 1,924,000 days in 1969, although they would more closely correspond to 1970 episodes, in terms of days per episode.

pitals—see next section). CMHCs were designed to provide a full range of services. Rather than creating new facilities, they usually provided services by contracting for them from already existing facilities (Regier & Taube, 1981; Thompson, Bass, & Witkin, 1982). When a CMHC provided inpatient care through a general hospital psychiatric unit, the issue arose of whether to count the facility as a general hospital psychiatric unit or as a CMHC. NIMH classified a unit as a CMHC when the entire unit was administered as a CMHC. If only part of the unit's clients were CMHC clients, NIMH counted both a unit and a CMHC. Further, AHA's count of psychiatric units probably includes what NIMH calls CMHCs.

Federally funded CMHCs are no longer funded with direct federal grants and ceased being surveyed as such after 1980. Therefore, the potential for duplicate reporting of episodes from CMHCs and the hospitals with which they are affiliated (primarily general hospitals) no longer exists. CMHCs that were freestanding (i.e., not affiliated with a hospital) were reclassified as "multiservice mental health organizations" when 1981 data were collected. In 1981, there were 292 that provided inpatient service, contributing 128,000 episodes.

General Hospitals [12]

People typically think only of state and private mental hospitals when they think of mental hospitalization. However, people are hospitalized for mental health problems in general hospitals, both in specifically designated units and, especially, in hospitals without such units. Table 3.6 compares data from NIMH, AHA, and the National Center for Health Statistics (NCHS).

NIMH and AHA define psychiatric units as physically separate areas of the hospital with beds that are set up and staffed specifically for providing mental health care. Both sources show a rise in the number of units over the last 20 years. In 1983 there were about 1,000, according to AHA. However, before 1980, AHA consistently recorded about 200 more units than NIMH, probably due to the overlaps with CMHC reporting that we alluded to previously (to be discussed more completely regarding rates of hospitalization in Chapter 4).

Table 3.6 presents two quite different and important surveys of general hospitals. The NIMH data shown on the left side of the Table are limited to psychiatric units in general hospitals. Inpatient episodes in psychiatric units of general hospitals increased 25% in the decade 1971–1980. This represents treatment in the specialty mental health sector—facilities specifically designed to treat only mental disorders (Regier et al., 1978).

The NCHS survey is quite a different matter. Their survey (specifically the Hospital Discharge Survey) is a study of the general health care sector. It consists of a probability sample of about 500 nonfederal hospitals out of a universe of about 6,000,[13] and samples roughly 200,000 discharge records from them.

Characteristics of each discharged person, such as their age, sex, and diagnosis, are recorded and then statistically inflated to represent all discharges from the national universe of hospitals. Whether the hospitals

TABLE 3.6
Number of Nonfederal General Hospitals with and without Separate Inpatient Psychiatric Units, Inpatient Episodes, Discharges, and Days of Care from Surveys by NIMH, AHA, and NCHS, 1955-1983

	NIMH			AHA	NCHS	
Year	No. of Nonfed. Gen. Hospitals with Inpatient Psychiatric Units[a]	Inpatient Episodes	Discharges	No. of Nonfed. Gen. Short-Term Hospitals with Inpatient Psychiatric Service Areas	Discharges with First-Listed Diagnosis of Mental Disorder[c]	Days of Care[d]
1955		265,934				
1956						
1957						
1958						
1959						
1960						
1961						
1962				582		
1963		349,654		622		
1964				659		
1965		519,328		685	678,000	9,038,000
1966		548,921		767	759,000	9,655,000
1967		578,513		734	753,000	9,329,000
1968	546	558,790[b]	325,832		799,000	9,760,000
1969	664	535,493	323,215	798		
1970				784	604,000	10,940,000
1971	653	542,642	519,926	831	1,050,000	12,341,000
1972				823	1,176,000	13,666,000

1973	684	487,787	468,415	871	1,227,000	14,176,400
1974				949	1,352,000	15,248,000
1975	791	565,696	543,731	996	1,494,000	16,496,000
1976				1,033	1,485,000	15,604,000
1977	843	571,725	551,190	1,056	1,625,000	17,606,000
1978				1,025	1,730,000	19,435,000
1979				1,045	1,723,000	18,983,000
1980	1,059ᵉ	676,941	648,205	1,075	1,692,000	19,578,000
1981				1,104	1,747,000	20,898,000
1982				1,141	1,746,000	21,115,000
1983				1,186	1,701,000	21,124,000

SOURCES: NIMH data: 1955, 1963-1968: Statistical Notes Nos. 21 and 23; 1969-1980: *Mental Health United States, 1983 and 1985.*
AHA data: Data from 1948 to 1970 appear in the journal *Hospitals* published in the following year; 1971 to 1983 appear in the annual editions of *Hospital Statistics.* NCHS (Hospital Discharge Survey) data: Discharges: 1965-1968, 1971-1983: Vital and Health Statistics Series 13, No. 6, 12, 16, 20, 25, 26, 31, 37, 41, 46, 60, 64, 72, 78, 82, respectively; Days of Care: 1974-1976: *Nation's Use of Health Resources, 1976 and 1979.* Other years: unpublished data from Hospital Discharge Survey.

NOTE: See Kiesler and Sibulkin (1983a) for further details on data collection and sources. Some statistics reported here differ slightly from the original article due to NIMH's revisions of their data. Both NIMH and AHA define inpatient psychiatric units as those having beds set up and staffed specifically for this service.

a From 1969-1977 NIMH reports the number of facilities as of January of the following year. They correspond to the utilitzation statistics for the year shown here.

b The drop in episodes from 1967 to 1968 is due largely to reclassifying about 50 general hospital units in 1967 to CMHCs in 1968 (Statistical Note No. 23).

c The first-listed diagnosis is intended to equal the principal diagnosis, which is "the condition established after study to be chiefly responsible for occasioning the admission of the patient to the hospital for care." In the absence of other information, the diagnosis listed first on the medical record is assumed to be the principal diagnosis (Kozak & Moien, 1985).

d Days of care are the total number of days spent in the hospital accumulated at the time of discharge by all discharges during the year including days spent prior to the beginning of the year.

e Not comparable to previous years due to the reclassification of some CMHCs into psychiatric units of nonfederal general hospitals (*Mental Health United States, 1985*).

sampled have a psychiatric unit or not is of no concern to the HDS. Only bed size and geographic region are used as sampling criteria.

The NCHS data in Table 3.6 show the number of discharges with a principal diagnosis of mental disorder. A principal diagnosis is the condition responsible for occasioning the admission to the hospital. The number with "mental disorders" is the number with codes for that classification in the International Classification of Diseases. This survey was first completed in 1965 and total discharges have increased from 678,000 to 1.7 million in recent years.

Since this survey is of all general hospitals, it includes those with psychiatric units—the ones surveyed by NIMH. That is, the NCHS data include both hospitals with psychiatric units and those without.

Therefore, the NIMH data for general hospital units are a subset of the HDS data for all general hospitals, and the difference between them should be a rough approximation of episodes in general hospitals *without* psychiatric units. Table 3.7 shows this comparison for each year of available data.[14] We see that in 1980 the number of episodes for mental disorders in general hospitals without psychiatric units was almost 60% more than the number in just hospitals with units. The last column shows that in 1980, there were 6 times as many inpatient episodes in general hospitals without units than in 1965. This is by far the most dramatic change of any type of inpatient facility.[15]

Our comparison of two different data sources shows that attention only to the specialty mental health sector obscures an important point. More people are hospitalized for mental disorders in general hospitals without a psychiatric unit than in any other site. Chapter 4 will discuss some controversy surrounding the inclusion of these episodes in national estimates.

Residential Treatment Centers

NIMH is the only agency that collects national data specifically for residential treatment centers (RTCs). Although RTCs generate inpatient episodes, NIMH considers them *nonhospital* as opposed to *hospital* inpatient episodes. Given the small number of RTC episodes, their inclusion or exclusion in a national count of inpatient episodes has little effect on the total.

According to Redick and Witkin (1983), distinguishing RTCs from boarding homes, halfway houses, foster care homes, and facilities for delinquent children is difficult. Beginning with the data collected for 1977, stricter criteria for inclusion as an RTC were used. Now RTCs

TABLE 3.7
Number of Inpatient Episodes for Mental Disorders in All General Hospitals, Those with Separate Inpatient Psychiatric Units, and Those without, 1965-1980

Year	Total—All General Hospitals [a]	General Hospitals with Psychiatric Units [b]	General Hospitals without Psychiatric Unit [c]
1965	703,000	519,328	183,672
1966	785,000	548,921	236,079
1967	779,000	578,513	200,487
1968	826,000	558,790	267,210
1969	826,000	535,493	290,507
1971	1,084,000	542,642	541,358
1973	1,266,000	487,787	778,213
1975	1,539,000	565,696	973,304
1977	1,673,000	571,725	1,101,275
1980	1,746,000	676,941 [d]	1,069,059

[a] Derived from NCHS (Hospital Discharge Survey) data. See Table 3.6. An average daily census was approximated by dividing discharge days by 365, which was added to discharges to approximate episodes.

[b] From NIMH. See Table 3.6.

[c] Approximated by subtracting episodes in hospitals with psychiatric units from those in all general hospitals.

[d] Not comparable to previous years due to the reclassification of some CMHCs into psychiatric units of nonfederal general hospitals. (See *Mental Health United States, 1985.*)

must not be licensed as psychiatric hospitals, must provide individualized mental health treatment under the direction of a psychiatrist, psychologist, social worker, or psychiatric nurse at or above the master's degree level, and must serve mostly children under 18 years. Also, at least 50% of the primary reasons for admission must be for mental disorders (excluding mental retardation and substance abuse) as classified by the Diagnostic and Statistical Manual. The most recent data show about 34,000 annual inpatient episodes since 1977, up from 21,000 in 1969.[16] RTCs tend to have very long-term treatment.

Other Sites for Inpatient Mental Health Care

We complete our count of the number of hospitalizations for mental health care by looking further into the general health care sector and presenting data on nursing homes, the Indian Health Service, and the military.

Nursing Homes. Nursing homes are argued to be replacing the state mental hospitals as places caring for the elderly with mental disorders (e.g., Goldman, Adams, & Taube, 1983; Redick, 1974; U.S. Senate, 1976). We will explore this hypothesis in detail in Chapter 7, as well as discuss the inclusion of nursing home data in national counts of mental hospitalization.

Characterizing the nursing home population is difficult, given the problems in distinguishing between primary diagnoses and chronic conditions. According to the National Nursing Home Survey, in 1977[17] about 122,000 residents were reported to have a primary diagnosis of mental disorder at their last exam (including mental retardation) and another 144,000 were judged senile. If we add in 126,000 discharges who had a primary diagnosis of mental disorder (including senility) at the time of their admission, we can roughly estimate 392,000 episodes in 1977. If chronic conditions (primary and secondary diagnoses) of mental disorders (including senility) is the criterion for the number of nursing home residents with mental disorders, the count increases to 750,000 (Goldman, Gattozzi, & Taube, 1981).

Including nursing home residents in counts of mental hospitalization is problematic, for the following reasons. First, the reliability of the diagnosis is suspect, given that nonpsychiatric physicians are likely to make the diagnosis. Second, categorizing senility as a physical or mental disorder is rather arbitrary, and good arguments can be made to include such patients in mental health statistics or not. We are uncertain ourselves. Third, assuming an accurate diagnosis of mental disorder is made, it is also rather arbitrary whether the mental health problem or a physical health problem is primary. The average number of chronic conditions per nursing home resident was 3.9 in 1977 (Hing, 1981). Fourth, the quality of nursing home data is probably lower than for other types of facilities, given that the survey is conducted by interviewing the staff at each nursing home about selected residents. The staff most familiar with each resident is supposed to supply the information, referring to the medical records when necessary. Quality of the data must vary widely, depending on how familiar the staff are with the cases and how systematically the medical records were consulted. Only a ballpark figure can be given for episodes for mental disorders, roughly between 400,000 to 800,000.

Indian Health Service. The Indian Health Service (IHS), a federal agency serving American Indians and Alaskan Natives, conducts an annual survey of its hospitals. The IHS operates about 50 general hospitals and abstracts diagnostic information from every discharge record. The IHS also tracks beneficiaries in several hundred community or "contract" hospitals with which the IHS contracts for service. However, we do not count these, in order to avoid any duplication of episodes between IHS and the other data sources we have reviewed.

Discharges from these hospitals with a principal diagnosis of mental disorder increased rapidly from 832 in 1959 to 4,390 in 1973, remained stable through 1981, then dropped in 1983. These are only discharges. To approximate episodes, we divided days of care by 365 to get an average daily census, which we then added to discharges to estimate episodes. Calculated in this way, the number of episodes reached a peak of 5,200 in 1975 and has gradually decreased to 3,900 in 1983, thus making up much less than 1% of total inpatient episodes for mental disorders.

Military hospitals. To count psychiatric episodes more completely in all types of inpatient facilities, we obtained data from the Army, Navy, and Air Force. The most currently available data show 10,512 discharges with a principal diagnosis of mental disorder in Army hospitals and 13,624 from Navy hospitals. The Air Force reports 8,506 discharges from their clinic service of psychiatry.[18] If we approximate episodes again by estimating an average daily census (total days divided by 365) and adding this census to the number of discharges, we obtain estimates of episodes of 11,007 for the Army, 14,373 for the Navy, and 8,900 for the Air Force. These sum to approximately 34,300 episodes comprising roughly 1% of the national total.

Summary of National Trends in Inpatient Episodes for Mental Disorders

(1) The target of deinstitutionalization efforts—the state hospitals—do show a decline in episodes over the last 25 years. However, the decrease in state hospital episodes is completely due to the decline in the resident population. While the number of people there on any given day continued to decline, the number of admissions simultaneously increased, but at a slower rate. The net result, when residents and admissions are added together to create episodes, is a general decline in episodes.

(2) In VA medical centers total inpatient episodes increased until 1976, before declining. Those episodes in what were VA psychiatric hospitals followed a pattern similar to state mental hospitals of a rapid decrease in residents.

(3) Private mental hospitals have had an increase in inpatient episodes, mostly accounted for by increasing admissions. However, the most recent data show an increase in residents as well.

(4) More inpatient episodes occur in general hospitals without psychiatric units than any other facility. Currently, over 35% of all inpatient episodes take place in general hospitals without psychiatric units.

(5) CMHCs handle a substantial number of inpatient episodes. Before they were recently redefined, more inpatient episodes occurred in CMHCs than private mental hospitals.

We have reviewed the trends in inpatient episodes for each type of facility, and Table 3.8 shows the most recent number of episodes at each site. Two important points are illustrated by Table 3.8.

(1) The total number of inpatient episodes is almost 3 million, about 60% more than the 1.8 million inpatient episodes reported by NIMH and widely cited in the literature (e.g., Goldman, Adams, & Taube, 1983; Goldman, Taube, Regier, & Witkin, 1983; Klerman, 1979a). (The total would be 400,000 to 800,000 more if nursing home episodes were included.) In Chapter 4 we will see that the difference is due to our inclusion of episodes in general hospitals without separate psychiatric units.

(2) The most frequent inpatient site for mental hospitalization is the general hospital. Within general hospitals, more episodes occur in those *without* separate psychiatric units.

A shift has occurred in where inpatient psychiatric episodes take place. Although the public may think of mental hospitalization as occurring in either state or private mental hospitals, Table 3.8 shows those two sites account for only 24% of the total national episodes, while general hospitals account for 62%. VA medical centers accounted for 7%, and all other sites combined accounted for 7%.

We agree with Goldman, Adams, and Taube (1983) that these shifts do not mean people who were formerly treated in state hospitals are now treated in other inpatient facilities. Chapter 7 will explore the evidence that the elderly have been transferred to nursing homes from state hospitals, and Chapter 8 will discuss evidence that general hospitals are seeing former state hospital residents.

The difference between our 3 million episodes and NIMH's most recent count of 1.7 million comes from our inclusion of episodes in general hospitals without psychiatric units. It has been argued that these episodes should not be included in national estimates, given that they do not occur in the specialty mental health sector and are probably not actually treated cases (Manderscheid, Witkin, Bass, Bethel, Rosenstein,

TABLE 3.8
**Estimates of the Total Number of Inpatient Psychiatric Episodes
in the United States by Site**

Site	Estimated Episodes	Source	Latest Year
State mental hospitals	499,000	NIMH	1981
Veterans Administration medical centers	198,000 [a]	VA	1983
Private psychiatric hospitals	177,000	NIMH	1981
General hospitals	1,759,000 [b]	NCHS	1983
Multiservice MH organizations [c]	128,000	NIMH	1981
Resident treatment centers	34,000	NIMH	1981
Indian Health Service	4,000 [b]	IHS	1983
Military	34,000 [b]	Army, Navy, Air Force	1982-3
TOTAL	2,833,000		

[a] Our calculation. See Table 3.3.
[b] Episodes were calculated by estimating an average daily census and adding in discharges.
[c] Many of these were formerly CMHCs.

and Thompson, 1984; Kiesler & Sibulkin, 1984a). There is also the problem of potential duplication from counting episodes in general hospitals and CMHCs. We will discuss these issues in Chapter 4, where trends in the *rate* of mental hospitalization will be presented.

Notes

1. This chapter is based on the following article by Kiesler and Sibulkin: "People, clinical episodes, and mental hospitalization: A multiple-source method of estimation" (1983a).

2. This category includes hospitals run by both states and counties. However, almost all are now state operated, and we refer to them as such.

3. AHA almost always shows a higher count of state mental hospitals, partly due to including hospitals for alcoholism and mental retardation in their

"psychiatric hospital" category, whereas NIMH excludes these hospitals from that category.

4. Residents in a previous year plus additions in a current year usually do not sum to episodes in Table 3.1. This results because NIMH derives episodes after reconciling data from different surveys.

5. Net releases are the people who actually left, derived by adding residents at the beginning of the year plus admissions and subtracting deaths and the number of residents at the end of the year.

6. Deaths continue to be a determining factor accounting for the shrinking state-hospital population. As Taube, Thompson, Rosenstein, Rosen, and Goldman (1983) point out, discontinuations (those discharged and placed on leave) were fewer than additions (those admitted and returning from leave) in 1978 and 1979, but deaths created a net loss of residents.

7. But recall that the meaning of episodes here is complex, since for years that statistic was composed of one increasing trend (admissions) and one decreasing trend (residents).

8. The AHA also collects VA data, but description of them would needlessly complicate this presentation.

9. The NIMH and VA counts should be similar, given that NIMH used VA's list of facilities to construct its universe.

10. Our VA episodes in Table 3.3 should not be confused with VA's own "episodes" and "patients treated" (neither are shown in Table 3.3). Beginning in 1977, VA "episodes" equal the patients treated (discharges plus remaining occupants) plus intrahospital transfers. Our episodes were constructed to resemble NIMH's. They differ from VA's in that admissions rather than discharges are used and both inter- and intrahospital admissions are included. "Total on rolls" are all residents (including those on leave) on the last day of the previous year, which we use as a substitute for residents on the first day of the current year. "Gains" equal admissions plus intra- and interhospital transfers.

11. AHA also collects data on private mental hospitals. However, they include those for alcohol dependence and mental retardation. Consequently, AHA data are somewhat of an overestimate and we do not present them here. The interested reader may consult Kiesler and Sibulkin (1983a) for presentation of these data.

12. This category is limited to nonfederal general hospitals; it excludes federally operated hospitals, such as VA or military hospitals.

13. Almost all of these nonfederal hospitals are general, as opposed to specialty hospitals. Therefore, we refer to them as general hospitals (National Center for Health Statistics, 1981).

14. Episodes for NCHS hospitals were approximated by dividing the days of care in Table 3.6 by 365 to approximate residents on a given day and adding these "residents" to the number of discharges, a proxy for admissions.

15. The number of episodes in general hospitals without units is only crudely approximated by subtracting the NIMH data for general hospital units from the

total mental disorder discharges reported by the Hospital Discharge Survey. The HDS represents the universe of all nonfederal short-term hospitals—both general hospitals and specialty ones, including psychiatric hospitals. Therefore, not all of the mental disorder episodes remaining after subtracting out those from general hospitals with psychiatric units are from general hospitals without units. Some are from psychiatric (and alcohol) hospitals. The number can not be estimated from the HDS data. However, based on independent AHA data for episodes in nonfederal, short-term psychiatric and alcohol hospitals, the correct estimate for hospitals without units should be about 200,000 fewer episodes in 1980. "Purifying" the HDS data base is part of our current research effort.

16. The change in definition resulted in 46 facilities in 1975 not meeting the criteria in 1977. Due to the change in definition, data for 1977 and 1979 are not directly comparable to previous years. There were 28,000 episodes in 1975, but 33,500 in 1977 even after application of stricter criteria.

17. The National Center for Health Statistics (NCHS) conducts the National Nursing Home Survey, which consists of randomly selecting a sample of records from about 1,700 nursing homes. At time of writing, data for 1977 were the latest available; the 1985 National Nursing Home Survey is now underway.

18. The Army and Navy maintain information systems in which all discharge records are abstracted. The Air Force abstracts discharge records and compiles data by clinic services, which are comparable to VA bed sections. Therefore, Air Force data correspond to psychiatric clinic services, rather than principal diagnoses of mental disorder.

CHAPTER 4

EPISODIC RATE OF MENTAL HOSPITALIZATION[1]

Has the rate of mental hospitalization been increasing or not in recent years? The answer is, yes, it has. However, the validity of that answer depends on how one regards a debated large number of inpatient episodes. Let us first provide some background, then the basic data, and lastly the debate and its context.

In Chapter 3, we saw that the number of inpatient psychiatric episodes increased over the last 25 years in all sites except VA psychiatric and state hospitals. The number of episodes, by any method of counting, would be expected to increase over time given the growth of the population (assuming a constant rate of incidence). An important statistic for assessing trends is the number of episodes per 100,000 population (i.e., the episodic rate). It is changes in the *rate* of hospitalization that more precisely reflect the nation's hospitalization practices, and we consider these now.

Experts in the field have generally accepted that the rate of hospitalization has been stable over the last 15 years or so. For example, based on NIMH data, Klerman has stated, "The number of inpatient care episodes per 100,000 population has remained relatively stable at about 800 since 1955" (1979a, p. 112). Goldman, Adams, and Taube (1983) came to the same conclusion. Bassuk and Gerson (1978) also used NIMH data to assert that the rate of inpatient episodes has remained constant in spite of the drop in the population of state mental hospitals.

We noted that our inclusion of episodes in general hospitals without formal psychiatric units puts the total sum at 3 million rather than NIMH's estimate of 1.7 million episodes. Our larger total obviously implies a larger rate as well. However, that does not mean that the change in the hospitalization rate over the years is any different by the two methods. Ignoring cases occurring in general hospitals without psychiatric units leads to an inference that the rate of hospitalization has been stable over recent years. Our method leads to a higher total (and rate), but has this adjusted rate also been stable over the same time period? That is the core question of this chapter. In order to determine whether our method of counting also leads to a conclusion of a stable rate of hospitalization, we will review the differences in the methods and the resulting differences in rates.

Sources of Data

First let us consider NIMH data. We saw in Chapter 3 that NIMH collects utilization statistics from state and private psychiatric hospitals, VA medical centers, psychiatric units of nonfederal general hospitals, community mental health centers, and residential treatment centers. Episodes are calculated by adding residents at the beginning of the year plus additions during the year. The rates are the number of inpatient episodes per 100,000 civilian population as of July 1.

Our method differs only in the use of two different sources of data—the Veterans Administration for statistics on their medical centers and the NCHS for statistics on all nonfederal short-stay hospitals (the general hospitals).

Rather than using NIMH's survey of VA facilities, we used the results from the VA's own information system that collects aggregate statistics on utilization of psychiatric bed sections in all VA medical centers (formerly divided into psychiatric hospitals and general hospitals with psychiatric bed sections). A more precise count of episodes is provided by VA data in that only psychiatric bed sections of both psychiatric and general medical hospitals are included, whereas NIMH includes the entire psychiatric hospital.

We calculated VA episodes according to NIMH's definition of residents at the beginning of the year plus additions. In VA terminology, these variables correspond to "total bed occupants" on the last day of the previous year plus all "gains" (admissions plus transfers) to the psychiatric bed sections.

As discussed in Chapter 3, NIMH and VA episodes (our calculation) are similar from the early 1970s to the present. However, for reasons not easily determined (but probably due to methods of accounting), the VA shows from 30,000 to 80,000 more episodes in previous years.

We also do not use NIMH statistics for general hospitals. Recall, NIMH surveys only (nonfederal) general hospitals *with* psychiatric units, a small minority of general hospitals. Their statistics therefore underrepresent the total episodic rate in general hospitals, to the extent that people are hospitalized for mental disorders in general hospitals *without* psychiatric units.

The National Hospital Discharge Survey (NHDS) data (collected by NCHS) were used for general hospitals, as discussed in Chapter 3. Episodes were approximated by a combination of average daily census plus discharges, a calculation that should be comparable to the NIMH definition of episode. We calculated general hospital rates by dividing our constructed episodes by the *civilian* population per 100,000.[2]

We constructed total episodes and rates by combining NIMH, VA, and NHDS data. Episodes reported by NIMH in state and private mental hospitals, residential treatment centers, and CMHCs were added together. Rather than adding in NIMH's episodes for the VA and general hospitals, we substituted our episode figures for these two sites. Therefore, our total episodes and rates differ from NIMH's only in the figures used for the VA and nonfederal short-stay hospitals. Since the last, but critical, statistic is based on the National Hospital Discharge Survey, we can only calculate total episodes and rates since 1965 when that survey began. However, rates based on NIMH data can be observed since 1955.

Table 4.1 shows the inpatient episodic rate per 100,000 civilian population for each type of facility. For state hospitals we see that the rate steadily declined from 420 in 1965 to 219 in 1981 (almost 50%).

The rate for private hospitals (including residential treatment centers) fluctuated around 60 in the late 1960s (after a decrease from 76 in 1955). Then it began to increase, reaching 93 in 1981, an overall increase of 43% from 1965 to 1981.

The episodic rate in psychiatric units of nonfederal general hospitals increased in the late 1960s and then remained stable at about 266 until 1979. The increase to 297 in 1981 is partly the result of counting former CMHCs as general hospital units. The total increase from 1965 to 1981 was 10% (however, the increase was 81% since 1955).

CMHCs show a consistent increase in rate since they began operating in 1967. The rate doubled from 1971 to 1977.

These are all NIMH data and their overall national estimate of rate of hospitalization is shown in Table 4.1. The NIMH rate in 1981 (based on a total of 1.7 million episodes) was 756 per 100,000 population. The rate has averaged 823 since 1965. Indeed, in 1955 the national rate of mental hospitalization, as calculated by NIMH, was 795 per 100,000, very similar to today. The stability in rate in recent years results partly from the decline in state hospital episodes being offset by a proportionate increase in CMHC inpatient episodes. These data form the basis of NIMH's statement that the rate of inpatient episodes was fairly stable from 1955 to 1977. Their statement is an accurate representation of the data on which they base it.

Now let us turn to the main difference between the two methods of calculation—the general hospital without a psychiatric unit. Recall that NCHS surveys all general hospitals including those with and without a unit. The rate based on that total is shown in Table 4.1. Recall that the survey was initiated in 1965 and no comparable data exist before then.

For all general hospitals, the rate of inpatient episodes with a principal diagnosis of mental disorder more than doubled from 1965 to 1981. The rate was 367 in 1965, reaching a peak of 824 in 1978 (not shown) and dropping slightly since then.

Our substitution of VA and NHDS figures results in rates for total episodes shown in the last column. The rate of total inpatient episodes across all sites was 950 per 100,000 civilian population in 1965 and it steadily increased to 1,343 in 1977 and then decreased to 1,251 in 1981. The overall increase from 1965 to 1981 was 32%.[3] The 1981 rate is almost 500 more per 100,000 than reported by NIMH. From the early 1970s to the present, our VA rates are similar to NIMH's estimates of VA rates. Therefore the much higher total rates are specifically due to the inclusion of episodes in all general hospitals, rather than only general hospitals with psychiatric units. Before 1970 this rate was only about 150 more episodes per 100,000 than NIMH's. The gap was narrower then because a much smaller number of psychiatric episodes took place in general hospitals without psychiatric units.

Figure 4.1 shows the rate for total inpatient episodes graphically, according to the two calculations, for the years 1965-1979.[4] One may see that the slopes of the best-fitting straight lines are quite different. The NIMH line has a slope near zero (−.20; $t = -.15$), meaning the rate has not increased (or decreased) over the years covered. The best-fitting line through the second set of points has a slope of 34.80, which is significantly different from zero ($t = 13.4$, $p < .001$).

The inclusion of episodes in hospitals without psychiatric units not only produces an increase in total number of episodes but also clearly shows an increase in rate across the years covered. Very rarely does one see such a dramatic trend line in national data on public policy.

THE PROBLEM OF DUPLICATION IN REPORTING

The problem of potential duplication can be described quite easily, but the effect or extent of the problem is more difficult to estimate. We have assumed, in adding up episodes to obtain a national total, that mathematically the NHDS results for all general hospitals includes the universe sampled by NIMH (those with psychiatric units), but without overlap with other categories of inpatient facilities. However, we know

TABLE 4.1
Number of Inpatient Episodes for Mental Disorders per 100,000 Civilian Population, Including and Excluding Episodes in General Hospitals without Separate Psychiatric Units, 1965-1981

| | NIMH | | | | | | Kiesler & Sibulkin Revised Estimates | | |
	State	VA	Private & RTC	Units	CMHCs	Total	VA	All General Hospitals	Total
1965	420	60	65	271		817	98	367	950
1966	414	64	54	283		815	101	406	975
1967	410	66	64	296	14	848	83	399	970
1968	401	68	60	283	14[c]	825	86	419	980
1969	385	94	62	269	33	843	96	419[c]	995
1971	365	87	62	266	64	843	94	529	1,114
1973	313	100	73	234	92	813	96	604	1,178
1975	283	101	78	268	117	847	99	720	1,297
1977	268	101	86	266	125	846	97	767	1,343
1979	236	101[a]	83	266[a]	114[b]	801	94	796	1,323

| 1981 | 219 | 90[b] | 93 | 297[b,e] | 56[d] | 756 | 91 | 792 | 1,251 |

SOURCES: NIMH data: 1965-1968: Statistical Notes Nos. 23 and 127; 1969-1981: Mental Health United States, 1983 and 1985; Kiesler and Sibulkin data: Total episodes were derived by summing the following: NIMH episodes for state and private (including RTCs) hospitals; CMHCs; episodes in VA psychiatric-bed sections (VA Annual Reports); episodes in general hospitals, with and without separate psychiatric units, derived from Hospital Discharge Survey data (from NCHS) by adding number of discharges to an estimated average daily census. Rates are per 100,000 civilian population (Statistical Abstract of the United States, 1985)

NOTE: The NIMH total rate is the sums of their reported rates for each inpatient site shown. The Kiesler & Sibulkin revised total rates were derived by summing the NIMH estimates for state and private hospitals, RTCs and CMHCs, and then adding in the substituted VA and General Hospital data shown. See sources of data below.

Rates differ from those reported in Kiesler and Sibulkin (1984b) due to NIMH's revisions of data and updating of U.S. population estimates.

[a] 1977 data.
[b] 1980 data.
[c] Previous year's data.
[d] Multiservice mental health organizations, most of which were former CMHCs.
[e] Not comparable to previous years due to the reclassification of some CMHCs into psychiatric units of nonfederal general hospitals (Mental Health United States, 1985).

NOTES: Rates differ from those reported in Kiesler and Sibulkin (1984b) due to NIMH's revisions of data and updating of U.S. population estimates.

FIGURE 4.1

Number of Inpatient Episodes for Mental Disorders per 100,000 Civilian Population, 1965-1979, Including or Excluding Inpatient Episodes in General Hospitals without Psychiatric Units

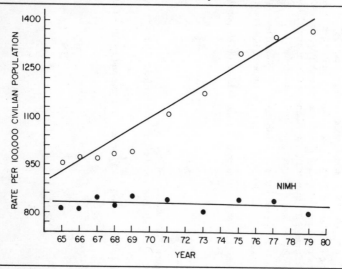

NOTE: Solid line represents best-fit line.
- Including episodes in hospitals without psychiatric units.
- Excluding episodes in hospitals without psychiatric units.

that the assumption is not completely true: There is at least some overlap of the NHDS data with CMHCs.[5]

Recall that the majority of CMHCs contract with or otherwise arrange for their inpatient needs to be provided by an existing inpatient facility, usually a general hospital psychiatric unit. For example, in 1976 about 70% of existing CMHCs claimed some affiliation with at least one general hospital (usually with a psychiatric unit) and another 19% were hospital based (in essence, functioning as the psychiatric unit), according to unpublished data from NIMH.

Data for CMHCs and those for psychiatric units are gathered (in separate surveys) by NIMH. Hospitals have been instructed to separate the data for CMHCs from other data for the psychiatric unit. However, hospitals have clearly varied in achieving this goal and some duplication has arisen, although it is difficult to say how much. The current NIMH survey program, which produced 1981 data, is designed to make this type of duplication very unlikely.

The question is, what happened when these hospitals (and those without units) responded to the NHDS before 1981. These hospitals with units presumably successfully separated their own cases from CMHC cases in order to comply with the requirements of the two NIMH surveys. What happened then in responding for the NHDS?

NIMH deals with aggregate totals. However, NHDS abstractors select individual discharge records for review and would have no reason to attend to CMHC status, even if CMHC records could be distinguished from non-CMHC records, which is unlikely. Therefore, CMHC data were probably reported twice in national totals: Once on the NIMH survey and again in the NHDS. Such duplication would inflate the national totals.

Such duplication is certainly possible, but how much of it in fact occurred is open to question. To provide a precise answer, we would have to check the three surveys (CMHC, psychiatric units, and the NHDS) completed by each hospital (or a sample of them)—something, for reasons of privacy and confidentiality, the federal agencies prohibit (we have tried).

To what extent does the duplication problem affect the more general conclusion of a rising episodic rate of mental hospitalization? When phrased that way, without specifying a particular degree of increase (but merely an increase), potential duplication does not affect our general conclusion at all. Consider the following line of argument. We do not know the extent of such duplication, but we certainly know the potential maximum. For example, in 1978, NIMH figures showed 299,000 inpatient episodes in its survey of CMHCs. The potential maximum duplication is that every case would be counted twice. This clearly could not be true since some CMHCs are not even affiliated with a general hospital and, further, not every hospital could possibly be confused in its reporting. It is a fairly outlandish maximum, but certainly the maximum.

However, suppose every potential duplication in fact occurred. Using 1977 as an example, Chapter 3 showed about 1.7 million inpatient episodes in general hospitals (with and without units) that year. Assuming every CMHC is duplicated, we should reduce that figure by 270,000 to 1.4 million in deriving both national totals and rates. If we did this calculation for each year, how would that affect the data shown in Figure 4.1? The resulting slope is less than Figure 4.1 now shows, of course, but it is still substantial and highly significant statistically.

In short, the general conclusion that the national episodic rate of mental hospitalization is increasing is undisturbed by any problems of duplication in reporting. The problem of potential duplication affects our ability to say *exactly* what the change in rate has been, but we can confidently conclude that it has increased substantially. We can further state what the range of possible true change is: True change is obviously somewhere between zero duplication and the arithmetic maximum duplication. Both endpoints of the range represent a substantial change in rate, however.

HOW SHALL WE REGARD CASES
IN GENERAL HOSPITALS WITHOUT UNITS?

Has the rate of hospitalization changed or not? The answer depends entirely on how one considers inpatient episodes in general hospitals without psychiatric units. If one excludes them, as NIMH does, the rate of hospitalization for mental disorders has been fairly stable over the 15-year period for which data are available. However, if one includes such cases, as we do, the answer is quite different: The rate of mental hospitalization has been increasing in a steady, approximately linear fashion.

The decision whether to include or exclude these episodes in the general health care sector must be based on knowledge of what types of people use these facilities and what happens to them there. The fact that more episodes occur in this site than in any other warrants investigation of these demographic and treatment characteristics.

We made an initial attempt to compare the characteristics of discharges from psychiatric units with those from general hospitals without units. We obtained distributions of discharges by age, sex, and diagnosis as reported by NIMH for units and NHDS for all general hospitals. We subtracted the data from discharges from units from those in all general hospital discharges to obtain an estimate of the number of discharges in general hospitals without units (using 1975 data). By subtracting NIMH data from NHDS data for each category of age, sex, and diagnosis, we derive a residual estimate for episodes occurring in general hospitals without units.

Patients in general hospitals with units tended to be under 35 ($\chi^2 = 70.1$, $df = 5$, $p<.001$) and female ($\chi^2 16.3$, $df = 1$, $p<.001$). The site of discharge was also highly related to diagnosis. Diagnostic categories cannot be compared precisely across published data sources, due to variations in how subcategories are defined. However, site of discharge appears highly related to diagnosis. Best estimates show that alcoholism and neuroses were far more prevalent in hospitals without units, whereas schizophrenia and personality disorders were overrepresented in the units.[6] These differences in patients' age, sex, and diagnosis between general hospitals with and without separate psychiatric units are of interest. However, they can be considered only very preliminary and some-what crude steps in the understanding of the changing pattern and episodic rate of psychiatric inpatient treatment. They are especially crude considering that the national totals we are subtracting are not population parameters, but rather estimates of them based on extrapolating from samples. Consequently, the reliability of these residual figures is not very high and the confidence intervals around them are rather wide. We will see in Chapter 5 that the average length of stay of psychiatric patients in general hospitals without units is approximately 8 days (estimated through our subtractive method), implying that they are not just being held a few days prior to transfer.

Subsequent Work

We are following up on this problem in two ways. We applied for and received a grant from NIMH to investigate the NCHS data base in some detail. We are currently (at the time of writing) working with the 1980 and 1985 national surveys, distinguishing hospitals according to whether they had a psychiatric unit or not, an alcohol/drug dependence unit or not, and whether there was an affiliation with a CMHC. This work is slow and laborious. NCHS, for reasons of privacy and confidentiality, will not identify which hospitals were in the surveys. Consequently, instead of categorizing the 500 hospitals in a survey, we have to categorize all 6,000, provide that information to NCHS, after which they will provide us with the basic data for analysis.

However, when finished, we will be able to offer some precise analyses instead of the crude subtractive approximations we have presented. Further, with this recategorization of NCHS data we will be able to complete a patient-by-patient analysis of hospitals both with and without psychiatric units. Assuming we are able to solve all the coding and identification problems in this research, this refined data base should provide a significant addition and research source to the literature.

A different and complementary approach to this set of issues is a more detailed local study of hospitals with and without psychiatric units. Friedman (1985), in a Ph.D. dissertation supervised by C. Kiesler, investigated a random sample of 426 medical records of patients with mental disorders in eight hospitals, four with and four without units. She found patients in units were more likely to be black, unmarried, middle-aged, and on public assistance than those in nonunits. There were few referrals from either site, but when referral occurred it tended to be from a *unit* and to a state mental hospital (probably when insurance expired). Units had substantially more psychotics than nonunits. However, when psychotics were treated in nonunits, they overwhelmingly were treated by a mental health professional, instead of a nonpsychiatric physician. These various differences are quite strong. In all of these differences described above the hospital was the unit of analysis and the data from the group of hospitals with units did not overlap at all with the group of hospitals without units. Further, in a multiple-discriminant analysis, a model derived from half her sample and based on diagnosis, gender, and funding source, she was able to categorize correctly (in unit or nonunit) over 75% of the cases in the other half of the sample.

Wallen (1985) also compared characteristics of people discharged with a principal diagnosis of mental disorder from hospitals with and without psychiatric units in 1977. Her data came from about 11,000 abstracts from 327 hospitals that subscribed to medical records abstracting services. Similar to Friedman, she found that the transfer rate was low for both hospitals with and without units. Only 11% of people leaving hospitals without units were discharged to another facility and only 6% of those discharged from hospitals with units were transferred.

Wallen's lower transfer rate from hospitals with units, relative to those without units, is partially accounted for by patients discharged from "scatter beds" (i.e., people who did not actually stay in the unit). These discharges may be the least likely to be transferred, and their inclusion would, therefore, lower the transfer rate for the hospitals with units.

Taken together, the national data, based on the substractive method, the Wallen study, and Friedman's local sample provide a clear case that the general hospital phenomenon is real. People with mental disorders are not being admitted to general hospitals without units by accident or as a holding action. Friedman's data are especially clear on this point: These patients are being actively treated in nonunits and then sent home (90% were sent home after treatment and another 3% to nursing homes).

Our general conclusions are that the episodic rate of mental hospitalization has been increasing over the last 15 years, and this increase is totally contained by general hospitals without psychiatric units. These two empirical facts have seemed to disturb many of our colleagues. They have suggested various explanations to us that seem worth sharing (partly because they may also be occurring to the reader). These alternative explanations for the observed effects have included the following:

(1) Potential duplication with other categories of reporting. This is really the CMHC issue and as we have discussed, even assuming maximum potential duplication, the basic conclusion is undisturbed. The

episodic rate of mental hospitalization has been increasing. The duplication argument addresses only *how much* it has increased. Regardless of duplication, the increase has been very substantial.

(2) The patients are really just sent to general hospitals without units as a holding ground for referral. This seems unlikely to us for several reasons. First, if referral were the primary goal, then the array of cases should be like that found in psychiatric units. As detailed above, the age, sex, and diagnoses are quite different. Two, if referral were the goal, then the length of stay should be very short, such as a day or two. In fact the length of stay is about eight days, which is not unusual for brief forms of treatment (e.g., Glick & Hargreaves, 1979) and is approximately equal to the average hospital length of stay for all disorders in general hospitals (National Center for Health Statistics, 1981). Both Friedman and Wallen found that only about 10% of people discharged with psychiatric diagnoses from hospitals without units were transferred to other facilities. Referral seems unlikely as the primary reason behind the increases in episodes in general hospitals without units.

(3) The patients are sent to general hospitals without units to avoid the stigma of incarceration in a psychiatric ward. This may be true, but begs the question. The notion that some patients are sent to units to avoid stigma has no implication for an increase in overall episodes. If such patients would formerly have been sent to units, then being sent to nonunits should decrease the national rate for units and keep the total national rate stable. That has not happened.

(4) A general hospital without a psychiatric unit is a healthier environment for an acute patient. This assertion begs the question in the same way 3 above did. Even if true this assertion has no necessary implication for an increase in overall rate, and therefore is not an explanation for an increase in overall rate.

(5) The increase in overall rate is due to the revolving door phenomenon (and where the cases became distributed is a separate issue). As we discuss in Chapter 8, there is very little evidence for the revolving door—an increase in the number of episodes per patient. Our data show a 57% total increase in inpatient episodes since 1965. As also described in Chapter 8, the most rational conclusion from the existing evidence is that the revolving door phenomenon does not exist. However, in no way could the evidence be distorted to account for a 57% increase in episodes.

(6) The advent of drugs has allowed more patients to live outside the hospital for longer periods with only short interval treatments inside, allowing one to use general hospitals more. This is really one implementation of the revolving door hypothesis. To the extent that it implies

more episodes per patient, it is undemonstrated; to the extent that it merely implies the shorter length of stay observed in general hospitals, it begs the question of why there has been an increase in rate.

In short, the national data base does not allow us easily to explain why there has been a steady increase in inpatient episodes over the last 15 years, nor why this increase has been specific to general hospitals without psychiatric units. We will return to this issue several times during the course of this book.

We have emphasized the *rate* of mental hospitalization in this chapter. However, the *absolute number* of episodes is also important. Indeed it is critical to public policy alternatives and particularly their funding. The absolute number of inpatient episodes has increased 57% or 1 million episodes in this time period (including some potential duplication). That is a critical piece of information for our society and we will return to it later when discussing the economics of mental hospitalization.

Notes

1. This chapter is based on the following article by Kiesler and Sibulkin: "Episodic rate of mental hospitalization: Stable or increasing?" (1984b).

2. The Hospital Discharge Survey used the civilian noninstitutionalized population before 1981, but began using the total civilian population in 1981 (Kozak & Moien, 1985).

3. During the same time period, there was an absolute increase in *episodes* of approximately 1 million, or 57%.

4. Figure 4.1 is reprinted from Kiesler and Sibulkin (1984b), which used slightly different rates than the updated rates reported here.

5. As noted in Chapter 3, some duplication also occurs with episodes from short-term state and private psychiatric hospitals. The HDS includes discharges from these facilities, which are also included in NIMH's broader category of long- and short-term hospitals. However, removing an estimate of these episodes from the total for each year (based on AHA data) has a negligible effect on the rising rate of mental hospitalization.

6. This is partly due to the fact that NIMH does not include units which exclusively treat substance abuse in its survey of psychiatric units. Therefore, the derived NHDS subsample contains episodes in this type of unit. A more refined analysis of these data would separately analyze these episodes. We note that the American Hospital Association reports a fluctuating trend in the number of alcohol/chemical dependency units in nonfederal short-term general hospitals. In 1975 (the first year of available figures) there were 322 such units and there were 354 in 1977 and 284 in 1980.

CHAPTER 5

TRENDS IN LENGTH OF STAY PER PSYCHIATRIC EPISODE[1]

One of the goals of the national de jure policy of deinstitutionalization is to minimize the length of stay once hospitalized. Therefore, we would expect national statistics to show a decrease in length of stay in recent years.

Given the unexpected findings that we have described showing an increase in both the absolute number and rate of total episodes, it was reasonable to study length of stay trends separately for the same facilities in order to obtain a more complete picture of the nation's institutionalization practices.

The question this chapter answers is "Has the average hospital stay for a mental disorder decreased or not?"

Definitions

The types of facilities to be studied were defined in Chapter 3. Before turning to the data we must define "length of stay."

Conceptually, the notion of a length of stay (LoS) in a hospital is simple. It is the elapsed time between when a patient arrives and is discharged. In practice, however, lengths of stay in hospitals for treatment of mental disorders are only rarely noted. Most national statistics published in the area of mental health do not reflect true lengths of stay.

A method typically used to calculate LoS, particularly for general medical care, uses the concept of inpatient days. There are serious distortions in LoS when inpatient days are used in the calculation, particularly so for mental hospitalization (as opposed to general medical care). Inpatient days represent the total days all patients spent in the hospital beds, during a given year, regardless of whether they were admitted or discharged during that year or not. Using this method, total inpatient days are divided by either admissions or discharges. However, the numerator includes all days spent in the hospital by people during the year: it does not include the days to be spent in the following year by those who have not been discharged; and it does not include days spent by discharges during the previous year(s). For example, a person discharged on January 1 would be counted as contributing one inpatient day (as well as one discharge and no admissions). If the patient had, in fact, spent the previous two years in the hospital, using one inpatient day in the calculation of LoS would seriously distort the true average.

In other words, inpatient days during a reporting period do not correspond to the actual admissions and discharges that contributed to these inpatient days. Therefore, dividing inpatient days by either the number of admissions or discharges does not result in a true average length of stay. If the true length of stay is constant over years (but less than one year) and the number of admissions/discharges is also constant, the ratio would be arithmetically equal to true length of stay. However, since hospital admissions for mental disorders have been increasing and our deinstitutionalization policy stresses shorter hospital stays, neither assumption is defensible.

To calculate an accurate average length of stay, the actual number of days spent in the hospital accumulated by a group of discharges is needed. Discharges must be used because it is not until people are discharged that the total number of days they were in the hospital is known. Further, the number of days accumulated by the discharges must include any days spent during the previous year(s). These days are called "total days," "discharge days," and "days of care" by various surveys. They should not be confused with "inpatient days," which is used only to mean total days spent *during* a specific year. Discharge days can only be obtained from actual individual discharge records. Aggregate national statistics within a single year are misleading and inaccurate. The difficulty (and expense) of inspecting individual records explains why national statistics for true length of stay are relatively rare.

The kinds of statistics that hospitals keep routinely include the numbers of admissions, discharges, residents, episodes, and total inpatient days. The average daily census (ADC), which is the average number of inpatients per day during the year, is also typically calculated (by dividing inpatient days by 365).[2] These statistics are kept because it is easy to do so from aggregate statistics without the labor of looking at files of individual patients.

It is important to note that these methods of calculating LoS produce less distortion in national statistics for general medical care than for psychiatric care. Mathematically, the degree of distortion depends partly on how long the true LoS is, and whether the true LoS or the number of inpatient episodes (admissions or discharges) is changing over time. The longer the true LoS, the greater the potential for systematic distortion;

the greater the change in admissions or discharges over years, the greater the distortion would actually be. If both true LoS and episodic rate are changing at the same time, there will be a substantial mathematic error in the calculated LoS.

General medical care has a fairly short LoS—about 8 days. Nationally, this LoS has been decreasing in recent years, but very slowly. Thus, using inpatient days and admissions or discharges to calculate LoS is not a serious problem for general medical care.

For psychiatric care, we have already shown that the episodic rate has risen sharply in recent years. Let us look now at what is known about average length of stay.

Sources of Data

The surveys we described in Chapter 3 vary as to how accurately length of stay figures are calculated. Following is a brief description of what the surveys provide and which we chose to use.

Most of the data NIMH collects are aggregate figures of admissions, discharges, and inpatient days, which do not provide true average length of stay figures. However, we will see that surveys of a sample of patient records provide a few figures for median length of stay. AHA does request discharges and discharge days (the critical statistics) from its hospitals but only publishes admissions and inpatient days, which is used to calculate average length of stay for nonpsychiatric hospitals.

Our best source of psychiatric hospital data was the National Center for Health Statistics (NCHS), given its availability and comparability with NIMH (both exclude hospitals treating primarily the mentally retarded and chemically dependent). NCHS obtains AHA's data tape on hospitals and publishes these hospital data as part of its National Master Facility Inventory (NMFI). We discovered that discharges and discharge days were published for two years and we subsequently obtained previously unpublished figures for seven additional years directly from NCHS. After 1978, we used unpublished AHA data. Therefore, our major source of the average length of stay for state and private psychiatric hospitals was NCHS's Master Facility Inventory.

For general hospitals, length of stay data cannot be derived from the AHA or NMFI surveys, because the hospital is the unit of analysis in those surveys. Since only a fraction of general hospital admissions or discharges are for mental disorders, any total utilization figures for general hospitals would include all health problems, not just mental health. Therefore, the other NCHS survey, the National Hospital Discharge

TABLE 5.1
**Discharges, Discharge Days, and Average Length of Stay in State
and County Psychiatric Hospitals from NCHS Surveys, 1969-1982**

Year	Discharges	Discharge Days [a]	Average Length of Stay
1969	436,695	183,818,098	421
1971	500,973	183,798,798	367
1972	480,010	167,161,427	348
1973	466,269	145,305,702	312
1974	457,721	119,715,721	262
1975	453,676	122,504,438	270
1976	443,874	114,544,086	258
1977	429,564	90,030,464	210
1978	392,121	74,164,396	189
1979	386,007	62,394,136	162
1980	376,428	61,936,491	165
1981	361,153	53,160,755	147
1982	352,556	50,499,458	143

SOURCES: NCHS data: 1973: Series 14, No. 16, 1971: Series 14, No. 12; all other years unpublished data from AHA and NCHS (National Master Facility Inventory). We calculated the average length of stay by dividing the discharge days by the number of discharges.

[a] Discharge days are the total number of days accumulated at the time of discharge by all discharges during the year, including days spent in the hospital prior to the beginning of the reporting period.

Survey (NHDS) was used for general hospital data. Since individual records are inspected, the number of discharges, discharge days, and true average length of stay for mental disorders alone can be obtained.

The VA's Patient Treatment File, which abstracts discharge records, was used to obtain true length of stay data for VA medical centers.

To summarize our major data sources, the VA's Patient Treatment File was used for all VA hospitals, the NCHS Master Facility Inventory was used for state and private mental hospitals, and the NCHS National Hospital Discharge Survey was used for general hospitals. Since NIMH is the only data source for CMHCs, we inferred what trends in length of stay probably exist, given that true length of stay data were not collected for CMHCs until the currently ongoing surveys.

Following the procedure we used for episodes and rates, we will first review the trends for each type of facility and then summarize the current state of affairs.

State hospitals. Table 5.1 shows data for state mental hospitals. In 1969, the average length of stay in a state mental hospital was 421 days, or approximately 14 months. In 1971 this had been reduced to approximately a year and then to six months in 1978. The average length of stay continued to fall to 143 days in 1982. NIMH has been widely quoted as stating that the stay in state hospitals declined from 44 to 26 days from 1971 to 1975, and the most recent sample survey showed a 23-day median in 1981. These are *median* lengths of stay obtained from systematically sampling records of new admissions during one month (Rosenstein & Millazzo-Sayre, 1981; Taube & Barrett, 1985). An infrequently cited survey of discharge records was done in 1969, and we calculated the median to be 47 days. Because both the mean and median have decreased, we can speculate that more than mere dumping out occurred.

In summary, both the mean and median lengths of stay have decreased in state mental hospitals, the mean very sharply. However, the average length of stay is still almost five months.

Veterans Administration. The Patient Treatment File provides counts of people categorized on the basis of their primary diagnosis at the time of discharge, based on inspection of their record. These data reported by the Veterans Administration are presented in Table 5.2 for most of the years from 1954 to 1983. For each year available, we report the number of discharges in a given year, which we saw in Chapter 3, the total of days in the hospital accumulated by the discharges, and the mean and median lengths of stay of the patients discharged. The VA also separates data for "psychotic" and "other psychiatric" diagnoses. (We will use the term "nonpsychotic" synonymously with VA's "other psychiatric.") Since the two distributions are substantially different, we present them separately here.

The means and medians are quite different for both the psychotic and other psychiatric distributions. For the nonpsychotic inpatients, one can see that the median length of stay remained relatively constant from 1954 through 1968. At that time it began to drop gradually from 25 days to 14 days in 1974 and has remained fairly constant to the present day. This suggests that a fairly substantial difference in the pattern of care at the VA occurred during those years. The mean of this distribution has a somewhat different array. The mean length of stay actually increased from the early 1950s through the late 1960s, and has subsequently decreased. Over the whole period covered, the median length of stay for nonpsychotics in VA hospitals has decreased from 23 days in 1954 to 16 days in 1983. The mean length of stay for the same patients has changed from 43 days down to 31. Over the 30 years we see about a

TABLE 5.2

Discharges, Total Days, Average and Median Length of Stay in All VA Hospitals, by Patient Type, from Surveys by the VA, 1954-1983

	Psychotic [a,b]				Other Psychiatric [a,b]			
	Discharges	Total Days [c]	Mean	Median	Discharges	Total Days [c]	Mean	Median
1954	22,896 [d]		445.0	66.0	29,568 [d]		42.8	22.7
1955	24,004 [d]		453.0	70.5	32,328 [d]		41.8	21.8
1956	22,520		526.0	82.5	31,852		42.8	22.5
1957	23,630		583.8	96.3	30,605		46.4	24.2
1958	25,020		671.9	99.0	29,155		51.9	25.7
1959	25,100		643.5	90.0	30,775		52.1	25.2
1960	28,910		647.3	87.0	30,790		60.6	26.7
1961	31,152		662.8	85.8	34,582		55.7	25.5
1962	34,253		633.1	81.0	35,795		53.5	26.4
1963								
1964								
1965								
1966								
1967								
1968	54,928	27,918,755	508.3	53.8	75,742	6,850,165	90.4	25.2
1969	57,851	26,986,958	466.5	48.4	87,100	8,008,886	92.0	22.7
1970	58,197	27,539,916	473.2	49.6	89,223	5,233,806	58.7	20.3
1971	66,603	29,801,010	447.4	48.4	100,186	5,732,808	57.2	20.0

1972	64,799	18,402,550	284.0	39.7	114,425	5,069,391	44.3	16.8
1973	66,838	13,610,474	203.6	35.2	128,252	5,179,094	40.4	15.7
1974	70,770	12,640,657	178.6	29.8	137,687	5,298,094	38.5	14.4
1975	73,026	11,614,048	159.0	27.6	145,752	5,269,606	36.2	14.0
1976	73,398	10,112,005	137.8	26.1	147,171	5,155,643	35.0	13.7
1977	75,149	9,231,886	122.9	24.9	139,983	4,824,591	34.5	13.8
1978	77,663	8,144,859	104.9	23.8	136,421	4,728,135	34.7	13.8
1979	78,524	7,777,489	99.1	22.0	134,032	4,390,282	32.8	13.5
1980	75,851	6,995,015	92.2	21.9	136,016	4,169,622	30.7	13.5
1981	78,538	6,944,803	88.4	21.7	129,853	3,927,811	30.3	14.1
1982	79,403	6,847,655	86.3	21.7	126,374	3,954,226	31.3	14.9
1983	79,163	6,816,381	86.1	22.4	123,609	3,859,929	31.2	15.8

SOURCES: VA Annual Reports. Medians for 1970-1973 are unpublished figures calculated from the frequency distributions. The means for 1968-1969 were calculated by dividing total days by the number of discharges.

a The "psychotic" and "other psychiatric" patient-type classification results from a recoding of the discharges with a principal diagnosis of mental disorder into these two groups. In condensing the several subcategories of mental disorder, as well as those in the other major diagnostic categories, into fewer patient types, the sum of the psychotic and other psychiatric discharges does not always equal the total discharges with a principal diagnosis of mental disorder.

b The VA defines "principal diagnosis" as the diagnosis "responsible for the major portion of the patient's length of stay as judged by the attending physician." This is different from the National Center for Health Statistics' criterion of the condition resulting in the admission.

c Total days equal the total number of days spent in the hospital by the discharges during the year, including days prior to the beginning of the reporting period.

d Include discharges of veterans from VA and non-VA hospitals.

one-third decrease in the length of stay reflected in both the mean and median.

For psychotics the pattern of treatment is changing much more dramatically. In 1954 the median length of stay was 66 days and rose to as high as 99 during the late 1950s and early 1960s. We see the same abrupt change in the length of stay from 1968 to 1974 (that we observed for nonpsychotics) and a gradual continued decrease since that time. The changes in the mean length of stay are more dramatic. In 1954 the average psychotic patient episode at the VA was about 15 months, increasing to almost two years in the early 1960s, and decreasing fairly sharply since then. Currently, the average length of stay for a psychotic patient is 86 days, with a median of 22. The median length of stay for psychotics has decreased by two-thirds (and the mean by over three-quarters) since the early 1950s.

Overall, the Veterans Administration shows the predicted pattern of decreased length of stay, reflected both for nonpsychotics and psychotics (but more dramatically for the latter). The decrease in the median length of stay suggests a changing pattern of treatment, and the change in the means suggests that an emptying out of long-term cases has also occurred.

In these published data, the changes in LoS cannot be traced to the site of hospitalization (psychiatric hospital versus a general hospital). However, the VA did provide us with five years of previously unpublished data, sorting the data described in Table 5.2 by site of hospitalization. We calculated the means from the overall data provided.

Table 5.3 shows a sharp difference among sites in average length of stay for both psychotic and other psychiatric patients. As can be seen, the LoS in VA general hospitals was stable 1974–1978 for both psychotic (approximately 75–80 days) and other psychiatric patients (28–29 days).[3]

The data for psychiatric hospitals are much different. Average LoS for both psychotic and nonpsychotic treatment dropped duringthe five-year period. Yet startlingly, the LoS at the end of the period was still twice as long for psychiatric hospitals than for general hospitals for both categories of patients.

The differences among sites and the recent stability of LoS in general VA hospitals suggest a serious qualification of our overall summary for the VA. We now know from Table 5.3 that the decrease in average length of stay for 1974–1978 reported in Table 5.2 is contained totally within psychiatric hospitals. The figures for treatment in general hospitals remained stable over that period. The extent to which changes

TABLE 5.3

Discharges, Total Days, and Average Length of Stay in VA Hospitals, by Patient Type and Type of Hospital, from Surveys by the VA, 1974-1978

Year	Psychotic [a,b]			Other Psychiatric [a,b]		
	Discharges	Total Days [c]	Mean	Discharges	Total Days [c]	Mean
General Hospitals						
1974	42,290	3,395,432	80.3	103,417	3,056,358	29.6
1975	47,587	3,445,097	72.4	114,635	3,315,370	28.9
1976	50,486	4,133,492	81.9	117,078	3,389,781	29.0
1977	52,201	4,293,029	82.2	110,359	3,169,582	28.7
1978	50,143	3,712,898	74.1	100,003	2,804,482	28.0
Psychiatric Hospitals						
1974	28,480	9,245,225	324.6	34,270	2,241,736	65.4
1975	25,439	8,168,951	321.1	31,117	1,954,236	62.8
1976	22,912	5,978,513	260.9	30,093	1,765,862	58.7
1977	22,815	4,923,858	215.8	29,461	1,649,066	56.0
1978	27,407	4,402,610	160.6	36,279	1,917,182	52.9

SOURCES: Discharges by patient type are published in the VA *Annual Reports* for those years. The breakdown of patient type by type of hospital shown here was obtained from the VA. We calculated the means by dividing the total days by number of discharges.

NOTE: Discharges and total days for the two diagnostic groups in 1977 and 1978 do not sum to those shown in Table 5.2. Data in Table 5.3 exclude cases with missing data.

[a] The "psychotic" and "other psychiatric" patient type classification results from a recoding of the discharges with a principal diagnosis of mental disorder into these two groups. In condensing the several subcategories of mental disorder, as well as those in the other major diagnostic categories, into fewer patient types, the sum of the psychotic and other psychiatric discharge does not always equal the total discharges with a principal diagnosis of mental disorder.

[b] The VA defines *principal diagnosis* as the diagnosis "responsible for the major portion of the patient's length of stay as judged by the attending physician." This is different from the National Center for Health Statistics' criterion of the condition resulting in the admission.

[c] Total days equal the total number of days spent in the hospital by the discharges during the year, including days prior to the beginning of the reporting period.

observed in other years are specific to site is unknown, but probably substantial.

The overall trends must be qualified by existing differences in average length of stay by site. Further, the overall figures are partly determined by variation in the proportion of total patients in each site. We know from admissions data that the proportion of total psychiatric cases admitted to the VA general hospitals (rather than psychiatric hospitals) has been rising (see Table 3.2). In 1970, less than half of the total of psychiatric patients were treated in general hospitals, whereas by the end of the decade over 75% were. When the LoS for general hospitals is much less than that of psychiatric hospitals, the overall mean is partly determined by the proportion of the former. In this case, at least some of the decrease in overall LoS in prior years is due to an increase in the proportion of patients treated in general hospitals (and hence who stayed a shorter time).

In summary, the LoS at VA general hospitals has been constant in recent years—about a month for treatment for nonpsychotics and about 2½ months for psychotics.

The LoS pattern is very different for VA psychiatric hospitals. LoS for nonpsychotics has decreased somewhat, but for psychotics it has fallen very rapidly in recent years. However, LoS for psychotics, at last report, was still over 5 months.

Private mental hospitals. Data from the National Master Facility Inventory are presented in Table 5.4, distinguishing between those hospitals run for profit and those not for profit.

For private mental hospitals run for profit, the average length of stay was 56 days in 1969, falling to 35 days in 1971 and remaining stable through 1982. For private mental hospitals in the nonprofit category, these data are much more variable. Over the 13-year period the average length of stay decreased from 74 days in 1969 to 44 days in 1973. It then fluctuated and reached a high of 56 days in 1976 and began fluctuating around 42 days since then. It is possible those fluctuations correspond to increases and decreases in the supply of beds. This hypothesis is indirectly supported by data showing a decrease of available beds from 1971 to 1973 and a corresponding increase from 1973 to 1976 (Sirrocco, 1974, 1976; Sutton & Sirrocco, 1980, and unpublished data). It is possible that the number of beds may have been increased to accommodate the press of patients or, alternatively, increased beds may have led to pressures to fill them. We can say, however, the length of stay began to drop again after 1976 while beds continued to rise (Strahan, 1981, and unpublished data). It is quite possible the bed supply and length of stay follow each other, with time lags of varying degrees.

TABLE 5.4
Discharges, Discharge Days, and Average Length of Stay in Private Psychiatric Hospitals from Surveys by NCHS, 1969-1982

	For-Profit Hospitals			Not-for-Profit Hospitals		
Year	Discharges	Discharge Days[a]	Average LoS	Discharges	Discharge Days[a]	Average LoS
1969	48,726	2,705,956	56	53,944	3,999,046	74
1971	54,864	1,938,132	35	50,254	3,270,442	65
1972	51,003	1,792,316	35	50,556	2,405,201	48
1973	63,932	2,259,160	35	51,696	2,252,881	44
1974	68,119	2,338,145	34	57,912	2,903,094	50
1975	76,021	2,361,208	31	63,679	3,025,789	48
1976	74,353	2,444,673	33	65,906	3,704,254	56
1977	76,436	2,527,421	33	62,901	2,701,822	43
1978	85,431	2,699,885	32	63,138	2,671,134	42
1979	87,596	3,085,376	35	66,402	2,530,237	38
1980	92,901	2,995,342	32	63,235	2,560,130	40
1981	101,601	3,404,124	34	63,687	2,689,493	42
1982	110,269	3,850,433	35	69,799	3,022,443	43

SOURCES: NCHS data: 1973: Series 14, No. 16; 1971: Series 14, No. 12; all other years: unpublished data from AHA and NCHS (National Master Facility Inventory). We calculated the average length of stay by dividing the discharge days by the number of discharges.

[a] Discharge days are the total number of days accumulated at the time of discharge by all discharges during the year, including days spent in the hospital prior to the beginning of the reporting period.

The data do not really allow us to be precise about explanations for these fluctuations. However, the fluctuations were not large from 1972 to 1982.

Similar to its survey of state mental hospitals, NIMH followed a cohort of admissions to private mental hospitals during one month in 1970, 1975, and 1981, providing median lengths of stay of admissions (but not the average lengths of stay for discharges).[4] Consistent with NCHS data, the medians hardly changed; they were 22 days in 1970, 20 days in 1975 and 19 days in 1981 (Rosenstein & Millazzo-Sayre, 1981; Taube, 1973a; Taube & Barrett, 1985). This suggests that treatment did not change and that LoS fluctuations reflect bed availability for long-term care cases.

In summary, average length of stay in private mental hospitals has decreased somewhat, but has been stable in recent years. The average length of stay for private, for-profit mental hospitals looks fairly similar to that found for nonpsychotics in the Veterans Administration. Perhaps the hospitals run for profit are more likely to take only patients that they feel they can treat more effectively, avoiding, perhaps, the more serious cases in the VA psychotic category.

Nonfederal short-term general hospitals. As previously mentioned, the major source of data on true length of stay is the National Hospital Discharge Survey (NHDS), conducted by the National Center for Health Statistics (NCHS). A true length of stay is obtained, since the date of admission and date of discharge are recorded for each discharge during the year.

Table 5.5 presents the mean length of stay from the National Hospital Discharge Survey for the years 1965 through 1983 and the medians for 1973–1983. As we saw in Chapter 3, the number of discharges has continued to rise over the years (678,000 in 1965 to 1,700,000 in 1983) but may be at the beginning of a decline. The mean length of stay has remained remarkably stable over those years. Length of stay in the mid-1960s was slightly over 12 days and has fluctuated around 11 to 12 days ever since. One can see that in recent years, the median LoS was very stable as well.

Let us compare these data with NIMH's on psychiatric units in general hospitals. Similar to the state and private hospitals, NIMH sampled discharges from nonfederal general hospital psychiatric units. This allows for a calculation of true length of stay from the date of admission to the date of discharge, as well as the median length of stay.[5] The average length of stay did not change between 1975 and 1981; it was 17 days, 6 days longer than the average for all general hospitals, with or without a psychiatric unit (Faden & Taube, 1977).

TABLE 5.5
Discharges with First-Listed Diagnosis of Mental Disorder, Days of Care, and Average and Median Length of Stay in Nonfederal Short-Stay Hospitals from NCHS Surveys, 1965-1983

Year	Discharges[a]	Days of Care[b]	Average LoS	Median
1965	678,000		12.6	
1966	759,000	9,655,000	12.7	
1967	753,000	9,329,000	12.4	
1968	799,000	9,760,000	12.2	
1969				
1970	604,000	10,940,000	18.1	
1971	1,050,000	12,341,000	11.8	
1972	1,176,000	13,666,000	11.6	
1973	1,227,000	14,176,000	11.6	6.8
1974	1,352,000	15,248,000	11.3	
1975	1,494,000	16,496,000	11.0	6.7
1976	1,485,000	15,604,000	10.5	6.5
1977	1,625,000	17,606,000	10.8	6.7
1978	1,730,000	19,435,000	11.2	6.7
1979	1,723,000	18,983,000	11.0	6.7
1980	1,692,000	19,578,000	11.6	6.9
1981	1,747,000	20,898,000	12.0	7.1
1982	1,746,000	21,115,000	12.1	7.0
1983	1,701,000	21,124,000	12.4	7.1

SOURCES: NCHS data: Discharges and Average Length of Stay: 1966-1967, 1970: unpublished data from the National Hospital Discharge Survey–the average length of stay was calculated by dividing the days of care by the number of discharges. 1965, 1968, 1971-1973: Series 13, Nos. 6, 12, 16, 20, 25, 26, 31, 37, 41, 46, 60, 64, 72, 78, 82, respectively; Days of Care: 1973-1976: *Nation's Use of Health Resources, 1976* and *1979* editions. All other years are unpublished data from the National Hospital Discharge Survey; Medians: Calculated from unpublished frequency distributions.

NOTE: Nonfederal short-stay hospitals are those having six or more beds and an average length of stay less than 30 days. Although the universe includes short-stay specialty hospitals, 94% of the nonfederal short-stay hospitals were general ones in 1978 (National Center for Health Statistics, 1981).

[a] The first listed diagnosis is intended to equal the principal diagnosis, which is "the condition established after the study to be chiefly responsible for occasioning the admission of the patient to the hospital for care." In the absence of other information, the diagnosis listed first on the medical record is assumed to be the principal diagnosis (Kozak & Moien, 1985).

[b] Days of care are the total number of days accumulated at the time of discharge by all discharges during the year, including days spent in the hospital prior to the beginning of the reporting period.

The median lengths of stay show little change between 1971 and 1975. In 1971 the median lengths of stay were 6.9 and 13.6 days, for psychiatric units in public and private nonfederal general hospitals, respectively. The medians were 8.1 and 13.6 days in 1975. However, in 1981 the medians for public and private hospitals were essentially the same—11 and 12 days. In 1971 and 1975 the median lengths of stay in psychiatric units in public hospitals were similar to those found in general hospitals without psychiatric units (approximately 8 days). Rather longer median stays were found in private general hospitals with psychiatric units. Little is known about the differences in type of patient served and treatment between general hospitals providing psychiatric care in a psychiatric unit versus the general medical ward and how these differences might relate to ownership.

In Chapter 4, we described a subtractive method used to separate hospital statistics into hospitals with and without units. Recall that we described some resulting differences in demographic characteristics and diagnosis. Using the same subtractive approach here we can calculate the length of stay for patients in hospitals without psychiatric units to be 7.9 days. We do so by subtracting NIMH discharge days from NHDS discharge days and dividing by the number of discharges, derived in the same way (1975 figures). This is a much shorter length of stay than for units. We discussed in Chapter 4 some of the difficulties in trying to discover who these patients are, who is treating them, and the like. However, recall that 7.9 days is approximately equal to the average length of hospital stay for all medical disorders.

Two points should be emphasized about treatment in general hospitals. The length of stay in these sites has remained stable over the years for which data are available. Further, the length of stay is also very short compared to other places of treatment.

Community mental health centers. NIMH has reported average length of stay in CMHCs as decreased (Vischi, Jones, Shank, & Lima, 1980), but the calculation is the number of inpatient days within a given year per episode treated. As we have suggested, this number is a distortion of true length of stay, if the number of admissions, discharges, or true length of stay actually vary across years. Table 5.6 shows the episodes and inpatient days we saw in Chapter 3 plus the length of stay in terms of inpatient days per episode. This number has fluctuated from around 13 to 18 days over the 9 years reported. The number of episodes has continued to rise, therefore the statistic is an underestimate of true length of stay, particularly in later years. This underestimate results because the numerator of inpatient days does not include the days the increased number of admissions will generate in the next year. Although there is not a

TABLE 5.6
Inpatient Episodes, Inpatient Days, and Number of Days
per Episode in Community Mental Health Centers from
NIMH Surveys, 1969-1980

Year	Inpatient Episodes	Inpatient Days	Inpatient Days/Episode
1969	65,000	1,923,720[a]	29.6
1970	110,622	1,923,720[a]	17.4
1971	130,088	2,225,396	17.1
1972	144,601	2,561,633	17.7
1973	191,946	3,275,630	17.1
1974	211,027	3,836,452	18.2
1975	246,891	3,948,466	16.0
1976	270,944	3,951,001	14.6
1977	268,966	3,818,497	14.2
1978	298,897	4,063,176	13.6
1980	254,288	3,609,000	14.2

SOURCES: Episodes and inpatient days: 1969, 1971, 1973, 1975, 1977, 1980: *Mental Health United States, 1983* and *1985*; other years: provisional data on federally funded community mental health centers, 1978-1979; inpatient days per episode: 1971 and 1975: Statistical Note No. 95 and Vischi, Jones, Shank, and Lima (1980). We calculated the length of stay for all other years.

[a] There is some ambiguity in the data sources as to whether these days occurred in 1969 or 1970. The most recent publications show 1,924,000 days in 1969, although they more closely correspond to 1970 episodes, in terms of days per episode.

great deal of variance across years in the number of inpatient days per episode, there is surely even less variance in the true length of stay, given the direction of the error underlying the reported statistic. One would suggest, therefore, that the true length of stay in CHMCs has been rather stable across the 11 years for which data are available. The LoS in CMHCs has hovered around 2 weeks from the beginning to end of their officially legislated existence.

Indian Health Service. The Indian Health Service (IHS) reports true average lengths of stay, calculated by dividing the actual number of days accumulated by the number of discharges.

The length of stay has been about a week for decades, slightly less in recent years. A substantial proportion of IHS discharges have diagnoses of alcohol dependency (40% in 1982).

Military hospitals. True average lengths of stay can also be calculated for military hospitals. The average length of stay in Army hospitals was of 17 days in 1982, identical to that of psychiatric units of general hospitals. The Air Force data also show an average length of stay of 17 days in 1982—the average fluctuated between 16 and 20 days since 1970.

The Navy trend data, on the other hand, show a fairly steady number of discharges between 1974 and 1982. However, the length of stay of steadily decreased from 25 days in 1974 to 8 days in 1981 (and then rose to 11 days in 1982). Some, but not all, of the differences may be accounted for by the fact that more Navy cases are alcohol dependent (42% in 1981) than the Army cases (approximately 20% in 1981).

Summary of Trends in Lengths of Stay

We have presented the available data on length of stay for inpatient treatment of mental disorders in the United States. Many of these data have been published in various federal sources, but a substantial proportion have not been published elsewhere. We have discussed trends across years within each site. In this section we present an overall summary of more recent trends in inpatient treatment. Table 5.7 summarizes our data by the major site of hospitalization, our representation of the trend in the last decade or so, and the actual latest figures in the year obtained.

As one can see, the largest change in trends of length of stay has occurred in the VA's treatment of psychotic patients in psychiatric hospitals and in the state mental hospitals. Both of these sites show very sharp decreases in length of stay over the decade. At the same time, however, both still represent substantially the longest lengths of stay of any inpatient site. While state mental hospitals have demonstrated sharp decreases in the average length of stay, the most recent data available indicate a still lengthy stay of 143 days on the average—over 4½ months. In the VA, the average length of stay for psychotics in psychiatric hospitals has also decreased substantially, but represents five months of inpatient care on the average in 1978.

One has to qualify the answer to the question of how long people stay in mental hospitals by the site in which one is hospitalized. Among possible sites, there is an 18:1 ratio between the shortest length of stay—in general hospitals without psychiatric units—and the longest—in state hospitals. Further, even though average length of stay, irrespective of site, has decreased, the total decrease is completely due to sharp decreases in the two sites that began with, and still have, the longest average length of stay. The shorter lengths of stay have stabilized in other types of hospitals.

We emphasize that all the data in Table 5.7 represent discharges and not people. To the extent that people are discharged and readmitted during a given year's reporting period, the figures presented in Table 5.7 represent an underestimate of average length of total *treatment.*

The only other changes in length of stay represented in Table 5.7 are the VA's treatment of nonpsychotic patients (but only in psychiatric hospitals) with a slight decrease of both mean and median in the 1970s, and the rather fluctuating data from private not-for-profit mental hospitals. All the other sites of mental hospitalization show stable lengths of stay during the past decade or so.

We can summarize Table 5.7 as indicating that for the seven major sites of mental hospitalization we surveyed, four have had fairly stable lengths of stay, one has fluctuated, and two have shown sharp decreases over the last decade or so. Those trends represent the sites of hospitalization, not patients, and only two of the seven sites show decreases. How are the patients arranged among sites? Phrased a slightly different way, we could ask, "What is the probability that, when a randomly drawn and hypothetical patient is hospitalized, the length of treatment would be less in 1980 than in 1970?" This question involves looking at the number of episodes in each site rather than just the sites.

The last column of Table 5.7 shows the most recent data on the number of episodes in each site. The number of episodes in private for-profit and not-for-profit hospitals are approximately equal over the years, although they fluctuate from year to year. For the purposes of our argument, let us assume that they are equal.

The outcome of this line of thought is as follows. The best estimate of the total number of episodes in these sites is 2.9 million. Of these episodes, 2,300,000 or about 80%, occurred at inpatient sites where the average length of stay has been stable (or fluctuated) over the last decade or so. Only 20% of the total number of episodes reported have occurred at sites where there has been a sharp decrease in average length of stay over the last decade or so.

In short, although there is some evidence that the average length of stay for mental disorders has decreased significantly at some psychiatric hospital sites, only increasingly small numbers of episodes nationally take place there. In that sense, if one were to be hospitalized now, one could expect to be hospitalized in a place where the average length of stay has not changed over the last decade.

If the deinstitutionalization effort is taken partly to mean getting people out of mental hospitals more quickly than before, then that picture is very complicated. Many people see the deinstitutionalization movement as specifically oriented toward state mental hospitals. To the

TABLE 5.7
Summary of Trends in Length of Hospital Stay for Mental Disorders and Current Number of Episodes by Site

Site	Trend of LoS during 1970s	Latest Figures Mean	Latest Figures Median	Year of latest LoS	No. of Episodes (Latest Year)[a]
VA Gen. Hosp.					
Psychotic	Stable	74.1		1978	155,179 (1978)[b]
Nonpsychotic	Stable	28.0		1978	
VA Psychiatric Hosp.					
Psychotic	Very sharp decrease	160.6		1978	56,790 (1978)[b]
Nonpsychotic	Slight decrease	52.9		1978	
Gen. Hosp.[c]	Stable	12.4	7.1	1983	1,759,000
State/County Hospital	Very sharp decrease	143	23[d]	1982	499,000 (1981)
Private (for-profit)	Stable	34.9	19[d]	1982	177,000
Private (not-for profit)	Fluctuating	43.3		1982	
CMHCs	Stable	14.2[e]	N/A	1980	254,000 (1980)

[a] Episodes do not equal the total shown in Table 3.8 due to reporting for different years. There is likely some duplication here between CMHCs, and other facilities, primarily general hospitals.

[b] These are episodes in the psychiatric bed sections of each type of hospital and are calculated as in Table 3.3. Figures differ from those reported in Kiesler and Sibulkin (1984c), which were calculated differently.

[c] Includes hospitals both with and without psychiatric units, based on NCHS Hospital Discharge Survey.

[d] From NIMH's 1981 survey of admissions (*Mental Health United States, 1985*).

[e] Approximate; see text.

extent that this is true, it has been a resounding success thus far. The average (or median) stay at a state or county mental hospital for a mental disorder is a fraction of what it was in the 1950s and 1960s. There is no question that such hospitals were the prime focus of deinstitutionalization, and that they represent the snakepits depicted film and literature. On the other hand, the average length of stay in a state hospital, in the most recent data available, is still almost five months.

The state mental hospitals have obviously not lost their custodial role in mental health treatment in the United States. The degree to which such a custodial role is needed (assuming one of high quality could be played) probably would be open to sharp debate among knowledgeable professionals. Further, others have argued that as a result of the deinstitutionalization movement, there has been a transfer of the elderly from state mental hospitals to nursing homes (Redick, 1974; but see Chapter 7 also). The number of patients in nursing homes with a diagnosis of mental disorder has increased through the same time period, but we will see in Chapter 7 that the majority of this increase is not due to transfers from state mental hospitals. Nursing homes may, but certainly do not necessarily, represent an advance in the treatment of the elderly who might otherwise in former times have been interred in a state mental hospital. If the custodial care of those mental disorders has only been transferred to nursing homes, then the nation's purpose of deinstitutionalization may not have been well served.

The state mental hospital may still be attempting to serve patients who are commonly regarded as incurable (and indigent) and whom other sites may not accept. There certainly is some face validity to that statement. The only other site, the length of stay of which has sharply decreased, is that of the VA psychiatric hospitals, particularly for psychotics. Average length of stay for such patients has decreased as sharply as for those in the state mental hospital, but the mean length of stay for psychotics in VA psychiatric hospitals is still five months. Presumably, the VA psychiatric hospital is serving the incurable and indigent as well.

The type of analysis that we have undertaken here ignores demographic and diagnostic differences among the populations of patients in the different hospital sites. It is surely true, for example, that patients in private mental hospitals are quite different than those in, say, state and county mental hospitals on such variables as diagnosis, income, education, family background, and the like. Some data are available on demographic and diagnostic categories for different hospital sites. However, to tease out adequately what the relevant variables are would demand that these variables be related to the true length of stay of a given patient. Since data are so sparse for several sites on true length of stay, it would be impossible to disentangle completely the intricacies at a national level. A detailed analysis of national data is clearly needed.

About 80% of inpatient episodes of treatment for mental disorder occur in hospital sites where average length of stay has been stable over the last decade or so. These sites of stable LoS are also those that tend to have the shortest average length of stay. Further, even though particular sites have stable lengths of stay over years, they are nonetheless reliably different from other sites that are also stable. For example, the original length of stay for mental disorders in a general hospital has hovered around 11 days for the past decade or so. The average length of stay in CHMCs has also been stable, but about three or so more days than that in the general hospital. Interestingly, the private for-profit mental hospital, while stable, has a length of stay approximately three times that at a general hospital. Both stability of length of stay in these sites and continuing reliable differences among them are fruitful areas for future research.

In summary, the average length of stay for a psychiatric inpatient episode has recently decreased only in state mental hospitals and VA psychiatric hospitals, which together handle only about 20% of the inpatient episodes. The length of stay in other mental hospitalization sites has remained relatively stable in recent years.

Notes

1. This chapter is based on the article by Kiesler and Sibulkin: "Episodic length of hospital stay for mental disorders" (1984c).

2. Given the long lengths of stay in some types of institutions, one could argue that the median, rather than the average, is the appropriate measure. There are problems with both the mean and the median in looking at statistics of this nature. The degree to which the mean is the best measure of some central tendency depends upon the degree to which the distribution of length of stay is skewed. When the distribution is highly skewed the median is probably a better measure of central tendency. The mean, on the other hand, allows one to calculate the total number of days spent in hospitals nationally, which can be used to calculate total public and private costs of inpatient care (see Chapter 11). The combination of the two statistics is illuminating. For example, if the mean and the median are substantially different, as they are in most cases in inpatient treatment for mental disorders, one can look at the differences between them as one measure of changing patterns of treatment over years. If the mean is decreasing

rapidly, while the median remains constant, one might suggest that institutions are pushing out long term patients without substantially changing patterns of treatment. If all treatments were simply improved or intensified, one might expect all patients to be discharged more quickly, affecting both the median and the mean. The best approach in summary statistics would be to report the mean, the median, variance, and frequency distributions. No source of data currently does that, however.

3. After 1978 the VA no longer distinguished between general and psychiatric hospitals; all facilities are called medical centers.

4. See Kiesler and Sibulkin (1984c) for details on the 1970 and 1975 sample surveys of private mental hospitals.

5. See Kiesler and Sibulkin (1984c) for details on the 1971 and 1975 sample surveys of general hospital psychiatric units.

CHAPTER 6

TRENDS IN THE PROPORTION OF TOTAL HOSPITAL DAYS THAT ARE FOR MENTAL HEALTH CARE

We have discussed trends in episodic rate of inpatient care and in average length of stay. But how do those trends translate into some sort of national total and how does mental health care fit into general health care in hospitals?

In this chapter we present one summary statistic—the total inpatient days for all mental disorders. We look at that trend over time and then compare it to the total inpatient days for all health care.

Because we include general hospitals without psychiatric units and because we have access to previously unpublished data, this analysis is both more extensive and accurate than any other attempted.[1]

This chapter answers the question, "How many total days are spent in hospitals for mental disorders, and how does that fit into general hospital utilization?"

In Chapter 4, we saw that the rate of mental hospitalization has increased in the last 15 years, if episodes in general hospitals without psychiatric units are included in the total. In Chapter 5, we noted that the average length of stay has remained relatively constant for most sites of hospitalization. The length of hospital stay has decreased only in state and VA psychiatric hospitals, but still remains about 4½ months in the former and about 5 months for psychotic patients in the latter.

We will review the data regarding the number of total inpatient days per year in each of these sites. "Inpatient days" are the number of days of care accumulated by patients during the year. For example, 10 patients staying 10 days would contribute 100 days to the year's count of inpatient days. Note that a one-to-one correspondence does not exist between the people admitted (or discharged) and the number of days they contribute during the year, because the inpatient days refer only to days during the reporting period. Therefore, someone admitted 5 days before the new year and staying 2 days during the new year contributes only 2 inpatient days. Similarly, someone admitted 2 days before the end of the year who is discharged 5 days into the next year also contributes 2 days to the current year. This is why inpatient days cannot be used to calculate an average length of stay. Inpatient days are, however, useful as a measure of resources consumed during a specified period of time. Because the days are limited to a one-year reporting period, inpatient days per year in one type of facility can be compared with those in another type.

Total inpatient days compared across years can be used to detect shifting national patterns of care and costs. The costs per day of mental hospitalization will vary across type of hospital (this will be discussed later). However, total direct costs of mental hospitalization will be a simple function of the total number of inpatient days within each site and totals can be summed across sites. Further, assessment of inpatient days for physical and mental disorders allows us to integrate mental hospitalization into discussions of hospital cost containment.

Hospital cost containment. The rising costs of health care in general and hospital care in particular have been a matter of extensive public discussion. The Health Care Financing Administration reports that in 1980, total United States health care expenditures came to $247 billion, more than 9% of the gross national product. Health care has taken an increasingly larger bite of the GNP since 1965 (Gibson & Waldo, 1981). Indeed the costs of medical services (1968 to 1978) rose almost 20% faster than the consumer price index (Jonas, 1981).

In 1980, hospital costs were estimated to be $100 billion and projected to be over $330 billion by 1990 (Freeland, Calat, & Schendler, 1980), almost 45% of the national health care bill.

These rising costs have led both the public and health care professionals to focus on ways to contain them. Some policy efforts have emphasized regulatory mechanisms. Prospective reimbursement has been the most recent popular technique (e.g., Schwartz, 1981). Diagnostic related groups (DRGs), the system for Medicare prospective reimbursement, is another.

Professional standards review organizations (PSROs) and certificate-of-need programs also have their advocates (see Melnick, Wheeler, & Feldstein, 1981; Saltman & Young, 1981). Alternative care outside the hospital has also received some attention (see Chapter 9).

These various strategies are designed to reduce the total number of days spent in hospitals. Unfortunately, most of the discussion has centered in nonfederal short-stay hospitals. In these hospitals the average length of stay for all disorders has decreased somewhat. However, the number of admissions has disproportionately increased. The outcome?

The total number of inpatient days has increased about 30% in general hospitals (AHA, 1981).

However, if one looks at all types of hospitals, as we shall in this chapter, the number of inpatient days has decreased. Our major goals of this chapter are to calculate the number of inpatient days for mental disorders over time and by site, and the proportion of all hospital days that are due to mental disorders. The proportion of total hospital days that are due to mental disorder would provide some insight into the role of mental health in the overall delivery system of health services. Let us first look at the sources of the data to be presented here.

Sources of Data

Total inpatient days for all disorders. As we have described, the National Center for Health Statistics (NCHS) surveys all hospitals, and all disorders treated in them, in conjunction with the American Hospital Association. These figures are shown in line 10 of Table 6.1. NCHS data were only available for 1969 and 1971–1978; unpublished AHA data were used for later years. NCHS/AHA surveys do not include either CMHCs or RTCs. Consequently, our independent estimates of those two sites were added to the NCHS total to obtain a revised, more complete national total of inpatient days for all disorders.

Estimates of inpatient days for mental disorders. The source used to estimate inpatient days for mental disorders varied by site. For the VA, inpatient days were taken from its AMIS survey of psychiatric bed sections in general and psychiatric hospitals. The use of data directly from the VA allows for identification of inpatient days in psychiatric bed sections of both general and psychiatric hospitals. Beginning in 1979, the VA no longer distinguished between psychiatric and general hospitals. Therefore, only one figure for the VA, representing total inpatient days in all psychiatric bed sections, is shown from 1979 on.

The Master Facility Inventory was used to derive totals for both state and private psychiatric hospitals. We could as easily have used comparable data from NIMH. MFI data were considered slightly preferable since the totals for all hospitals are also MFI data and therefore provide a more comparable universe.

The other NCHS survey, the National Hospital Discharge Survey (NHDS) was used for general hospitals. As described in Chapter 3, discharge records from a probability sample of nonfederal short-stay hospitals listed in the MFI are systematically selected, based on the terminal digits of their medical record numbers, and the principal diagnosis is recorded. A problem with NHDS data for our purposes is that we must use discharge days, because inpatient days are not collected. However, the distortion is probably slight given the fairly constant average length of stay for mental disorders in the last ten years in general hospitals.

To complete our universe of sites for inpatient mental health care, we must include community mental health centers (CMHCs) and residential treatment centers for emotionally disturbed children (RTCs). NIMH is the only data source for inpatient days in these sites. As mentioned, days for these sites were also added to the NCHS total to create the total base for all disorders.

To summarize our sources of data, the Veterans Administration was used for VA hospitals, the NCHS Master Facility Inventory was used for the state and private mental hospitals, and the NCHS National Hospital Discharge Survey was used for general hospitals. NIMH was used for CMHCs and RTCs.

Results

Table 6.1 shows the inpatient days spent in each of eight hospital sites, their total, and a comparison with total hospital inpatient days in the United States for all health care. The first eight lines of Table 6.1 show the number of inpatient days accumulated in each site for the years 1969 to 1982.

For example, line 3 shows the inpatient days in state mental hospitals. It shows a total of over 131 million days in 1969, steadily dropping to a total of about 44 million inpatient days in 1982. The last column shows the percentage changes in days from 1969–1982, in this case a decrease of 66%.

Line 9 shows the total psychiatric inpatient days for all sites in a given year. Line 10 shows NMFI data for the total number of inpatient days spent for all health care. Line 11 shows the results of adding the days for CMHCs and RTCs to the total NCHS figures, since they are not covered by the NMFI. This effectively adjusts the national total inpatient days.

Line 12 shows the result of dividing line 9 by line 11, i.e., the percentage of all inpatient days accumulated for psychiatric care.

Psychiatric inpatient days. Let us first inspect the trends of each site over the decade and then the trend of the total psychiatric days. We can then look at trends in total hospital days and compare the two data sets. The two sharpest downward trends in psychiatric days are VA psychiatric hospitals and state mental hospitals, as would be expected.

Between 1969 and 1978 the number of inpatient days dramatically decreased 77% in the psychiatric sections of the VA psychiatric hospitals (read across line 2). Days in all psychiatric bed sections continued to decrease through 1982, creating an overall decrease of 54%. The decrease in state mental hospitals was 66% between 1969 and 1982 (line 3). This is consistent with the equally dramatic decline in length of stay for these two sites, as described in the last chapter.

In contrast to these two traditional sites of inpatient care, the number of inpatient days increased 92% in the psychiatric sections of the VA general hospitals (1969–1978) and 116% in general hospitals (line 6). This is consistent with the large increase in episodes we have shown in these two sites.

Inpatient days in private mental hospitals run for profit (line 4) almost doubled in this time period (a 92% increase). On the other hand, nonprofit private hospitals show a slight decrease (line 5). Ignoring profit orientation, total inpatient days in private mental hospitals showed a 28% increase during this time. RTC inpatient days increased 35%.

Summing the figures from the separate sites, the net result is a decrease in total psychiatric inpatient days from 169 million in 1969 to 88 million in 1982 (line 9). This represents an annual "saving" of 81 million hospital inpatient days per year. This 48% decrease is more than accounted for by the large decreases in the sites where most of the days were accumulated—government psychiatric hospitals. The two VA hospitals and state mental hospitals alone decreased inpatient days by over 95 million from 1969 to 1982. Consequently, all other sources together showed an *increase* of over 14 million inpatient days.

The state mental hospitals still account for the majority of all psychiatric days—50%. However, general hospitals (with and without units) account for the next largest percentage—24%. Private mental hospitals, the VA, CMHCs, and RTCs each handle less than 10% of the total psychiatric inpatient days nationally. Recall that state mental hospitals now account for a small percentage of total episodes. However, their long length of stay results in half of the total psychiatric inpatient days occurring there.

Total hospital inpatient days. The total number of inpatient days for all diagnoses, including mental, decreased about 18%, from 469 million in 1969 to 386 million in 1982, an annual saving of 83 million days per year (line 11). Note that total inpatient days for all disorders continued to fall only until 1978–1979. More recently they have increased somewhat.

Total versus psychiatric inpatient days. The percentage of all inpatient days due to mental disorders was 36% in 1969 and gradually

TABLE 6.1
Number of Inpatient Days (in millions) Recorded at Various Types of Facilities According to National Center for Health Statistics (NCHS), VA, and NIMH Surveys, 1969-1982

Facility	1969	1971	1972	1973	1974	1975	1976
1. VA general hospital, psychiatric section	2.726	3.731	4.504	4.536	4.650	5.166	5.277
2. VA psychiatric hospital, psychiatric section	13.283	10.021	6.966	5.697	5.145	4.345	3.789
3. State mental hospitals	131.555	113.821	100.604	89.246	77.868	69.119	61.217
4. Private mental hospitals (for profit)	1.987	1.991	1.786	2.174	2.216	2.343	2.380
5. Private mental hospitals (nonprofit)	3.272	2.488	2.251	2.137	2.357	2.457	2.453
6. General hospitals [a]	9.760[b]	12.341	13.666	14.176	15.248	16.496	15.604
7. CMHCs	1.924	2.225	2.562	3.276	3.836	3.718	3.951
8. Residential treatment centers (RTC)	4.528	6.356	6.356[c]	6.338	6.338[c]	5.900	5.900[c]
9. Total psychiatric days	169.035	152.974	138.695	127.580	117.658	109.774	100.607
10. Total NCHS inpatient days	462.360[d]	434.290	416.066	408.858	400.070	391.437	384.461
11. Total NCHS, CMHC, and RTC inpatient days	468.812	442.871	424.984	418.472	410.244	401.285	394.312
12. Total psychiatric inpatient days as percent of total hospital days	36%	35%	33%	30%	29%	27%	26%

continued

TABLE 6.1 Continued

Facility	1977	1978	1979	1980	1981	1982	% change 1969-1982
1. VA general hospital, psychiatric section	5.207	5.247	7.892 [c]	7.692 [c]	7.479 [c]	7.444 [c]	−54 [g]
2. VA psychiatric hospital, psychiatric section	3.364	3.088	—	—	—	—	—
3. State mental hospitals	56.582	51.458	49.847	48.102	45.782	44.347	−66
4. Private mental hospitals (for profit)	2.474	2.630	2.911	3.021	3.430	3.807	+92
5. Private mental hospitals (nonprofit)	2.482	2.816	2.834	2.915	2.909	2.940	−10
6. General hospitals [a]	17.606	19.435	18.983	19.578	20.898	21.115	+116
7. CMHCs	3.818	4.063	4.063 [c]	3.609	2.472 [f]	2.472 [c,f]	+88 [h]
8. Residential treatment centers (RTC)	6.546	6.546 [c]	6.531	6.531 [c]	6.127	6.127 [c]	+35
9. Total psychiatric days	98.079	95.283	93.061	91.448	89.097	88.252	−48
10. Total NCHS inpatient days	376.792	370.930	370.692	377.140	378.732	377.120	−18
11. Total NCHS, CMHC, and RTC inpatient days	387.156	381.539	381.286	387.280	387.331	385.719	−18
12. Total psychiatric inpatient days as percent of total hospital days	25%	25%	24%	24%	23%	23%	

SOURCES: VA hospitals: 1969-1976, 1979-1982: Average daily census for each year from the VA Annual Report (published in the following year) multiplied by 365 to estimate inpatient days; 1977-1978: Unpublished average daily census figures from the VA, multiplied by 365; State and private mental hospitals–1969, 1972, 1974, 1975-1982: Unpublished data from American Hospital Association/NCHS Master Facility Inventory; 1973: Series 14, No. 16; 1971: Series 14, No. 12; General hospitals, 1976: *Nation's Use of Health Resources, 1979*; 1973: *Nation's Use of Health*

Resources, 1976, (both published by NCHS); all other years are unpublished data from NCHS National Hospital Discharge Survey; CMHICs and RTCs: *Mental Health United States, 1985* and *1983* editions, NIMH; Total NCHS inpatient days, 1969, 1971, 1973, 1976, 1978: Series 14, Nos. 6, 12, 16, 23, 24; 1977, 1979-1982: unpublished data from American Hospital Association/NCHS Master Facility Inventory; 1972, 1974, 1975: *Health Resources Statistics,* 1976-1977 editions (published by NCHS).

a Discharge days, not inpatient days

b Discharge days in 1968; medical data are not available for 1969.

c Previous year's data.

d Approximated by multiplying the number of patients present on the last day of the reporting period by 365.

e Total days in psychiatric bed sections. Beginning in 1979, the VA no longer distinguished between general and psychiatric hospitals.

f Multiservice mental health organizations, most of which were former CMHICs.

g This is the percentage change across both types of hospitals. Between 1969 and 1978 days in general hospitals increased 92% and days in psychiatric hospitals decreased 77%.

h This is the percentage change for CMHICs from 1969-1980.

decreased during these years to 23% in 1982. Although mental health problems are not the most common in terms of episodes, they account for a disproportionate number of inpatient days. Total inpatient days for all disorders decreased by 83 million between 1969 and 1982, and psychiatric inpatient days alone decreased by 81 million. Therefore, practically all of the decrease in total days for all disorders is accounted for by the decrease in psychiatric days.

Viewed a different way, total days fell by 83 million, of which mental disorders accounted for 81 million. Total hospital days for nonmental disorders, therefore, dropped only 2 million days.

Older data. A precise analysis of psychiatric inpatient days as a percentage of total inpatient days could not be accomplished prior to 1969, because the Master Facility Inventory did not exist in the same form and psychiatric episodes in general hospitals could not be estimated. However, we can still confidently assert that in 1955, inpatient days for mental disorders comprised over 50% of the total days. Using American Hospital Association data (the original source of MFI hospital data), federal, state, and private psychiatric hospitals alone accounted for 54% of the total hospital days in 1955. This does not include psychiatric episodes in general hospitals and therefore represents a minimum. The decrease in the proportion represented by psychiatric days that we have documented in detail is only part of a continuing trend over a 25-year period.[2]

About one-quarter of all inpatient days are currently for psychiatric care, a substantial reduction from the 36% in 1969, but still surprisingly high. Cost containment policies based on these findings must be site specific. However, the reduction in expenditures at each site depends on the cost of a psychiatric day of care at that site, relative to other sites, and to other health care in the same site. For example, only 7% of the discharge days in general hospitals are for psychiatric care. However, the cost of a day of psychiatric care there is not well known (Greenhill, 1979; see Chapter 11). One-half of all psychiatric inpatient days occur in state mental hospitals but the overall average expenditures per day are less than at other sites (Rubin, 1982). Further, costs of care (and savings) depend on the intensity of the treatment; custodial care being clearly less expensive than active treatment. A thorough analysis of the cost of psychiatric care in various sites must also distinguish between acute and chronic care. For example, the cost per day in a state hospital is surely more for an acute admission than for a chronic resident. These issues will be discussed further in Chapter 11.

Inpatient days for mental disorders decreased 48% from 1969 to 1982. The potential for further decrease, particularly in VA psychiatric and state mental hospitals seems substantial. For example, Chapters 9 and 10 describe the results of experiments showing the effectiveness of alternative care programs for the deinstitutionalized and the noninstitutionalized patients. Of course, reductions in length of stay and in the resident census in these facilities at a national level would require policy changes in funding mechanisms and an increase in the availability of alternative care, as we discuss later.

These data demonstrate the need to distinguish carefully in national statistics between health and mental health. Mental hospitalization accounts for a substantial part of total hospitalization days, yet is relatively absent from general discussions of hospital cost containment. Further, although total United States hospital days decreased 83 million days between 1969–1982, 98% of the decrease was accounted for by changes in treatment of mental disorders.

Notes

1. Excluding, of course, our article (Kiesler & Sibulkin, 1983b) on which this chapter is based.

2. This could be even a longer trend. Grob (1983) says that in the 1930s in Massachusetts, the State Department of Mental Diseases absorbed about 25% of the state's income.

CHAPTER 7

NURSING HOMES AND DEINSTITUTIONALIZATION[1]

The issue of nursing homes has arisen several times, in most detail in Chapter 3 where we discussed their impact in trying to count the number of inpatient episodes for mental disorders. In this chapter, we go into some detail regarding the care of the mentally ill in nursing homes.

The care of the mentally ill in nursing homes has played an important role in the thinking of both the detractors and advocates of deinstitutionalization. Both sides believe that the decline in residents in state mental hospitals and the increase in residents in nursing homes represent the same people—"a true shift in the population of chronic mental patients . . . . Clearly, a large proportion of current nursing home residents would have been state mental hospital patients prior to deinstitutionalization" (Goldman, 1983, pp. 35–36). "The increased utilization of nursing homes can be largely attributed to the deinstitutionalization movement" (Cicchinelli, Bell, Dittmar, Manzanares, Sackett, & Smith 1981, p. 91).

We ask here: What is the relationship between the decrease in residents in state mental hospitals and the increase in nursing homes? Are they really the same patients? Would current residents in nursing homes be placed in state mental hospitals under pre-deinstitutionalization practices? If so, is it true of only the elderly or all patients?

We will see that direct evidence is difficult to come by. We will approach the problem by basing assumptions on our detailed analysis of a national survey. We will also look at trends over time based on other surveys. We admit our approach here represents detective work as much as science, but readers may judge for themselves the merits of the conclusions.

Table 7.1 shows the overall picture of nursing homes, beds, and residents from 1963 to 1977. All have increased substantially. There has been over twice the number of nursing homes as hospitals since national data collection on nursing homes began. On average, nursing homes have doubled in size; in 1963 the average number of beds per home was 35, and it was 74 in 1977. The number of residents in 1977 was 2½

TABLE 7.1
Number of Nursing Homes, Beds, Residents, and Deaths, 1963 to 1977

Year	Number of Nursing Homes[a]	Beds	Residents	Admissions	Discharges (including deaths)	Deaths
1963	16,370[b]	568,546	505,242	402,896	378,326	147,900
1964	17,400		554,000			
1968	19,533	894,162	813,335	801,013	756,289	223,100
1969	18,391	880,700	815,100	968,750	900,521	298,000
1973	15,749[c]	1,177,300	1,075,800	1,110,800	1,077,500	327,600
1977	18,900	1,402,400	1,303,100	1,367,400	1,117,500	289,800

SOURCES: Vital and Health Statistics Series, published by the National Center for Health Statistics, as follows: 1963: Series 12, Nos. 2, 16, and 23; 1964: Series 12, No. 8; 1968: Series 12, No. 16; 1969: Series 12, No. 23; 1973: Series 13, No. 28: 1977: Series 13, No. 43.

NOTE: Statistics do not match those reported by the National Master Facility Inventory (MFI). The National Nursing Home Survey data, reported here, are based on a sample from the MFI universe and were collected at a different point in time. Admissions, discharges, and deaths occurred during the previous year.

[a] Nursing homes include nursing homes, personal care homes with nursing, and personal care homes. Geriatric hospitals and nursing wings of hospitals are also included. Homes providing only room and board are excluded.
[b] Excludes hospitals or units of hospitals.
[c] Personal care homes were exluded.

times what it was in 1963. The increase in residents (61%) during the period 1963 to 1969 might be attributable to Medicaid coverage. However, the number of residents has continued to grow, with another 60% increase in residents in 1969–1977.

Although the number of deaths has almost doubled, they have declined as a percentage of all residents, from 29% in 1963 to 22% in 1977.[2]

National Data on Nursing Homes and State Mental Hospitals

We saw in Chapter 3 that the total number of state mental hospital residents has declined sharply since the 1950s. In this section we will look more closely at this trend and the corresponding trend in nursing-home utilization, in order to infer the extent to which state hospital residents or potential residents have been transferred to nursing homes.

Trends in state hospital residents. The Senate Subcommittee on Long Term Care of the Special Committee on Aging (United States Senate, 1976) noted that the elderly were being "pushed out" of state hospitals at an even faster rate than the younger residents. This observation was based on the data for 1969 through 1974, during which time the percentage decrease in elderly residents was larger than for the total resident population.

Table 7.2 shows the number of residents and deaths in state mental hospitals from 1964 to 1981. According to these data from NIMH, the percentage decrease for the elderly (50%) was indeed greater than for the under 65 group (38%) during 1969 to 1974, as the Committee on Aging asserted. However, when viewed over the longer time period, we see that the data points for 1969 and 1974 are only fluctuations within an overall trend. The under-65 and 65+ groups both decreased about 75% between 1964 and 1981. Clearly, the elderly have not been "pushed out," at least not more so than the nonelderly.

We also note the dramatic decline in the number of deaths in state mental hospitals; from 44,800 in 1964 to 7,100 in 1980. This percentage decrease is even greater than the decrease in the resident population. Deaths obviously decrease the pool of people available to be discharged to a nursing home, and we will consider them again regarding estimated transfers to nursing homes.

Table 7.2 also shows separate data for residents with organic brain disorders, given that this condition describes over one-third of the elderly state hospital population, and over one-half of nursing home resi-

TABLE 7.2

State Mental Hospital Residents End of Year, Those with Organic Brain Disorders, Net Releases by Age and Deaths According to NIMH Surveys, 1964-1981

	Residents		OBD[a]		Deaths	Net Releases	
	Under 65	65+	Under 65	65+		Under 65	65+
1964	346,616	143,833	39,633	56,525	44,824	252,499	16,117
1965	334,872	140,330	40,872	59,823	43,964	271,093	17,304
1966	317,379	134,710	36,011	51,984	42,753	291,748	18,622
1967	297,972	128,337			39,608	312,596	19,953
1968	279,012	120,140			38,677	333,696	21,300
1969	258,549	111,420	40,632	52,407	35,962	435,255	16,884
1970	238,532	99,087	35,810	45,811	30,804	439,461	21,608
1971	220,601	88,382	32,528	40,498	26,835	454,958	21,766
1972	196,358	78,479	28,332	35,107	23,282	447,682	23,615
1973	177,903	70,615	24,085	30,592	19,899	427,105	21,845
1974	160,922	54,664	20,144	23,037	16,597	419,237	31,443
1975	137,196	54,195	16,770	22,109	13,401	426,699	17,609
1976	122,008	49,489	11,331	18,821	10,922	403,639	20,922
1977	113,136	45,683	10,359	17,430	9,716	388,590	20,392
1978	104,417	42,866	9,155	16,075	9,080	374,794	18,088
1979	99,234	40,312	8,360	14,767	7,830	363,059	17,219
1980	95,872	37,678	7,422	13,362	7,108	358,788	18,082
1981	92,696	33,663	6,017	12,416			

SOURCES: Residents: 1964: Statistical Note No. 112; 1965-1975: Statistical Note No. 146; 1976-1981: Survey of Patient Characteristics for each year, unpublished; residents with OBD: 1964-1966: Patients in Mental Institutions; 1969-1975: Statistical Note No. 146; 1976-1981: Survey of Patient Characteristics for each year, unpublished; deaths: Reprinted in Goldman, Adams, & Taube (1983); net releases: Total net releases are reprinted in Goldman, Adams & Taube (1983). We estimated net releases by age by adding Residents at the beginning of the year plus additions and subtracting Residents at the end of the year and deaths separately for each age group. (All deaths were assumed to be 65+.) Residents at the end of the previous year were substituted for Residents at the beginning of the year. We used additions (which include returns from long-term leave) rather than admissions, because additions are available by age. For 1964 to 1968 additions by age were not available. Therefore, net releases were calculated by estimating that 6% of NIMH's total net releases were 65+ and 94% were under 65. (This ratio was used because the 65+ groups were 6% of our estimated net releases in 1969-1975.) Hence, net releases for 1964 to 1968 are low relative to later years, because they are based on admissions rather than additions.

NOTE: The total number of residents do not always agree with those in Table 3.1, the results of different surveys.

[a] Organic Brain Disorders (OBD) exclude those conditions due to alcohol and drug use, except 1969 to 1975, which include them.

dents. The under-65 state hospital group with organic brain disorders decreased at an even faster rate (about 85%) than residents in general.[3] In absolute numbers, the elderly in state mental hospitals dropped from 144,000 in 1964 to 34,000 in 1981. However, the number of residents at the end of any particular year is the net result of admissions, discharges, length of stay, and deaths. Therefore, the difference in the number of state hospital residents at two points in time does not represent all the people released who could have entered nursing homes. We calculated "net releases" according to the NIMH formula of adding the number of residents at the beginning of the year plus admissions, and then subtracting out deaths and residents at the end of the year.[4]

Table 7.2 also shows the number of net releases who were under and over 65 from 1964 to 1980. Note that before 1971, it was more likely that those over 65 would die in the hospital than be released, whereas in 1981 over twice as many elderly were released as died there. This is consistent with a hypothesis that the elderly are being transferred somewhere rather than remaining until death. We will try to estimate how many might have been transferred to nursing homes, after reviewing trends in nursing home residents with mental disorders.

It is important to note the difference in size of the two age groups. The under-65 resident group has consistently been about 2½ times as large as the 65+ group. Further, the difference between the age groups in net releases has always been much larger than that for residents. There has consistently been 15–25 times as many net releases for the under-65 group than for the 65+ group. There is an important point to be made here. In the years covered, the state mental hospital has not been a haven for the elderly—not in terms of residents, but especially not in terms of net releases.[5] Keep this in mind, for this will be a central feature in our later discussions.

Trends in nursing home residents with mental disorders. The number of nursing home residents with mental disorders must be separated from the total number of residents for comparison with state mental hospital data. Table 7.3 shows trend data on the number of residents with mental disorders and senility, both as "primary diagnoses" and as "chronic conditions." The primary diagnosis is the "major diagnosis noted at the resident's latest medical examination." Chronic conditions and impairments "include those long-term physical and mental problems of the resident" and are selected from a list of conditions on the interview form. Only one primary diagnosis is assigned to each resident. Therefore, the total number of primary diagnoses will equal the total number of residents for any given year. However, several chronic conditions could be assigned. Obviously, more residents will have a chronic condition of mental illness or senility than will have these as a primary diagnosis. Although the primary diagnosis category would be more comparable to our statistics from other sites, the count of chronic conditions is not inappropriate when dealing with an elderly population. They are likely to have several chronic conditions, both physical and mental as a result of aging. In 1977 61% of all nursing home residents had one or more chronic mental conditions and the average number of chronic physical conditions was 3.5.

When dealing with an elderly population, the problem of classifying "senility" becomes central. The National Nursing Home Survey distinguishes between senility and advanced senility. Senility is a more general term referring to the deteriorating effect of age on mental functioning. Advanced senility is the result of several conditions, such as chronic brain syndrome, and involves psychoses. Given the difficulty in distinguishing between senility and advanced senility, we have combined the two categories and refer to them as "senility." The NNHS uses "mental illness" or "mental disorder" to indicate all mental disorders except senility.

Table 7.3 shows that the number of residents with a chronic condition of mental illness or senility increased dramatically between 1964 and 1977, from about 101,000 to 394,000 for mental disorders and from 148,000 to 741,000 for senility. As mentioned, these figures represent some duplication. The number of residents with primary diagnoses of mental disorders at last exam also increased, particularly for senility. Of course, we would expect an increase, given the increase of the elderly in the general population, and we will discuss the change in rates shortly. We will first look at the prevalence of mental disorders in the resident population.

Table 7.3 shows that the percentage of total residents with a *primary diagnosis* of either mental disorder or senility has been stable at about 20% (total) since 1969, the first year of data on principal diagnoses. However, the percentages with *chronic conditions* are quite different. The percentage of total residents with chronic senility doubled between 1964–1969 from 27% to 56% and has remained at that level. The percentage with a chronic condition of mental illness began to rise in 1969 from 18% to 30% by 1977.

Cicchinelli, et al. (1981) provide an extensive reanalysis of the 1977 National Nursing Home Survey. They claim that 789,000 nursing home residents are chronically mentally ill, sufficiently to warrant hospitalization for that reason alone. However, these patients average 3.5 physical problems, and consequently their primary diagnosis may be somewhat arbitrary. Later, we argue that the estimates of Cicchinelli et al. are

TABLE 7.3

Number of Residents in Nursing Homes and Number of Residents with Mental Disorders as a Chronic Condition and as a Primary Diagnosis at Last Examination, 1963-1977

	Total Number of Residents	Chronic Conditions[a] Mental Illness	Senility	Primary Diagnosis at Last Exam Mental Disorders	Senility
1963	505,242				
1964	554,000	100,700 (18%)	148,400 (27%)		
1969	815,100	147,705 (18%)	459,700 (56%)	84,600 (10%)	77,200 (9%)
1973	1,075,800	273,200 (25%)	627,200 (58%)	115,800 (11%)	146,800 (14%)
1977	1,303,100	394,200 (30%)	741,100 (57%)	121,900 (9%)	144,200 (11%)

SOURCES: Vital and Health Statistics Series, published by the National Center for Health Statistics, as follows: 1963: Series 12, No. 2; 1964: Series 12, No. 8; 1969: Series 12, No. 22 and Series 13, No. 29; 1973: Series 13, No. 29; 1977: Series 13, No. 51.

NOTES: Percentages of total residents are in parenthesis.
Senility includes advanced senility and chronic brain syndrome. Mental illness and mental disorders include mental retardation. In 1977, alcohol and drug addiction and insomnia were included. Earlier surveys do not list them separately; 1973 data do not include personal care homes.

[a] Each resident can have more than one chronic condition.

preferable to base discussion and intensive analysis on, rather than the primary diagnosis.

We would expect some increase in the absolute number of nursing home residents, given the greater number of elderly people in the population. As people age, their risk of having any type of chronic physical or mental condition becomes greater. That is, we would expect that people over 85 would enter nursing homes at a higher rate than people between 75 and 85, who in turn would enter at a higher rate than those between 65 and 75 years. In order to observe more rigorously the trends in nursing home residents with mental health problems, we calculated the rates per 100,000 civilian population for males and females in four age categories: under 65, 65 to 74, 75 to 84, and 85+. Table 7.4 shows these rates for chronic conditions of mental disorders and Table 7.5 shows them for senility.

The first column in Table 7.4 shows a clear increase in the nursing home resident population, beyond what would be expected by the increase in the number of the nation's elderly alone. The rate in 1977 (607) was twice what it was in 1964 (293). The rate for mental disorders increased even faster; between 1964 and 1977 it increased 3½ times (the absolute number quadrupled). As expected, the rates are higher for older age categories, and the rates are generally higher for women than men.[6] However, the overall increases in rate from year to year were similar for men and women in each age group.

Table 7.5 shows the rates for nursing home residents with senility as a chronic condition. The rate for senility increased about four times between 1964 and 1977, twice the increase for total residents. Since over half the total residents are labeled as senile, the diagnosis is not very discriminating, particularly with older age groups. There has been a large increase in senility rate in the under-65 group; a diagnosis of senility for them barely existed in 1964. However, the under 65 senile is a small group (40,000) and represents a very small proportion of the total of senile residents (5%).

The number of nursing home residents per 100,000 population has gone up rapidly during 1964–1977, but the number of senile and mentally disordered in such homes has gone up much more rapidly.

Comparisons of nursing home and state mental hospital trends. The only direct evidence at the national level that people are transferred to nursing homes from mental hospitals comes from the question in the National Nursing Home Survey that asks the prior living arrangement of the resident. In 1977 only 6% of all residents lived in a mental hospital immediately before entering the nursing home (Hing, 1981). Given that the question asks where the resident was staying ''immediately before

TABLE 7.4
Number of Nursing Home Residents and Number and Rate with a Chronic Condition of Mental Disorder by Age and Sex, 1963-1977

	Total Residents	Total Mental Disorders	MALE					FEMALE				
			All Ages	Under 65	65-74	75-84	85+	All Ages	Under 65	65-74	75-84	85+
1964	554,000 (292.9)	100,700 (53.2)	40,200 (43.8)	16,700 (19.9)	10,600 (200.2)	9,100 (403.9)	3,800 (981.9)	60,500 (62.2)	14,600 (16.8)	14,900 (230.5)	21,300 (692.7)	9,700 (1485.5)
1969	815,100 (409.3)	147,705 (74.2)	54,064 (56.4)	23,431 (26.8)	14,852 (275.2)	11,838 (485.2)	3,943 (859.0)	93,641 (90.6)	27,859 (30.3)	23,038 (333.6)	27,869 (767.5)	14,875 (1754.1)
1973	1,075,800 (517.0)	273,200 (131.3)	95,300 (94.8)	36,500 (39.8)	24,700 (429.6)	20,700 (826.0)	11,400 (2091.7)	177,900 (165.4)	42,800 (45.0)	38,500 (515.6)	56,100 (1411.0)	40,500 (3732.7)
1977	1,303,100 (606.9)	394,200 (183.6)	145,800 (140.6)	66,500 (70.6)	39,300 (619.9)	27,600 (1070.2)	10,300 (1565.3)	247,300 (222.8)	73,200 (75.4)	51,500 (624.2)	69,200 (1626.7)	50,100 (3513.3)

SOURCES: Vital and Health Statistics Series, published by National Center for Health Statistics, as follows: 1963, 1964, 1969: Series 12, Nos. 2, 8, and 22, respectively; 1973: Series 13, No. 29; 1977: Series 13, No. 51.

NOTES: Rates per 100,000 civilian population appear in parentheses. Rates based on population estimates in Current Population Reports, Series P-25, Nos. 519 and 800, U.S. Bureau of the Census. Each resident can have mroe than one chronic condition; 1973 data do not include personal-care homes. Mental disorders include mental retardation. In 1977 alcohol and drug addiction and insomnia are included. Earlier surveys do not list them separately.

TABLE 7.5
Number of Nursing Home Residents and Number and Rate with a Chronic Condition of Senility, by Age and Sex, 1963 to 1977

	Total Residents	Total Senility	MALE All Ages	Under 65	65-74	75-84	85+	FEMALE All Ages	Under 65	65-74	75-84	85+
1964	554,000 (292.9)	148,400 (78.5)	43,400 (47.3)	1,400 (1.7)	7,100 (134.1)	21,000 (932.1)	13,900 (3591.7)	105,000 (107.9)	2,300 (2.6)	12,400 (191.9)	47,300 (1538.2)	43,000 (6585.0)
1969	815,100 (409.3)	459,700 (230.8)	130,600 (136.3)	7,093 (8.1)	23,977 (444.4)	55,102 (2258.3)	44,414 (9676.3)	329,000 (318.3)	7,240 (7.9)	38,541 (558.2)	142,333 (3919.9)	140,972 (16,624.1)
1973	1,075,800 (517.0)	627,200 (301.4)	169,900 (169.0)	8,929 (9.7)	31,404 (546.2)	62,996 (2513.8)	66,549 (12210.1)	457,300 (425.1)	12,690 (13.4)	47,246 (632.7)	176,851 (4448.0)	220,615 (20,333.2)
1977	1,303,100 (606.9)	741,100 (345.1)	182,000 (175.5)	19,300 (20.5)	32,300 (509.5)	74,100 (2873.2)	56,300 (8556.2)	559,100 (503.6)	20,700 (21.3)	62,200 (753.9)	225,700 (5305.6)	250,400 (17,560.0)

SOURCES: 1963-1969: NCHS: Vital and Health Statistics Series, Series 12, Nos. 2, 8, 22; 1973, 1977: NCHS Vital and Health Statistics Series 13, No. 29, 51.

NOTES: Rates per 100,000 civilian population appear in parentheses. (Rates based on population estimates in Current Population Reports, Series P-25, Nos. 519 and 800, U. S. Bureau of the Census.) Senility includes advanced senility and chronic brain syndrome. Each resident can have more than one chronic condition; 1973 data do not include personal care homes.

entering this facility," the count is an underestimate of the number who were recently in mental hospitals. People going home from a mental hospital for a few days while a nursing home placement was found were probably counted as coming from home, if the question is taken literally. However, this same underestimate presumably occurs in counting those from general hospitals. A brief stay at home might follow a discharge from a general hospital until a nursing home placement is found.

Cicchinelli et al. extensively reanalyzed the 1977 data. They derived a definition of chronic mental illness, which included serious disorders irrespective of whether they had been otherwise categorized as primary at the last examination. They concluded that 789,000 (or over 60%) of nursing home residents have chronic mental conditions. There are several reasons why one might wish to use this more liberal estimate of prevalence for further analysis rather than primary diagnosis. One, a patient could be transferred from a state hospital because of a deteriorating physical condition. Indeed, 71% of all admissions of chronic mental patients to nursing homes were primarily due to the physical condition of the patients. Further, mental patients in nursing homes averaged the same number of physical disorders (3.5) as did patients there because of physical disorders. Two, Medicaid policy places a 50% limit for mental patients in a nursing home population, leading to underdiagnosis of mental disorders as primary.[7] Three, there is a strong tendency for physicians in nursing homes to miss psychiatric diagnoses, even of serious disorders (Zimmer, Watson, & Treat, 1984).

In the analysis to follow, we use Cicchinelli et al.'s estimate of 789,000 chronic mental patients in nursing homes. Of those, they found 9.5% (or 75,000) of their chronically mentally ill were transferred from a "mental hospital." They also tried to investigate the placement prior to that, and found 20.2% came from a "health facility." If mental hospitals were proportionately similar for second prior placement as first, this would account for another 3.4% (or 27,000). This would imply a total of 102,000 nursing home residents who had come from a mental hospital immediately prior or once removed.

If we assume that all of our estimated 102,000 residents who previously lived in mental hospitals would have a primary diagnosis of mental disorder or senility, they account for a modest percentage of nursing home residents with these primary diagnoses. We see how few of these residents are accounted for by former hospital residents. Although 266,100 residents had a principal diagnosis of mental disorder or senility in 1977, only 38% of them would be accounted for if all the residents who lived in mental hospitals prior to the nursing home had these primary diagnoses at their last exam in the nursing homes.

Although the total number of nursing home residents with primary diagnoses of mental disorders (including senility) far outnumber former mental hospital residents, we now ask to what extent state hospital discharges could be accounted for by transfers to nursing homes. In other words, former mental hospital residents may account for a minority of nursing home residents with mental disorders, but they may account for a large or small percentage of people leaving mental hospitals.

These statistics on nursing home residents do not address the dynamics of transfer from mental hospitals. The residents in a nursing home at a particular time do not reflect people who are admitted and either die or are discharged during the year. Therefore, the 102,000 former mental hospital residents in 1977 is an underestimate to the extent that people were admitted from mental hospitals during 1977 but either died or were discharged. On the other hand, the number of residents at a particular time is an accumulation of people entering in previous years and staying until the current year. It is much higher than the number entering nursing homes that year. Therefore, we estimated the number of former mental hospital residents who entered nursing homes in 1977 in two steps. We first approximated the number entering based on their length of stay distribution and then approximated the number of live discharges and deaths of former mental hospital residents that year.

The National Nursing Home Survey data show the distribution of length of stay of nursing home residents who came from mental hospitals. Only about 16% of the former mental hospital residents had been in the nursing home less than a year (Van Nostrand, Zappolo, Hing, Bloom, Hirsch, & Foley, 1979). The largest percentage (36%) had been there 5 years or more, and the median number of days for former mental patients was 1,299. Using Cicchinelli et al.'s estimate of 102,000 former mental hospital inpatients, we estimate that approximately 16,000 of them were admitted during the previous year.

Cicchinelli et al. also found that 83% of CMI residents were over 65. However, only 53% of residents previously living in mental hospitals were over 65. Applying that estimate to recent admittees, 8,500 of the 16,000 entering residents were over 65 and 7,500 were under 65.

Some people had presumably been admitted that year but died (without being surveyed). We estimate these to be 2,270 for the 65+ group.[8] Some patients also would be admitted and discharged during the year. However, only 2.3% of the Cicchinelli et al. group were expected to be discharged within the next 6 months. This percentage is also factored in.

In summary, assuming 102,000 nursing home patients were former patients in a mental hospital, we estimate new admits to nursing homes in 1977 as follows:

	Over 65	Under 65
Number surveyed	8,500	7,500
Deaths prior to survey	2,270	—
Discharges	196	173
Total	10,966	7,673

Those are our estimates of people entering nursing homes from state hospitals (actually *all* mental hospitals.) Now we may compare them to the available pool of state hospital releases. For the age 65+ group, we estimate approximately 11,000 new admissions in 1977 from state hospitals; they may be compared with the 20,400 net releases from state hospitals in 1977.

The reliability of our estimates is unknown. Certainly there are a number of important assumptions we have made, and our estimate of 11,000 admissions to nursing homes from mental hospitals could be off substantially. However, the two figures seem intuitively in the right range: 20,400 elderly patients were released from state hospitals in 1977 and we estimate that 11,000 elderly mental patients were admitted to nursing homes from mental hospitals. If accurate, over 50% of released elderly state mental hospital patients went to a nursing home immediately or with one intervening stop.

However, for the group under 65, the situation is very different. We estimate that 7,700 of the under-65 group were admitted to a nursing home in 1977. However, 390,000 were released that year from state hospitals. *Clearly, given the number of released patients, nursing homes play little or no role whatsoever in handling former state hospital patients who are under 65.*

It is important to remember that 95% of the releases from state hospitals that year were patients under 65. Consequently, it cannot be said that nursing homes play a substantial role in custodial care of all patients discharged from state hospitals. They clearly do not. However, nursing homes do play an important role for that fraction of patients who are over 65.

There is one important proviso here regarding the elderly patient from state hospitals and those from other mental hospitals. Our estimate (1977) is that 11,000 elderly new admissions were from mental hospitals. We have discussed this number as if all came from state hospitals but that may not be true. One clue is income; state hospital patients are poor, and would be more likely to be on Medicaid or Medicare. However, for Cicchinelli et al.'s (1981) CMI patients, 36% had their own income as their principal source of payment. This subgroup paid an average of $588 a month for their own nursing home bill (or 87% of the total charge). The people in this subgroup are unlikely candidates to have been state mental hospital patients previously. If 36% of our estimated new admits are in similar circumstances, our maximum estimate should decrease accordingly, to the 7,000 range. The impact of this adjustment, if valid, questions whether the simple majority of the elderly state hospital releases (N = 20,000 +) do go to nursing homes.

Trend analysis. Our analysis here concentrates on one year (1977) for which more data exist than for other years. In that year, clearly nursing homes accepted only a very small percentage of total net releases from state hospitals. The percentage is necessarily small because most releases from state hospitals are under 65, but most admits to nursing homes are over 65. Indeed, two-thirds of the CMI residents in nursing homes are over 75!

However, a different level of question concerns deinstitutionalization as a change in practice over time. This question asks, *could the increase in number of nursing home residents, particularly CMI residents, be people who would have formerly been sent to a state mental hospital?*

The answer is complicated, but also age linked. Over 70% of the state hospital residents and over 90% of the net releases have always (since 1964 at least) been under 65. Only 5% or less of the total nursing home residents have been under 65, but the under-65 group represents 17% of Cicchinelli et al.'s CMI group.

Some of the increase in nursing home residents is due to the increased number of the elderly in the total population, but not very much. For example, diagnoses of chronic mental illness in nursing homes increased from 100,000 to 394,000 (1964–1977). Only about 16% of that increase can be accounted for by the increase in number of the elderly in our country. The residual is due to a change in rate of admission to nursing homes. Further, that increase is equal to twice the decrease in residents in state mental hospitals in the same time period (for the elderly).

That analysis refers only to a diagnosis of a chronic condition of mental illness. An analysis of chronic senility would reveal even more dramatic differences.

These analyses reveal a special conclusion about the elderly mentally ill in nursing homes: There are many more of them than would be expected either from releases from state hospitals or from a change in former institutionalization practices.

The data for the under-65 group are complicated as well. The number of residents under 65 in state mental hospitals went from 347,000 in 1964 to 113,000 in 1977, a decrease of 234,000. In nursing homes, the number of residents with a chronic condition (not primary) of mental illness went from 31,000 in 1964 to 140,000 in 1977 (Table 7.4). In this case, estimates converge. Cicchinelli et al. find 17% of their 789,000 CMI group, or 134,000, to be under 65. The number of younger mental patients in nursing homes has increased, although not nearly as much as the number of younger residents in state mental hospitals has decreased. Recall further that the number of nursing home admissions who came from mental hospitals is a small fraction of the number released from state hospitals in a given year. This strongly suggests a diversion of the younger patients from state hospitals to nursing homes—potentially an outcome of change of national practice.

Phrased a different way, ignoring age, only a fraction of the increase in the mentally ill in nursing homes can be accounted for by either releases from state hospitals or changes in institutionalization practices. For the elderly, about half or less of the increase of their mentally ill in nursing homes could be accounted for by both sources. For the non-elderly (under 65) who largely are and have been the residents of state mental hospitals, nursing homes have played little role for the recent mental patient. However, there is a clear and substantial increase in younger nursing home residents who have not come from a mental hospital, which suggests that it could be due to changes in national practice.

Phrased yet a third way, the increase of the older mentally ill in nursing homes is at least twice that which might be expected by changes in practice or releases from state mental hospitals. The bulk of incidence of mental illness of the elderly in nursing homes is a new national phenomenon.

In Chapter 4, we described an increase in the rate of mental hospitalization. To that rather dramatic increase must be added a new and increasing population of the institutionalized mentally ill—those in nursing homes. The "new" part of this refers to those older residents who have not been, nor would have been in former times, in mental hospitals. However, the change in national practices could, at least numerically, account for the increase in younger nursing home residents with mental disorders.

Let's look at some general conclusions from all these data.

(1) State mental hospitals are not a haven of the elderly. The proportion of *residents* who are elderly is small (25%–30%), and has not

changed since 1964, at least. The proportion of net *releases* who are elderly is tiny, only about 5%. The number of elderly releases has been fairly constant for years.

(2) Nursing homes are the next step for many elderly who are released from state mental hospitals. This proportion may be substantial, and it may be a majority.

(3) Nursing homes do not play a role in care of the nonelderly patient (under 65) who is released from a state hospital. The number of younger patients in nursing homes has increased, but still is a small fraction of the total. It is almost inconceivable that more than 5% of nonelderly released state hospital patients go to nursing homes. However, the number of younger mentally disturbed residents who have not come from a hospital has increased substantially.

(4) The number of patients with chronic mental disorders in nursing homes is increasing very rapidly. A substantial majority of all nursing home patients are chronic mental patients (although they average 3.5 physical problems as well).

(5) Only a small fraction of the increase of the mentally ill in nursing homes is due to their increase in the number of elderly in the general population. Most of the increase represents a change in *rate*.

(6) Of the change in the rate for the elderly, only half or less can be accounted for by either releases from state hospitals *or* a change in institutionalization practices. The remainder represent a new phenomenon in the United States.

(7) Mental patients in nursing homes are not treated well. Cicchinelli et al. (1981) found such data as: a time of 37 days since the last physician visit; only 6% had received any psychotherapy in the previous month; only 9% had any kind of leave in the previous year (even overnight); and they averaged only 2.5 hours of physical and recreational therapy a week and only about one hour for all other kinds (see also Shadish, Silber, & Bootzin, 1984; Shadish, Straw, McSweeny, Koller, & Bootzin, 1981).

(8) For the elderly, deinstitutionalization did *not* cause the increase in patients in nursing homes, nor even that subpart with mental disorders. It did not cause it either in the sense of patients released from mental hospitals or in the sense of changed hospitalization practices from the deinstitutionalization movement. Both sources together do not account for even a majority of the increased number of elderly mental patients in nursing homes.

(9) For the younger patient, deinstitutionalization practice has apparently affected the increase in nursing home residents. However, those

with mental disorders do not go to nursing homes from mental hospitals; they appear to be going there instead of mental hospitals.

Notes

1. Thanks to William R. Shadish, Jr. who extensively reviewed an earlier draft of this chapter.

2. A likely cause of the decreasing percentage of deaths is that residents are more frequently taken to hospitals during an acute illness and then die there.

3. Organic brain disorders (OBD) include conditions due to several causes, one of the most frequent being cerebral arteriosclerosis, usually leading to "senility." This subgroup of OBD is almost exclusively a condition of those 65 and over.

4. We approximated net releases by using additions instead of admissions, because the former are available by age. Additions include people returning from long-term leave. Therefore, our total net releases are higher than those reported by NIMH. Also, all deaths were assumed to be 65 and over.

5. At least in terms of overall number. However, there is a press to keep the elderly in the state hospital (a smaller proportion are released), implying a haven of a different sort.

6. However, the rates for men and women are very similar below age 75.

7. More than 50% of residents with a primary diagnosis of mental disorder is a criterion for reclassifying the nursing home to an "institution for mental disease" (IMD). People 22–64 years are excluded from coverage in IMDs.

8. The deaths were derived as follows: There were 30,400 deaths of people who had a primary diagnosis of mental disorders or senility at admission. This is an underestimate, given that a duplicated count of 158,000 deaths with one or more chronic conditions were reported. This is a duplicated count which we tried to convert to people in the following way. A total of 789,000 people (Cichinelli et al., 1981) had 1,135,000 chronic conditions, the former representing 69.5% of the latter. If we assume that the 158,000 figure is a similar duplicated figure this leads to an estimate of 110,000 people dying (with a duplicated count of chronic conditions of 158,000). Of these, 16% or (17,600) are assumed to have been there one year or less; 12.9% of these (or 2,270) are assumed to have come from a mental hospital immediately or prior. This means an estimate of 2,270 deaths during the year of former mental patients with chronic conditions who had been in the nursing home less than one year. As before, we assume these deaths are totally with the over-65 group. Since the number is small, otherwise dividing them into the two age groups would not change the following discussion much.

CHAPTER 8

READMISSIONS

Thus far in this book we have focused on psychiatric inpatient episodes. For individual patients, an episode consists of an admission to a hospital, some treatment, and a discharge from the hospital. In aggregate data, episodes (always plural) are defined as the number of residents at the beginning of the year plus all new admissions (and readmissions) during the year.

Whether discussing individual or aggregate data, we have ignored the question of whether it is a person's first inpatient experience (first admission) or whether he or she has been an inpatient before (a readmission, or rehospitalization), either once or perhaps even several times.

There is good reason for previously ignoring the question of readmission: In almost all of the research literature on mental hospitalization that we have discussed, the status of the patient is not known. If it is an individual episode, we typically don't know if the episode is the person's first admission or fifth. In aggregate data, we do not know the proportion of first admissions, second, and so forth.

Admission status is an important issue for mental health policy, for national planning, and for questions of treatment effectiveness and cost. However, it is a datum not commonly recorded and often of uncertain reliability when it is.

Yet there is a lively debate about its influence on national statistics, and a commonly held belief about the relationship of admission status to deinstitutionalization. To wit, it is commonly believed that deinstitutionalization has led to shorter lengths of hospital stay but more stays in the hospital per patient. This is the so-called "revolving door phenomenon," in which patients are alleged to be in and out of hospitals frequently, and specifically because of the current shorter stays.

This chapter focuses on three questions:

(1) Does the revolving door phenomenon really exist? Meaning, have the shorter stays implied by deinstitutionalization led to a larger number of inpatient episodes per patient? Recall, however, lengths of stay have become shorter only in state and VA psychiatric hospitals.

(2) Given the recent large increase in inpatient episodes, has the number of people hospitalized increased, or just the number of episodes per patient?

(3) What generally do we know that enables us to predict whether a given discharged patient will subsequently be readmitted or not?

Methodological Problems

There are a number of rather serious methodological problems in this research literature that make it difficult to draw firm conclusions. Because they pervade the journals, they are worth some discussion.

(1) *Reliability.* Mental illness is not a glamorous illness, and patients are often reluctant to admit having been treated before and particularly so when the inpatient treatment has occurred several times (Cannel, 1965; Karon & VandenBos, 1981; Strauss, Carpenter, & Nasrallah, 1978). Yet often it is the patient's verbal report that provides the critical information about whether the episode in question is a first admission or not.

Further, many investigators of readmission rates have no way of ascertaining prior or subsequent readmissions, other than at the hospital at which they work. Sometimes, investigators at state hospitals have access to data from other state hospitals, but not other kinds of hospitals. Since only a small minority of inpatient episodes occur in state hospitals, this represents a major methodological problem.

(2) *Insufficient time span and data points.* To develop a solid empirical base for a national trend, one needs to follow that trend over a number of years and a number of data points. Too many studies of readmissions either cover only two or three years, or only have two data points (or both). Take the following example—the figure from Chapter 4 on episodic rate of mental hospitalization. On the bottom line, look at the rates for 1969 and 1973. The rate for 1969 is greater than that for 1973. There was once a well-cited article (we will not reference it) that by chance investigated those two years and concluded that the rate of mental hospitalization was decreasing! That research is a prime example of insufficient time span and an inadequate number of data points. There is a difference between those two years, granted. However, each represents a minor statistical fluctuation (in the opposite direction) from what is clearly a flat trend line. This sort of methodological flaw is a common problem in research on readmission.

(3) *Research design flaws.* These are almost too numerous to mention. *Replicability* is one: Many studies track readmission rates for only

one hospital. That datum is of interest, but the reader has no way of ascertaining which idiosyncratic aspects of that hospital influenced the rate. The only way that source of error can be reduced is to investigate a number of hospitals simultaneously. Lack of *random assignment* is another typical flaw. This is typically a problem when investigating the effect of a treatment or aftercare on readmission rates. Without random assignment, there is little to be concluded from such a study (see the next chapter). Knowledge of *other important variables* is often lacking. For example, one study (Silverman & Saunders, 1980) found 40% of the variance in admission rates to a mental hospital in the province of Ontario was predictable by a simple knowledge of the geographical distance to the hospital—a simple variable, obviously an important one, but seldom ascertained. Details of the *patients' past or future environment* are typically insufficient. For example, we would like to know if the patient is married and whether the spouse looks forward to the return, whether the patient was committed voluntarily or involuntarily, whether the patient has access to various "aftercare" programs, and whether he or she uses them. We typically do not know the patients' *psychiatric status at discharge*. Is the patient judged to be capable of functioning on his or her own? Hold a job? Have a close friend?

Serious methodological problems are typical in the research literature on readmission rates. This makes firm, scientifically based conclusions difficult to draw.

National Needs

From the perspective of national mental health policy, it is essential to know not only how many people create how many episodes in the aggregate but also the actual frequency distributions of readmissions. The ultimate goal of policy analysis is to provide alternative policies from which to select the best one, based on appropriate criteria (e.g., cost-effectiveness, humanitarian goals). In the case of national mental health policy, knowledge of what the distributions are and what causes these patterns is required for formulating effective policies.

As mentioned, concern with readmissions originated with the deinstitutionalization movement and the consequent rapidly decreasing resident census of the state mental hospitals. It appeared to many that residents were discharged after a briefer length of stay, to communities where they did not receive adequate aftercare and were therefore readmitted again. As mentioned, the term "revolving door" is used to describe this phenomenon. It refers to a rising readmission rate, meaning the same people are rehospitalized more frequently during a specified period of time than previously. Speculation began as to what accounted for the revolving door phenomenon, without at the same time demonstrating that it existed. Were people discharged before thay were ready, or were aftercare services inadequate to maintain them in the community (e.g., Altman, Sletten, & Nebel, 1973; Bassuk & Gerson, 1978; Ozarin & Sharfstein, 1978)?

Although readmissions became an issue due to the policies of deinstitutionalization and community care, the literature considers the problem more in the context of treatment effectiveness rather than in a policy context. The questions addressed are whether readmissions imply ineffective hospital treatment and what can prevent readmissions, rather than identifying long-term patterns of readmissions.

A substantial literature on readmissions does exist, but it is terribly flawed scientifically. In addition, it grows out of a different set of questions than we are interested in. The majority of articles on readmissions attempts to identify what percentage of a sample of discharges are readmitted within a specified time and what demographic, diagnostic, treatment, and environmental variables correlate with readmission.

Most of the research on readmissions has focused on predicting readmission from a knowledge of: (1) base rates, (2) characteristics of the patient, (3) types of prior treatment, (4) types of aftercare, and (5) characteristics of the patient's environment. Additional studies assess the relation of other variables to readmission, such as staff expectations and legal changes.

We will briefly discuss some of these data in this chapter, but let us focus first on issues surrounding the revolving door.

The Revolving Door?

NIMH has collected some national survey data on readmissions in its sample surveys of state and private psychiatric hospitals and psychiatric units of general hospitals. These are the same surveys providing the data on length of stay. For state and private hospitals, records from a sample of admissions during a sample month are selected, and information is abstracted. In 1975 the survey form asked whether the patient had any earlier professional mental health care as an inpatient or outpatient. The inpatient categories were care in (a) the same hospital, (b) another hospital of the same type, (c) another type of inpatient facility, or (d) previous care unknown. All that applied were checked.

The results for state mental hospitals showed that in 1962 48% of admissions had no previous inpatient care at any type of facility. This percentage slowly fell to 35% in 1972 and in 1975 only 31% had no previous inpatient care. Most of these peoples' previous admissions were to state hospitals (Meyer, 1973; Taube, 1974). This increase in readmissions was taken as evidence of a revolving door phenomenon.

Various NIMH staff (Klerman, 1979b; Taube, 1974), urged caution in interpreting these data. They noted that the percentage of admissions that are readmissions should rise as the pool of potential readmissions increases. The more previously hospitalized people there are in the community, the more people there are at risk of being rehospitalized. As Taube (1974) illustrates, the increase in percentage of admissions who were readmissions between 1969 and 1972 primarily resulted from a large increase in the population at risk (We clarify this below.) New admissions actually decreased 4%. The number of readmissions per 1,000 "net live releases" in the previous three years actually decreased 16% between 1969 and 1972. NIMH staff further pointed out that the number of readmissions also increased due to a definitional change. Placement on long-term leave status has been decreasing in favor of regular discharge status. Whereas a person on leave who is rehospitalized would not be counted as a readmission, those with regular discharge status would be.

Let us illustrate these points more specifically with a nice analysis of New York State data by Weinstein (1983). He noted that the New York increase in the readmissions percentage in state hospitals was even greater than the national trend reported by NIMH, and that this "fact" had received much attention in the popular press.

Weinstein points to two major artifacts explaining this apparent change in readmission rates from the mid-1960s to the 1970s. First, the ability to identify readmits was improved, because more strictly defined catchment boundaries (and adherence to them) made patients more likely to return to the same hospitals—and hence be so identified. In addition, there were better computer systems and more thorough checking.

More important, there was a significant change in administrative law and practice governing discharges and therefore readmissions. Before the mid-1960s, patients were more likely to be placed on leave (convalescent care) than they were to be discharged outright (this has actually been true since the nineteenth century—Grob, 1983). There were two major reasons for the prior practice: (1) A patient on leave did not need a new court certification to return; (2) patients on leave could receive treatment in state aftercare facilities (while discharged patients could not).

A state legislative change in 1965 undid the need for these two practices and changed the official readmission rates dramatically. Consequently, from 1965–1980, discharges rose from 10,000 to 28,000, while placements on leave fell from 23,000 to 1,200. The sum of these—what Weinstein calls "gross releases"—was 33,000 in 1965 and 29,000 in 1980.

"Readmissions" were modified by Weinstein to mean both readmissions after discharge plus returns from "leave," called readditions. He then used the NIMH category of "net live releases" to form a readmission index: the total number of readditions divided by the number of discharges during the previous three years (times 1,000). The latter is the population at risk.

This index of readmission was quite stable, varying between 202 and 256 over those years and at last report was 237. In short, the readmission rate, more completely defined, fluctuated but it did not vary systematically over a 16-year period.[1]

In short, both the NIMH studies and Weinstein's clearly demonstrate that readmission rates in state hospitals have not increased, providing one takes into account the population at risk (i.e., the people eligible to be readmitted) and does not ignore returns from long-term leave. Indeed, the NIMH data, thus corrected, show a slight decrease in readmission rate.

That the readmission rate in state mental hospitals is either stable or declining is quite surprising. Surprising partly because the opposite view is widely held, but surprising also because the patient population is changing. The number of admissions is down in state hospitals (Chapter 3). The number of readmits as a proportion of the total patient population in state hospitals is up (this fact having caused all the confusion in the first place).

Weinstein (1983) describes the changing mix of patients in New York State: From 1968–1980, the number of first admissions for the elderly (over 65) fell by 88%. Patients under 65 have decreased somewhat but they are different: "Sicker, more aggressive, more difficult to treat" (p. 335). The total decrease represents voluntary admissions: the number of involuntary admissions has remained constant. In spite of these rather dramatic changes in patient population, the readmissions rate, properly qualified, has *not* increased.

Two other important studies of readmissions rates have been carried out with state and county registers. The data that have been discussed most frequently over the years is a study by Bahn, Gorwitz, Klee,

Kramer, and Tuerk (1965) on the first-year data for the Maryland State Psychiatric Register. Such registers attempt to track all psychiatric episodes, whether inpatient or outpatient, within a given year. They typically underestimate the number of outpatient episodes and visits, since the state or county registers tend to track the practices of only psychiatrists and exclude such other mental health professionals as social workers and psychologists. On the other hand, one would expect them to be substantially more accurate for inpatient episodes. Bahn et al. found each hospitalized patient to account for 1.2 inpatient episodes during that year. Thus one could multiply the reciprocal of that number (.83) by the number of episodes to derive the actual number of people involved. We note that their study was for one year only, did not track people beyond that time period, was derived over 20 years ago, and covers only one specific geographical region of the United States.

More recently Goldberg and Allen (1981) completed a multiple-year study of the Monroe County (New York) Psychiatric Case Register. Some of the comparisons lack reliability because of changes in record keeping over the years. However, Goldberg and Allen were able to study one five-year period intensively. They found an average of approximately 1.35 episodes per person during each year leading to a correction factor of .74. This is a slightly higher readmission rate than the Maryland data of 15 years earlier.

The alleged revolving door phenomenon demands such a difference in readmission rates. However, it is difficult to disentangle, in these two studies, whether the difference between them reflects changed national treatment practice or rather some other mechanism based on differences between the two regions or the difference in time. Several things should be noted. The readmission rate found by Goldberg and Allen is only about 12% higher for the mid-1970s than Bahn et al. found for the early 1960s. Consequently, this slight change in the readmission rate could in no way be used to explain the much more dramatic increase in number of total inpatient episodes nationally.

There is another problem with these data in attempting to use them to support a revolving door hypothesis. Even though the average readmission rate found by Goldberg and Allen was 12% greater than that found by Bahn et al., Goldberg and Allen found no difference in readmission rate across the five-year period they studied very intensively. That is, if one wished to infer that the difference in readmission rate between these two studies is real, then one must also conclude that the readmission rate is no longer rising.

Looked at a different way, a slight increase in readmission rate would not necessarily be cause for alarm. We saw in Chapter 5 that during the time period covered by these two studies the average length of stay at hospitals decreased substantially more than the difference in readmission rates found in the two studies. Assuming the difference in readmission rate to be reliable, valid, and reflective of the nation at large, the inference would be that we put people in mental hospitals slightly more often but for much less time each episode, making for a substantially decreased total number of inpatient days per person.

The Bahn et al. study was for one year only. We emphasize that the Goldberg and Allen study, even though reflecting multiple years, deals with data that are within-year only. We have no way of ascertaining whether people hospitalized in year 1 were also hospitalized in years 2, 3, and 4. The data were not gathered in a way that allows such an analysis. There is some evidence that one should track individuals across years, rather than simply within years. An NIMH study over a 10-year period with Monroe County data clearly demonstrates this point (NIMH, 1976). NIMH reported the number of psychiatric inpatient days spent in the first year in which a patient was admitted, and a total for the 10-year period. (They do not break the data down year by year.) In that study, in the first year that patients were hospitalized, they spent an average of 86 inpatient days. The same patients over the course of the 10-year period spent an average of 332 days. Thus, only about a quarter of the total inpatient days in the 10-year period occurred during the first year following admission. This finding suggests very strongly that we should be tracking patients over years, and cannot easily evaluate the outcomes of our national inpatient policy without such data.

With the same constraint in mind, it is still possible that the national readmission rate for inpatient care has risen much more dramatically than the difference between Bahn et al. and Goldberg and Allen. That is to say, we may have a revolving door phenomenon, but simply now have a longer period of time between a given discharge from a hospital and the next readmission. A hypothesized increase in readmission rates might presumably be detected if one went beyond the one-year data period.

The data on the revolving door phenomenon are surprisingly sparse. No national data allow one to make such an inference. The best data existing are those accumulated by Goldberg and Allen. However, they reflect one county only and are stable over an intensively studied five-year period. Goldberg and Allen do find slightly higher readmission rates for the mid-1970s than Bahn et al. (1965) found for the early 1960s. However, other differences between the two places where the data were gathered could easily account for the difference.

Even the data from state hospitals do not support the notion of a revolving door. If one takes due account of the increased population at risk (of ex-patients), the NIMH data suggests the readmission rate has decreased. Weinstein's careful analysis of New York data suggest a flat line.

Many of our professional colleagues are firmly convinced that a revolving door phenomenon exists. We do not have the data to rule out the possibility, but there are no impeccable data clearly supporting it. The most rational conclusion from the existing data base is that the revolving door phenomenon does not exist. Readmission rates have not risen in the last 15 or 20 years.

Other Data

In a 1972 review of studies conducted during the 1960s, Anthony, Buell, Sharratt, and Althoff reported the "recidivism rate," defined as the percentage of discharged psychiatric patients who are subsequently rehospitalized. That is, a cohort of discharges was tracked over time, and this group formed the base of the percentage rehospitalized.

The studies reviewed by Anthony et al. are of "traditional hospital treatment," consisting of drugs and possibly some form of individual or group therapy. The studies covered different types of institutions and geographic locations. The findings across studies were similar, showing a recidivism rate for a one-year period of about 40% to 50%.

Generally, an increase in the recidivism rate occurred with time from discharge. Other studies reviewed by Anthony et al. have found rates of 30% to 40% by 6 months and 65% to 75% at 3 to 5 years.

In a subsequent review article, Anthony, Cohen, and Vitalo (1978) added additional studies with varying lengths of follow-up to the first review. Follow-up studies done in the 1970s should show higher rehospitalization rates than those done in the 1960s, if the revolving door hypothesis were valid. Only one of the additional studies with a one year follow-up was done in the 1970s, and the rate was about the same—37%. Five additional studies were done in the 1960s and showed rates of 35% to 41%. For follow-ups of less than one year, studies done in the 1970s showed generally lower rates than one-year follow-ups, as was the case in the first review. Studies done in the 1970s with longer than one-year follow-ups again generally showed higher recidivism rates with greater time since discharge. Studies that were added but done in the 1960s had results similar to the first set of 1960s studies.

These review articles do not show an increase in percentage of readmissions during one-year follow-ups from the 1960s to 1970s. The studies cover the time span of 1960 to 1975, but most years are represented by only one study and none was intended to be nationally representative.

Baseline rates of the percentage of discharges who return in a specified length of time or the percentage of admissions who are readmissions serve as preliminary documentation of readmission rates. However, a problem with many studies is the absence of information on whether all readmissions to any inpatient facility are tracked or only to the facility from which the person was discharged. Our impression is that unless otherwise stated, only readmissions to the hospital under study are counted. This represents a substantial methodological limitation, as we have discussed.

Characteristics of the Person Related to Readmissions

Concomitant with the literature on baseline rates is literature on correlates of readmissions. In this section we will review findings on demographic variables, diagnoses, and number of previous hospitalizations.

Buell and Anthony (1975) reviewed studies on the relationship of person characteristics to probability of readmission and found that the only variable consistently related to rehospitalization was the number of previous hospitalizations. Other authors, reviewing additional work, have reached the same conclusions (Braff & Lefkowitz, 1979; Kirk, 1976; Rosenblatt & Mayer, 1974). Buell and Anthony (1975), Braff and Lefkowitz (1979), and Kirk (1976) also found that length of prior hospitalization was consistently positively related to readmission.

In their own study and replication Anthony and Buell (1974) and Buell and Anthony (1973) used multiple-regression techniques to analyze the unique contributions of 10 variables in predicting readmissions of state hospital patients. Controlling for all other variables, the number of previous hospitalizations was the best predictor at 6 months since discharge in the first study, but was not the best predictor until 12 months in the replication. (Marital status was the best predictor at 6 months in the replication.) It should be noted that all 10 variables together only accounted for 24% to 30% of the total variance of readmissions. Although the number of previous hospitalizations uniquely accounted for 19% in the first study of a six-month follow-up, it accounted for less than 5% in the replication study. Length of last hospitalization did not account for a significant amount of unique variance in any of the three tests.

Diagnosis itself, independent of such chronicity measures as number of previous hospitalizations, is consistently unrelated to probability of rehospitalization (Anthony & Buell, 1974; Buell & Anthony, 1975; Buell & Anthony, 1973; Braff & Lefkowitz, 1979). Gender, age, and marital status have not shown consistent relationships with rehospitalization (Braff & Lefkowitz, 1979; Anthony & Buell, 1974; Buell & Anthony, 1975; Buell & Anthony, 1973).

Characteristics of the
Treatment Related to Readmissions

In this section we summarize findings on the relation of hospital treatment to readmission rates. Reviewing one study of each of four types of traditional hospital treatments of various types of therapies, Anthony et al. (1972) concluded that none was superior to another; each showed similar rehospitalization rates. Therapies that structured the total hospital environment toward therapeutic ends typically improve patient functioning in the hospital, but there have been few tests of their effectiveness in keeping people out of the hospital. Two comprehensive programs that did follow up patients found lower than base line rehospitalization rates, but it can not be concluded whether the effect was due to aspects of the treatment or the posthospital environment. A later review (Anthony et al., 1978) came to essentially the same conclusion.

When we review the evidence from true experiments comparing the effectiveness of nonhospital treatment with active inpatient care (Chapter 9), we will see that some inpatient programs resulted in low rehospitalization rates, but the groups receiving alternative care had even lower rates of ever being hospitalized.

Relation of Aftercare to Readmissions

The type and intensity of professional mental health services received by people in the community after their discharge from inpatient psychiatric care vary greatly. Services range from the dispensing of drugs to intensive involvement in all aspects of the discharged person's life. Anthony et al. (1972) concluded in their review that rehospitalization rates are lower for those who attend aftercare clinics, but the effect cannot necessarily be attributed to aftercare. In these nonexperimental studies, it is quite plausible that people who attend are those who have the necessary skills and environmental supports to keep them out of hospitals.

Studies of transitional facilities (e.g., halfway houses) generally report lower than base rate rehospitalization rates while the person is still participating. After leaving the facility, the rehospitalization rates often increase up to the base rates.

Aftercare is not always available and when it is, discharged people do not necessarily attend, or they stop after a few visits. Anthony et al. (1978) and Kirk (1976) report studies showing varying rates of receiving aftercare ranging from 10% to over 50%. The rates of receiving aftercare, including whether or not any contact is made, depend on how people are referred, if at all, and how aggressively they are followed up (e.g., Stickney, Hall, & Gardner, 1980; Kovacs, 1981; see Meyerson and Herman, 1983 for additional work).

Further evidence that the existence of aftercare does not mean that all discharged people necessarily receive it is given by Zeldow and Taub (1981). They investigated the aftercare procedures for all 196 discharges from the two psychiatric wards of a VA hospital during an 8-month period. Although 97% were thought to need some kind of aftercare, only 70% were referred to one of the VA's services. Of the 47 patients referred to the mental hygiene clinic, only 26 had any contact.

In a true experiment with random assignment to groups and a 9-year follow-up, Beard, Malamud, and Rossman (1978) showed that attendance at aftercare services, as measured by number of visits, was higher for the groups receiving 2 years of outreach than for a control group with the same services available but who received no outreach. Attendance remained higher after the outreach process ended.

The existence of aftercare servcies does not mean that discharged patients are necessarily using them. Tessler and Mason (1979) studied a sample of 146 patients admitted to a Massachusetts state hospital. The modal length of stay was 3 to 4 weeks and most had previous hospitalizations. The clinics to which the people were referred on discharge were contacted to determine whether they attended. Of the 100 people referred to community clinics, only 55% continued attending beyond one meeting. Twelve percent refused the referral, 21% had not had contact as of 1 month after discharge, and 11% had one contact. (It is unknown whether people contacted community services other than the ones to which they were referred.)

Kirk (1976) also reviewed some conflicting findings on the effect of aftercare on readmissions, concluding that the more rigorous studies evaluating experimental projects tend to show lower rehospitalization rates than studies of routine aftercare. Some studies, such as Franklin, Kittredge, and Thrasher (1975) show an inverse relationship between amount of aftercare received and readmissions, possibly because the staff of aftercare services arranged for rehospitalization (see also Beard, Malamud, & Rossman, 1978; Tessler & Mason, 1979).

Meyerson and Herman (1983) reviewed aftercare studies published between 1977 and 1981. They note that since there has been little controlled research on the effects of psychosocial rehabilitation on rehospitalization, employment, and level of functioning, its benefits are in doubt, particularly regarding what type of treatment works for whom. They also reviewed day treatment studies, which show some effect of day treatment in improving functioning after discharge and lowering rehospitalization rates, but none had proper comparison groups or allowed for identifying what aspects of the programs worked (e.g., drugs, therapy).

Meyerson and Herman (1983) concluded that many studies report an association between participation in general aftercare services and reduced rehospitalization, but effects cannot be attributed to aftercare per se, due to self-selection of participants and other uncontrolled factors, such as medication.

In general, this research literature is replete with design flaws. Many studies start with an assumption that the revolving door exists and try to investigate why—a questionable approach at best. Other studies have problems with patient self-selection, inadequate description of inpatient treatment, note whether or not a discharged patient had an aftercare contact, but not what it consisted of and whether or not it could be expected to be effective. At minimum one can conclude that aftercare in general delays rehospitalization. Whether aftercare prevents rehospitalization has not been demonstrated, but it also has not been tested by reasonable scientific criteria.

Shift in Locus of Inpatient Care

We have seen that much attention has been given to national statistics that show a higher proportion of inpatient episodes occurring in facilities other than state mental hospitals, whereas in the 1950s the majority of inpatient episodes occurred in state hospitals. This phenomenon has been referred to as a shift in locus of inpatient care, but as Thompson, Bass, and Witkin (1982) pointed out, it cannot be inferred that the same people who would have been hospitalized in state hospitals are now hospitalized elsewhere.

In their 1977 report, the General Accounting Office concluded that federally funded CMHCs and mental health clinics had only a limited effect in reducing unnecessary admissions to state hospitals. Although the report does not provide direct evidence, a major reason cited for the lack of success is the development of CMHCs without a formal link with the state hospitals. This is a quite plausible hypothesis. According to one study reported by the GAO, CMHCs themselves did not view reduction of state hospital admissions a primary goal. In one study by an NIMH contractor, 175 CMHCs ranked the goal of decreasing state hospital utilization next to last out of 10 goals.

Several studies show decreased admissions to state mental hospitals following the opening of community services but the decrease cannot be unequivocally attributed solely to the community services (Wolford, Hitchcock, Ellison, Sonis, & Smith, 1972; Dyck, 1974; Doidge & Rodgers, 1976; Barnes & Adams, 1974).

As part of NIMH's evaluation of CMHCs, Windle and Scully (1976) analyzed both resident rates and admission rates for state mental hospitals in 16 states. The data were reported by county, each classified as to whether it was in the catchment area of an operating, federally funded community mental health center and if so, when the center opened. Between 1964 and 1971 all counties showed a decline in the number of hospital residents per 100,000 population, regardless of when their center opened or whether they had one at all. The same analyses for admission rates showed some tendency for counties with centers to have lower rates than those without. The authors note that working relationships between centers and state hospitals usually do not exist, which may partly account for the lack of impact of the centers on state hospital utilization.

Using Monroe County psychiatric case register data, Babigian (1977) tracked the use of all hospital facilities in the four catchment areas in Monroe County, New York. Only two had federally funded centers (although beds in other facilities were available), thus allowing for comparisons within counties before and after the centers opened, while using centerless counties for base rate comparisons. Hospitalization rates are reported for 1963 through 1973. Catchment area A's center opened in 1968, and B's opened in 1967. Areas C and D had no center. Unlike the data reported in previous studies, the admission rates reported are unduplicated within each year; only one hospitalization per person is counted.

The hospitalization rate for area A was already decreasing but dropped more precipitously in 1968. Rates in Area B rose until 1967 and began to drop in 1968. Rates in centerless area C also dropped sharply in 1968, and centerless area D showed a steady decline, apparently unaffected by new centers in other areas, probably due to its distance from any mental health facilities.

The declines in hospital rates occurred while total rates for all types of care simultaneously rose. Hospitalization rates for new admissions rose until 1967 for Area B and then began to decline, and Area A showed the same peak and decline in 1968 when its center opened. However, the first admission rate for centerless Area C also began to decline in 1968 but rose back to its original level in 1973. Centerless Area D showed a gradual decrease in first admissions; its rate was much lower than the other three areas. The author concludes that despite the addition of new beds at the centers, hospitalization rates declined due to the increase in ambulatory care. It seems to us that the centers accelerated an already decreasing trend in hospital admissions, given declines in the centerless areas. The ongoing decrease was probably due to lower admission rates in the state hospital; the national trend in state hospital admission rates show a decline between 1963 and 1973.

Although Babigian did not describe the interagency relationships among the centers and other inpatient facilities, it seems likely that formal liaisons existed, at least for Area A, given that the center was developed by the medical school of the University of Rochester. This assumption makes the results consistent with previous findings that suggest more impact of centers occurs when coordination for patient care exists among facilities.

Shaeffer, Schulberg, and Board (1978) studied the effect of community mental health centers on state hospital admissions and analyzed admissions by clinical and demographic characteristics. They note that the composition of state hospital admissions may change without an overall decrease. They compared the admissions to the same state hospital from two counties; Beaver County had a comprehensive center since 1970 and Lawrence County did not have substantial outpatient and partial hospitalization services until 1973, but these were not as extensive as in Beaver County. Data were collected for 1966, 1969, and 1970 through 1977. Both counties showed an increase in proportion of admissions with previous hospitalizations (either at the state hospital or elsewhere) during these years, and both counties showed an increase in proportion of diagnoses of schizophrenia. Therefore, these two characteristics of admissions could not be attributed to expanding community services; the trend began before community services were available.

The authors did conclude that expanded community mental health services were associated with decreased state hospital admission rates, because the rate for Beaver County declined after the opening of the 1970 center while the rate for Lawrence County did not change. Also, the rate for Lawrence County sharply decreased after 1973 when its community services were expanded. They also found that the center in Beaver County was screening potential admissions to the state hospital. Between 1971 and 1977 at least 90% of county applicants were screened before admission to the state hosptial, presumably to determine whether local care was possible.

All these results are consistent with the idea that CMHCs can reduce state hospital admissions, but perhaps only if they coordinate with the state hospitals. (See also Spearly, 1980; Billings, 1978.)

Summary. The best evidence is that the revolving door does not exist. The main evidence in favor of it was the increasing percentage of inpatients in state hospitals who have been there before. As Taube (1974) and Weinstein (1983) clearly demonstrate, this is an artifact and it occurs because there is now a substantially larger number of ex-inpatients at risk. The NIMH data even suggest that the national readmission rate to state hospitals, more properly calculated, had decreased.

There was never good reason to believe the revolving door existed in the first place. Perhaps the effect existed in the late 1950s and early 1960s when deinstitutionalization first began. However, many patients were discharged then who had spent the better part of their lives in a state hospital. To take that argument to its logical extreme, discharged patients must obviously have a higher readmission rate than those never discharged!

If the readmission rate has not increased (and it is increasingly difficult to argue otherwise), then the implications of this for interpreting the data on episodic rate are clear: The increase in inpatient episodes nationally consists of new people in the hospitalization system. Indeed, if the NIMH conclusions of a decreasing readmission rate are valid, then the number of new psychiatric inpatients is even greater than the increase in episodic rate would imply.

As we have discussed, nothing correlates very strongly with readmission, except number of previous admissions. What we are to make of that fact is the topic of the next two chapters.

Note

1. We note that it is important to take into account the population at risk. If one does not and simply looks as the proportion of all patients admitted who are "readmits," that percentage increases steadily from 49% in 1965 to 67% in 1980. However, this statistic does not really address the question of whether the *rate* of readmission has changed over time.

SECTION III

ATTEMPTS TO TREAT THE HOSPITALIZED AND HOSPITALIZABLE

In previous sections we have looked at national practices in the hospitalization of people with mental disorders. In summary we have found that the total number of people hospitalized currently in the United States consists of approximately 3 million episodes; that the episodic rate of mental hospitalization has been increasing quite rapidly over the last 15 years; that the length of stay for most hospital sites has been relatively stable over the last decade; that the readmission rate probably has not changed recently; and that the percentage of total hospital days in the United States that are for mental disorders is about 25%.

Mental hospitalization is a substantial and economically important feature of health and mental health care. In the next two chapters, we attempt to assess studies of the effectiveness of mental hospitalization. In this section, we separate research on mental hospitalization into two basic questions: that focusing on mental health treatment *instead of* mental hospitalization (nonhospitalization or the prevention of hospitalization); and hospital treatment that decreases the length of stay or lowers the recidivism rate once released. Chapter 9 focuses on experimental studies of nonhospitalization and compares it to the effect of hospitalization. Chapter 10 focuses on deinstitutionalization research, comparing various forms of hospital treatment, and particularly community treatment following (or integrated with) hospital treatment.

Chapter 9 compares the effectiveness of inpatient treatment of mental disorders with alternative care outside a hospital. There are a variety of reasons, discussed below, for separating care instead of hospitalization from studies comparing forms of hospitalization. Our definition of include overnight stays. However, studies that include, say, more than a day or two are reviewed in Chapter 10 (e.g., the study of Endicott, Herz, & Gibbon, 1978, which starts patients out with approximately a week of hospitalization).

We break down the research in this way for a variety of reasons. One, it is a finer grained analysis. If there were really little or no difference between the types of studies as we group them separately in Chapters 9 and 10, we could regroup them later. In the interim, we may at least determine whether such differences exist.

There is also a long tradition in the mental health movement of separating institutionalization from other forms of treatment. In part, this tradition is based on values rather than research; values that prefer freedom to confinement, personal choice to close supervision; and independence to dependence (see Estroff, 1981). Such spokesmen as Thomas Szasz (1963) are morally opposed to any form of involuntary commitment.

In addition, there is a good deal of research and theory that suggests the effects of mental hospitalization can be negative and antitherapeutic. Erving Goffman (1961) sees mental hospitals as one type of total institution, which shares certain characteristics with other total institutions, such as prisons, the military, and monasteries. He defines (p. xiii) a total institution as "a place of residence and work where a large number of like-situated individuals, cut off from the line of society for an appreciable period of time, together lead an enclosed, formally administered round of life." Goffman's original work on mental hospitals as a form of total institution was based on a year's field work in St. Elizabeth's, a federal mental hospital in Washington, DC.

Since Goffman's original work, a rather sizable literature has developed in sociology on the effects of total institutions. Recently McEwen (1980) has reviewed the literature on the potentially debilitating effects of total institutions in general, and Goldstein (1979) has reviewed the literature on mental institutions as a subcategory of total institutions. The effects of total institutions are often seen as fostering institutional dependence in various ways. Such dependence progressively leads to loss of social and vocational competencies, thereby undercutting one's ability to manage one's life and deal independently with the world outside the institution. The confinement also involves loss of meaningful contact with others who could provide social and other forms of support.

Various studies have found that the amount of active treatment in a mental hospital can be quite minimal. Rosenhan (1973) employed eight people to pose as patients in various mental hospitals. By training these participant observers to fake certain symptoms, each was admitted as a regular inpatient in a mental hospital. Rosenhan describes that the volunteers emphasized in their participant reports they felt very powerless and depersonalized. He asserts that among the factors contributing to the feeling of depersonalization was the lack of interaction between patient and staff. Indeed the staff seemed to be going out of their way to avoid interacting with the patients. In a number of instances the patient observers were instructed to keep daily records of actual contact with psychiatrists, psychologists, nurses, residents, and physicians, regardless of any context. He found that contacts averaged 7 minutes per day per patient. Aside from the potential effect of depersonalization, the lack of interaction with therapeutic professionals may have an independent but additional negative effect.

Further, in many mental hospitals—and particularly state hospitals—the quality of care is suspect. It is well known that over 50% of the psychiatrists who work in state and county mental hospitals did not receive their medical training in the United States. Many of these foreign-trained psychiatrists are not sufficiently proficient in English and lack a deep understanding of the American culture. If one of the primary aspects of treating mental disorders is the treatment of deviant behavior, then some deep understanding is necessary of the culture from which the behavior is presumed to deviate.

In addition to low quality and quantity of care, and the potential debilitating effects of a mental hospital as a total institution, theorists point to other reasons why care alternative to a mental hospital might be more effective. Theorists such as Bandura (1978) and Stein and Test (1980) emphasize that a patient who is perceived by a professional to need hospitalization has essentially lost the ability to deal with his or her environment. Consequently, they say the most effective treatment must include some significant relearning, and that relearning is better conducted in the very environment in which the patient will ultimately have to cope. Although such relearning could on theoretical grounds occur after hospitalization rather than instead of hospitalization it is an empirical question about which is most effective. To other more sociological theories (e.g., Schur, 1971), the effects of stigma and self-labeling lead to potentially negative effects of mental hospitalization. In this view, the self-label such as ''crazy'' interferes with subsequent rehabilitation. Further, these theories say, such self-labeling is more likely to take place if one is hospitalized for treatment than if one is treated outside a mental hospital.

These considerations all argue that preliminary evaluation of research dealing with the effectiveness of mental health treatment should distinguish hospital treatment (and subsequent treatment) from treatment that is alternative to a hospital. Further, the deinstitutionalization movement in the United States, which involves treatment after hospitalization, is highly controversial. It is commonly accepted that the general approach and treatment of the deinstitutionalized mentally ill has been badly organized, without effective treatment programs or other resources available to the patient following hospital treatment (General Accounting Office, 1977). We should not routinely compare the deinstitutionalized with the nonhospitalized.

Much of the public debate regarding mental hospitals and their positive or negative effects on patients is philosophical in nature and neither scientific nor empirical. On the one side are those who accept the "hospital syllogism": people who are seriously ill should be treated in hospitals; mental illness is a serious illness; ergo, people with mental illness should be treated in hospitals. To the extent the syllogism is accepted unthinkingly without an openminded acceptance of new data and questions, that view is unscientific—indeed, antiscientific. In its extreme form, it becomes a matter of belief, rather than science.

At the opposite end of the belief continuum are the Marxists, who insist that mental hospitals are inherently repressive. "In their eyes, mental illness was not an objective description of a disease within the conventional meaning of the term; it was rather an abstraction designed to rationalize the confinement of individuals who manifested disruptive and aberrant behavior" (Grob, 1983; p. ix). Such scholars discussed in Chapter 2 as Foucault, Rothman, and Scull have a rather hostile view of psychiatry in general and mental hospitals in particular. In their view mental hospitals have not only failed, but that failure is, was, and will be inevitable.

Readers who accept either of these extreme positions will probably not like what is to follow. We will take a critical and thorough look at the best available scientific data, comparing treatment in a mental hospital with treatment outside a hospital. We urge the reader to keep a priori beliefs in abeyance in order to take a dispassionate look at the data. The data are necessarily complicated, but reasonably consistent and quite interesting.

Given the controversy surrounding mental hospitalization and the accepted premise that deinstitutionalization has been badly managed with inadequate programs, it seems wise to separate the studies of the deinstitutionalized from the noninstitutionalized. If mental hospitalization has the negative effects that many claim, then one should separate the effects of treatment following hospitalization from treatment instead of hospitalization. However, this premise holds even if mental hospitalization has no negative effects. Treatment following mental hospitalization can be seen as "a follow-up" to primary treatment. But alternative care is a form of primary treatment. It does not necessarily follow that effective alternative care and follow-up care should have the same variables determining their effectiveness.

We now move to Chapter 9 where we discuss experimental studies of treatments alternative to hospitalization, and then to Chapter 10 where we discuss the research related to variations in hospital treatment or treatments following hospitalization. Chapter 10 also includes some discussion of the homeless and chronic patient.

CHAPTER 9

ALTERNATIVE TREATMENT: NONINSTITUTIONALIZATION

In this chapter, we present research involving random assignment to treatment condition and comparing the effectiveness of mental hospitalization to that of some alternative treatment. The array of alternative treatments considered are not all the theoretically possible ones. They are the set of particular alternative treatments, the effectiveness of which has been tested against mental hospitalization. In reviewing this literature, the reader should be careful not to assume that some treatment process not reviewed here is thereby ineffective. We are reviewing the best literature that compares mental hospitalization with some alternative treatment. There easily could be wonderful alternative treatments (or forms of mental hospitalization) which have not been tested using the rigorous criteria that we use in this chapter.

Good research in this area is difficult to accomplish, and drawing conclusions can be a chancy business indeed. Let us first look at some of the requirements for a reasonable research design and some of the difficulties one has in making such comparisons. We will then look more closely at the principle of random assignment, and why we have adopted this as the essential design requirement.

Research Design Requirements

Most of the research that we have discussed in this book is not directly relevant to the question of whether mental hospitalization or some alternative form of care is the most efficacious form of treatment for the seriously mentally disturbed. For example, Lorei and Gurel (1973) followed up a large cohort of 957 schizophrenic patients discharged from 12 VA hospitals, trying to discover the demographic, psychological, and medical factors that precipitated readmission to the hospital. They included a large number of potentially important factors in their study, but found that the best predictor of readmission was not any treatment, personal, or environmental factors, but rather simply the number of times that the patient had been hospitalized before.

Should we conclude from such a study that the effects of hospitalization are negative? The answer is clearly NO. The design of such a study does not allow such a conclusion and should not be considered a test of hospitalization per se. There are other easily available alternative explanations for the effect obtained. Most obviously we would expect that the most seriously ill patients would be in the hospital at any given instant, or if out of the hospital would be the most likely candidates for readmission. If so, the number of readmissions (as a predictor of subsequent hospitalization) could easily be a measure of the seriousness of the case rather than any effects of hospitalization per se.

Further, research showing that hospitalization can have negative effects is not necessarily germane to a discussion of other forms of care. That is, a given patient could experience negative effects from a hospital treatment (and even feel thoroughly depersonalized), but still have that experience be more positive than any other treatment modality (including not being hospitalized at all). That is, even if the patient deteriorates within the hospital environment, it does not preclude the possibility that he or she would have deteriorated even more outside that environment.

We review here experimental studies of the effects of mental hospitalization compared to some fairly well specified alternative method of care outside a hospital. Again, we emphasize that we are not including research specific to the issue of alternative care *following* hospitalization. As we have discussed in the introduction to this section, that research may or may not be germane to the issue of alternative modes of care *instead* of hospitalization.

Let us discuss for a moment the scientific requirements of a study comparing mental hospitalization with some alternative form of care. First, the patient should be sufficiently mentally disturbed so that mental hospitalization would be the usual form of care. Second, given that level of disturbance, we argue that the next research requirement would be random assignment to condition. Thus, a good study involves a pool of patients, who would ordinarily be treated in a mental hospital, being randomly assigned to be treated either in the hospital or with some alternative form of care outside the hospital. We discuss this critical condition somewhat more completely below. Third, we prefer some fairly detailed specification of the patient population, including symptomatology, age, race, sex, and other demographic variables, recent psychiatric history, family characteristics, and the like. Fourth, we would like to see the details of each treatment, including level and amount of drugs prescribed and taken, degree and content of interaction with mental health professionals, and the like. Fifth, we need details on outcomes of such treatment, including psychological testing, psychiatric symptomatology, behavioral patterns and deviations, perceptions of the family and significant others of the patient, employment, and variables related to emotional independence (such as establishing relationships with other people and the ability to live independently). Last, we would like to see whether the treatment effects endure over time, including fairly detailed follow-ups over a good length of time following the treatment. As one potential outcome of such treatment, we would want to ascertain whether the patient was readmitted to the hospital (for the hospitalized group) or ever admitted to the hospital (for the alternative care group).

Random Assignment

We would argue that a necessary (but obviously not sufficient) condition for a minimally adequate study in this area is random assignment to treatment condition. There are a number of reasons for this. To begin with, if one wants to test the effects of mental hospitalization as a treatment modality, one has to have something to compare it with. To study mental hospitalization or some alternative form of care without another condition for comparison tells us very little. That sort of study should be regarded mainly as a demonstration, in which the feasibility and *potential* usefulness of the approach are the only conclusions to be drawn. Similarly, random assignment to condition or some form of precise matching is necessary to ensure comparability of the populations being studied. Without comparability of the samples, one cannot conclude that any posttreatment differences between them were due to the treatment or to the potential noncomparability of the samples.

In an area as undeveloped as outcome research for psychiatric intervention, we argue that there is no real alternative to random assignment to treatment condition. In research generally, other forms of control of potential pretreatment differences are possible, such as covariance techniques or matching. Both are decidedly riskier than random assignment in an undeveloped research area. Take covariance for example. Covariance is a statistical technique designed to lessen the impact on the outcome measure of some important pretreatment difference between conditions. The effects of the covariance and the need for it depend both upon the difference between the conditions on the variable prior to treatment and on the correlation of the variable with the dependent measure. However, if the difference between conditions is reasonably large prior to treatment, then covariance as a technique will undercorrect the effect of this variable on the dependent measure (Campbell & Erlebacher, 1970). That is, one would conclude that the treatment had a greater effect on the outcome variable than in fact was the case. This under-correction can lead to thinking a treatment was effective, when it was not.

In addition, the correlation between the pretreatment variable and the dependent variable is affected and limited by the reliability of the measurements. In psychiatric outcome studies, we would argue that we have insufficient information to say on a priori grounds what the dif-ferences in pretreatment variables might be. Further, the reliability of the measures often taken in psychiatric outcome studies is not terribly high.

Consequently, in using covariance technique for psychiatric outcome studies we might be deceived in two ways. Because of substantially large differences prior to treatment, the covariance technique may be underestimating the effect of the prior variable on the dependent measure. Second, the reliability of the measuring instruments may be such that we are underestimating the true correlation among variables. If either of these premises hold, the covariance technique is an unreliable method of assessment in psychiatric research. To get around these two obstacles, we would have to have independent and objectively reasonable evidence that the differences on related variables are not large and that we are not underestimating correlations of covaried vari-ables and dependent measures due to unreliability.

The principle of matching is also often a good technique in experi-mental research. However, to use matched pairs implies that we have some knowledge of the relevant variables on which to match. Since such diverse variables as genetic background, age, sex, race, social class, and even geographical residence seem to have somewhat independent effects on psychiatric outcome (and incidence), it would be impossible to state on a priori grounds that one has matched on all the proper variables. Until we know more about mental illness and health, random assignment to condition is a necessary prerequisite to good outcome research, and much preferred over either covariance techniques or matched pairs as forms of pretreatment control.

Of course, random assignment to condition is not a magical solution, and does not guarantee that the two samples thus obtained are com-parable. Comparability of the samples depends partly on their size, partly on the standard error of measurement on whatever is being measured, and partly on the true variance of the population at large. We will return to some of these issues and problems later in the chapter after presentation of the data that we were able to find.

True Experiments Involving Random Assignment
to Either Mental Hospitalization or Alternative Care

Kiesler (1982a) reviewed research studies that compared mental hospitalization with some alternative form of care, and in which there was true random assignment to treatment condition. He was able to find 10 such studies, each having a hospital condition (H condition) and a comparison condition involving some alternative method of care (AC condition).[1] The number of subjects in each treatment condition across the 10 studies ranged from 10 to 189, and the total for each condition across all experiments was about 650. The various studies are outlined in Table 9.1 and are consecutively numbered from 1 to 10.

Several other reviews of comparable literature were appearing at the same time although not specifically oriented toward experimental studies. Braun, Kochansky, Shapiro, Greenberg, Gudeman, Johnson, and Shore (1981) reviewed the literature on what they categorized as alternatives to hospital admission, modifications of conventional hospitalization, and alternatives to continued long-term hospitalization. Obviously, their first category overlapped with that of Kiesler, although they did not limit their review to studies involving random assignment. Their category of "alternatives to continued long-term hospitalization" includes studies that we discuss in the next chapter. Their category of "modifications of traditional hospitalization" includes some studies that are discussed in the next chapter and some that were reviewed by Kiesler. Several studies that they review under modifications of traditional hospitalization included studies of day hospital treatment, with random assignment, and some involved no hospitalization. These studies were also reviewed by Kiesler and are included in Table 9.1.

Greene and De La Cruz (1981) published a general review of comparative studies of day treatment as a modality alternative to traditional full-time hospitalization. They also did not limit themselves to random assignment but the studies they review with random assignment are included in Table 9.1. Straw (1982) in his Ph.D. dissertation did a meta-analysis of studies of "deinstitutionalization," one category of which was alternatives to traditional hospitalization. Braun et al. and Greene & De La Cruz present detailed study-by-study analyses of the literature. Straw presents some rather detailed meta-analyses, but does not break his review down into a case-by-case basis, and does not break out a sub-analysis of that group of studies with random assignment. In addition, Test (1981) provides a general critique of issues in this area, while also not limiting herself to studies involving random assignment.

As we have discussed, it is important to present an analysis of individual studies involving random assignment comparing traditional hospitalization with alternative care. Our approach in this chapter is to build on the review published by Kiesler. We carefully inspected each of the other reviews, looking for additional studies of alternative care involving random assignment. In doing so we were able to find four more studies, and they are labeled numbers 11 through 14 in the material to follow. We have organized this material in the following way. To assure comparability with materials of the earlier Kiesler article, we have reproduced his descriptions of the 10 studies he was able to find. The first 10 studies listed in Table 9.1 are reproduced from that article. Additional material gained since that publication is clearly marked (e.g., 1a, 4a). The presentation of the four additional studies (no. 11–no. 14) is presented descriptively in the text in a manner similar to that originally used by Kiesler, and the summary statistics have been added to Table 9.1 (nos. 11–14, accordingly). In this manner, it is easy for the reader of the original article to see what material has now been added as a result of a close inspection of other reviews of this literature.

As the reader will be able to see, the intent of each study was originally to test some pet alternative care project. Although several of the studies are well known, they are individually known for the specific method of alternative care rather than the fact that random assignment to condition allowed a true experimental test of the effects of hospitalization. One piece of evidence that these investigators were primarily interested in a specific alternative treatment is that they almost uniformly refer to the hospitalized patients as "the control group." Across the 14 studies, the total for each condition of care was about 880 patients.

THE EXPERIMENTAL STUDIES

(1) The program investigated by Stein, Test, and Marx (1975) was designed to help patients acquire the coping skills and autonomy necessary for reasonable community adjustment. Patients were assigned either to a "community-living model" or to regular inpatient care at Mendota Mental Health Institute; patients were between the ages of 18 and 62 with any diagnosis other than severe organic brain syndrome or primary alcoholism, and they had previously served an average of 14 months in other institutions. The inpatient care involved "progressive treatment aimed at the preparation for return to community" and entailed a median length of hospital stay of 17 days. In the community-living approach, which lasted 14 months, the therapeutic staff assisted the patients in their homes and neighborhoods and trained them in such

TABLE 9.1

Summary of Experimental Studies of Hospital Versus Alternative Treatment for Mental Disorders

Study	N	Patients	Excluded	Type of AC Treatment	Type of H Treatment
1. Stein et al. (1975)	60 each	18 to 62 years	Alcoholism OBS	Coping skills/ independence training	Inpatient mental health institute
1a. Test & Stein (1978)	Same as 1; One-year follow-up				
2. Mosher & Menn (1978)	AC = 33 H = 30	Young, first admission, Schizophrenia	All other	"Soteria"	"Good inpatient unit"
3. Brook (1973)	49 each	All	None	"Hostel"	Inpatient unit, mental health clinic
4. Flomenhaft et al. (1969)	150 each	All	None	Family crisis therapy	Psychiatric hospital
4a. Langsley et al. (1971)	Same as 4; One-year/18-month follow-ups				
5. Herz et al. (1971)	45 each	Not "too healthy" Not "too ill"	78%	Day care	Regular inpatient
6. Pasamanick et al. (1967)	57 drug 41 placebo 54 H	18 to 62-year old schizophrenics; no homicidal or suicidal tendencies; cooperative families	All others	(a)Drug/public health visits (b)placebo	Regular inpatient
7. Levenson et al. (1977)	10 each	Acute schizophrenics	All others	Drugs/daily therapy	Regular inpatient
8. Washburn et al. (1976)	H = 30 AC = 29	Female, not suicidal, not homicidal; capable of treatment	58%[a]	Day care	Regular inpatient
9. Wilder et al. (1966)	189 each	All	34%[b]	Day care	Regular inpatient
10. Krowinski & Fitt (1978)	H = 50 AC = 51	Not too healthy/ill, suicidal, violent, disorganized, drug dependent	38%[c]	Day care	Regular inpatient
11. Polak & Kirby (1976)	AC = 37 H = 38	All	10 excluded	Total community care	Regular inpatient
12. Rittenhouse (1970)	AC = 35 H = 37	U	No family	Family unit therapy	Therapeutic community
13. Goodacre et al. (1975)	AC = 87 H(1) = 38 H(2) = 48	All	Age <16,>69 No alcohol, drugs	Home treatment	H(1)=hospital & home[d] H(2)=regular inpatient
14. Fenton et al. (1979)	AC = 76 H = 79	>18, willing family, No OBS, alcohol, drug, suicidal, violent	45%	Home, community care	"Short-term" with follow-up

NOTE: H = hospital setting; AC = alternative method of care; OBS = organic brain syndrome; U = unknown.

[a] In addition, 27% refused to participate.

[b] 34% of AC patients were transferred immediately to inpatient status.

[c] 12% suicidal; 19% "too well"; 7% refused assignment.

Initial H Stay (days)	% or ratio AC Ultimately Hospitalized	% or Ratio H Readmitted	Costs	Outcome/Comments
22.9	6/60	14/60	Less for AC	No difference in symptoms; greater employment in AC and more time spent in independent settings.
		34/60	Less for AC	Average total days in hospital, H = 46, AC = 7.7; AC greater sheltered employment, greater income, more contact with friends and social groups, more satisfaction, less symptomatology
28	53%	67%	$4,400 each	2 years later: AC group had higher occupational level, more living independence; 1-year differences: AC group was more likely to be working, in school, have a long-term friend, less psychopathology
U	1/49	6/49	$410/month	Less remission of symptoms in AC after 6 mos., more medication given; no differences on 11 other outcome measures
26.1	19/150	39/150	Less for AC	H group stayed twice as long when readmitted as the AC group stayed when admitted
	17/126 15/126	22/121 17/99	U	Two figures are 6-12 months and 12-18 months; groups similar on social adjustment; AC better re: family problems, crisis management; Total inpatient days H = 5,121 AC = 1,859
138.8	30%	50%	U	Substantial difference after 4 weeks, favoring AC group; less after 2 years
83	13/57 drug 27/41 placebo	25/54	U	Drug/public health group better after 2.5 years; erosion of differences after 5 years; savings of 4800 inpatient days by AC over H within 2.5 years
U	U	U	$3,330 (H) $565 (AC)	Remission (not manifestly psychotic): 90%—AC (M = 12.5 days); 70%—H (M = 19.5 days)
U	U	U	$21,916 (H) $13,824 (AC)	Differences on subjective distress, community functioning, family burden, cost, days of attachment to program, with AC better
20	40%	45%	U	Patients excluded from AC still included in evaluation sample and data; few differences between groups
16	20%	38%	Less for AC	Greater improvement of AC on psychiatric scores; somewhat more AC considered to have improved
U	U	U	Less for AC	Follow-up after 4 months: AC clients more satisfied, had greater goal attainment and self-disclosure
U	1/35	16/37	U	Readmission at 3 months are major data; few other differences
Med=42	67%	H(1) = 13% H(2) = 17% AC = 12%	No difference*	Severely ill patients: 43% AC patients admitted immediately, or within week; only outcome difference is 33% of AC patients never hospitalized
28.3	29/76 f	19/79		Outcome measures at 1, 3, 6, 12 months. No difference between H & AC on clinical symptoms, role functioning, or family burden; both groups significantly improved; during second six months H group received 3 times as much outpatient care.

d A second hospital plus home treatment condition was run but without random assignment.

e Note that the AC condition was not fully implemented.

f 30% spent an average of 1.8 days and 8% averaged 177 days; see text.

daily living activities as doing laundry, shopping, cooking, grooming, budgeting, and the use of public transportation. Dependent measures included a demographic data form, a short clinical rating scale, a community adjustment form, the family burden scale, and the like. All interviews were conducted by an independent research team.

The study tracked the patients for four months after their initial interviews. In general, the psychiatric dependent measures were similar for both sets of patients. Ultimately, 6 of the 60 AC patients were hospitalized. During the four-month period, 14 of the 60 H patients had already been readmitted after being discharged once; that is, more hospitalized patients were rehospitalized than those undergoing alternative care were ever hospitalized. There was a highly significant difference between the two groups in the amount of time they spent in independent settings during the four-month observation period (greater time by the AC group). Further, the AC group had a smaller percentage unemployed at the end of four months than did the H group, although the difference was mainly in sheltered nonfull-time employment. The 6 AC patients who ultimately were admitted to the hospital spent a mean of 13.8 days there, whereas the original H group spent a mean of 22.9 days in the hospitals during their first admission. No data were given for the length of stay for the 14 H patients who were subsequently readmitted to the hospital. The authors do not describe costs, but an economic cost-benefit analysis (Weisbrod, Test, & Stein, 1980) involving a number of assumptions and approximations suggests increased initial costs for the AC group, but a longer term savings of $400 per patient per year (compared to the H group).

(1a) Stein et al. (1975) concentrated on the first four months of treatment in their study. Test and Stein (1978) report a one-year evaluation, when treatment was still continuing for both groups. By that time the readmission rate of the H group was 57% (34/60). They do not give the admission rate of the AC group at this point, but the readmission rate was 6%. Over the course of the year H patients spent an average of 46 days in hospitals; the AC group 7.7. The AC patients spent significantly less time in unemployment, more in sheltered employment, and earned more income. AC patients had more "contact with trusted friends" and more contact with social groups. At 12 months AC patients were more satisfied with their life situations (but also had higher self-esteem at base line). AC patients showed less symptomatology on 7 of 13 scales. Although a similar number of people were taking medication in the two groups, the AC group showed greater compliance.

The TCL treatment lasted 12 months. After that period TCL patients had to rely on traditional community programming. Stein and Test

(1980) report a follow up 16 months after the cessation of treatment (28 months after the initiation of treatment). They found a steady increase in the use of hospitals following cessation of AC treatment. Over the course of the 16-month posttreatment phase, AC patients averaged 26.5 days in hospitals, H patients 54.1 (although during the last 4 months, the figures were 9.56 and 11.32, respectively); the differences for sheltered employment and unemployment decreased, but not money earned. The higher involvement in social groups was maintained but the difference in contact with close friends disappeared. The differences in life satisfaction, symptomatology, and medical compliance also all disappeared by the end of the 16-month posttreatment period.

We will discuss economic issues in Chapter 11, but this experiment has received rather extensive cost-benefit analysis by Weisbrod et al. (1980) and Weisbrod (1983), and some of their effort should be reported here. They find that in terms of costs, the AC group was more expensive than the H group over a one-year period. They include under costs not only direct treatment but the use of other services (e.g., sheltered workshop, other hospitals) and maintenance costs. For reasons related to ease of quantification, they do not include such things as families reporting physical illness or emotional strain due to the patient, both of which favor the AC group (25% versus 14%; and 48% versus 25%, respectively). Under benefits they include only earnings. The enhanced earnings of the AC group produce a net cost-benefit difference of $400, favoring the AC group. That is, the AC treatment cost (in total) $800 more per patient, but led to a benefit of $1200 more per patient; a net of $400 in a cost-benefit analysis. We note that the generally more positive outcomes for the AC condition (symptomatology, social relationships, and patient satisfaction with life) are left out of the benefit calculation, because of difficulty in quantifying a dollar equivalent for benefit.

Weisbrod (1983) also finds a startling result by extending his cost-benefit analysis to diagnostic groups. He sorts the patients into three groups: schizophrenics, nonschizophrenic psychotics, and personality disorders. The cost-benefits differences for AC and H patients are quite different for these three categories. For schizophrenics and other psychotics, there is a clear cost-benefit net favoring AC: $1046 and $2281, respectively. For personality disorders there is a substantial difference favoring the H group: $2649. The difference between the two sets of outcomes is disproportionately due to decreased inpatient treatment costs for the H group. Apparently the hospital was unwilling to keep the patients with a personality disorder in treatment very long. They were discharged rather quickly (and are often seen as untreatable), although they continued in AC treatment. Weisbrod does not discuss the comparative effectiveness of treatment by diagnostic category.

(2) Mosher, Menn, and Matthews (1975) compared outcomes in two groups of young first-admission schizophrenics: one receiving usual treatment, including drugs in the wards of a good community mental health center; the other being treated by a nonprofessional staff, usually without drugs in a small homelike facility called Soteria. Staff and residents shared responsibility for the maintenance of the house, preparation of the meals and cleanup, and at least two staff members were on the premises at all times. Residents were discharged when the total group informally reached a consensus that they were ready to be discharged. The hospital group received a half-hour of psychotherapy daily, 1½ hours of occupational therapy daily, plus a daily living community meeting led by a member of the treatment team. In addition, within the H condition a crisis group met for 1½ hours five times per week; a couples group for 2 hours a week; and a women's group, 2 hours a week. Thus the hospital group was clearly an unusual and highly intensive method of inpatient treatment.

Mosher et al. report various outcome measures at discharge, six months after discharge, and one year from admission. Soteria residents had significantly lower psychopathology scores than the hospitalized patients at all measurement intervals. Substantially more of the Soteria patients were working in full-time or near full-time employment both six months after discharge and one year after admission. Significantly more Soteria patients were able ultimately to live alone or with peers, whereas hospital patients tended to reside ultimately with their parents or relatives.

Mosher and Menn (1978) report a two-year follow-up. Generally the difference between conditions reported at one year continue, but are smaller. Matthews, Roper, Mosher, and Menn (1979), in a more detailed study of relapse, found that AC patients had about a 20% better chance of not ever being hospitalized at any point in time over two years following completion of the program.

(3) Brook (1973) described an opportunistic study that, although not a true random design, is so close as to warrant inclusion in this review. For several months the inpatient unit at Fort Logan Mental Health Center was closed. All patients who ordinarily would have been hospitalized in this unit were instead put in a "hostel." Forty-nine residents who underwent this hostel systems intervention treatment were compared with the last 49 patients admitted to the inpatient unit when it was still open. Since all patients presenting themselves for treatment were included, this comes very close to a true randomized design. Most of the

patients were acutely ill; almost half were diagnosed as at moderate to high suicide risk; half were schizophrenic, and half of those, chronic; one-fourth were depressive reactive; the remaining fourth involved alcohol or drug abuse, adjustment reaction, marital maladies, or excessive compulsiveness. Of the 49 AC cases, 11 had previously been hospitalized. The hostel had no residential staffing and neighbors helped with meals and occasionally other problems. The overall approach to treatment was intervention by the crisis staff in whatever part of the resident's social system was seen as the source of the crisis, typically the family. Some sessions with patients were held at the hostel, including some with the family; other sessions were held at the patient's home. Individual therapy occasionally supplemented these social systems interventions. When not in evaluation or therapy sessions, patients continued normal activities as far as possible. The mean stay was 5.75 days. Patients were then transferred to outpatient status and scheduled for six to eight more sessions of family or individual therapy.

There were no outcome differences between the two groups on 11 difference measures, although the hostel group had less remission of symptoms. On the other hand, the hostel group also received much more medication than did the inpatient group (perhaps reflecting the staff's anxiety about the adequacy of the treatment in the hostel). Of the 49 hospitalized patients, 6 were subsequently readmitted within six months (3 of them twice), whereas only 1 of the 49 patients in the hostel was admitted to hospitalization within six months after discharge.

(4) Flomenhaft, Kaplan, and Langsley (1969) randomly assigned 150 patients to family crisis therapy and another 150 to regular inpatient care in the Colorado Psychiatric Hospital. The inpatient group stayed an average of 26 days in the hospital; the family crisis therapy group was seen by a team for 2.5 weeks. The typical AC outpatient care consisted of five office visits, one home visit, and three telephone contacts. "The team's aim is to restore the confidence of the patient and family sufficiently so that they can manage their own problems, cope more adaptively with expected future problems, and perceive less need in the future to exclude a member" (p. 41). The team worked with all members of the patient's immediate family and significant others and was available 24 hours a day. The team took the unusual step of home visits and conducted the first visit at the patient's home within four hours after the initial contact. In an analysis of half of the experimental and half of the control subjects six months after admission, the AC patients were doing as well as the H patients on "two measures of functioning, and the experimental (AC) returned to prestress functioning much more rapidly than did control (H)" (p. 43).

(4a) Langsley, Machotka, and Flomenhaft (1971) report a more complete analysis of the 6-month data, as well as a 12-month and 18-month
follow up. In the more complete 6-month analysis, they found twice as
many (39) H patients had been rehospitalized as AC patients (19) for the
first time.[2] When H patients were rehospitalized they stayed twice as
long as AC patients. Over the 18-month period, H patients spent a total
of 5121 days in hospitals, whereas the AC patients spent 1859 (with the
former being a relative underestimate, since the data for only 99 of 150
patients are reported in the third 6-month period).

Both groups at 18 months show substantial but similar improvement
on social adjustment and personal functioning. The AC condition shows
greater ability to handle family problems and crisis management.

(5) Herz et al. (1971) compared day-care treatment with regular
inpatient treatment. Their study is unique in that essentially the same
treatment occurred for all patients. "Patients in both groups were treated
by the same staff and participated together in the same activities during
the day" (p. 108). An initial evaluation and three follow-up evaluations
of psychopathology and role functioning were made at two weeks, four
weeks, and an average of almost two years. The main evaluation instruments were the Psychiatric Status Schedule and the Psychiatric Evaluation Form. Unfortunately the researchers eliminated from consideration
patients who were either "too healthy" or "too ill" to be included in
the study. Thus, 78% of the total pool of patients were eliminated from
consideration prior to the random assignment to conditions. This design
is not inadequate, but the generalizations that can be drawn from it are
more limited.

The average number of days from randomization until the patient was
discharged from inpatient or day care and lived in the community full
time for at least one week, was 48.5 days for the day patients and 138.8
for the inpatient (opposite to the usual finding). The data in Table 9.1 of
the percentages of people in the H condition readmitted to the hospital,
and those in the AC condition ultimately hospitalized, are approximate
and are estimated from a figure presented in the original article. The difference between conditions of cumulative percentages of patients discharged from initial hospitalization are consistent and sizable, with more
day patients being discharged at all points across a 7.5 month period.
Indeed, about 25% of the inpatients had never been released after
7.5 months.

At all the outcome points measured in the study, the day patients
showed better results on both evaluation forms, although differences
between the two groups on these forms persisted only on two subscales
at the end of the two-year measurement period. Although costs were not

described, we note that the difference in length of treatment is so substantial (90 days more care for the H group) that had costs been calculated, they would have favored the AC group by a substantial amount.

The authors observed considerable apprehension and resistance among staff members concerning the wisdom of placing acutely ill patients on day care. Even as the study progressed and clear differences were being shown in outcome in favor of day care, "the antagonism and apprehension lessened but the staff continued to prefer inpatient care" (p. 116).

(6) Pasamanick, Scarpitti, and Dinitz (1967) had three treatment groups in their study: a regular inpatient group in a state hospital and the psychiatric unit of a general hospital, a group that received only placebos and visits from public health nurses, and a group that combined the public health care with regular medication (AC). Although a psychologist, a psychiatrist, and a social worker were involved in the study, public health nurses were the principal treatment agents, and they regularly visited the patients' homes. There were four requirements for a patient to be included in the study: diagnosis of schizophrenia, age between 18 and 62, no evidence of homicidal or suicidal tendencies, and a family willing to provide supervision and information on patients and family at home. Thirty months later, all three groups had improved, with very small differences among conditions on psychiatric evaluations. Comparisons between conditions are reported infrequently, but the authors say that "in all of the many specific measures, home care (AC) patients were functioning as well or better than the hospital control (H) cases" (p. 251). H patients, however, were much more likely to be rehospitalized than AC patients ever were. Pasamanick et al. report a cumulative savings of 4,818 hospital days by the AC group over that experienced by the H group (over 2½ years). Davis, Dinitz, and Pasamanick (1972) report that after a five-year period, there were small differences among the three conditions on problem behaviors, vocational performance, domestic performance, or psychiatric status. If anything, the placebo group tended to be worst on outcome measures, with the drug-public health condition the best, and the hospital condition intermediate.

(7) Levenson et al. (1977) compared regular inpatient treatment of acute schizophrenics with a specially designed, city-county hospital outpatient clinic. The outpatient group was given a regimen of pharmacotherapy, supportive individual psychotherapy, and family counseling within the context of daily appointments lasting approximately 20 minutes. This intensive treatment continued until the patient entered remission (i.e., was given a global rating of not manifestly psychotic) or

was transferred to another less intensive treatment setting. Nine of the 10 clinical patients and 7 of the 10 ward patients successfully attained remission (not a statistically significant difference). As indicated in Table 9.1, the average time to remission was 12.5 days in the ward group (again, not statistically significant). The authors give no indication of what happened to the patients who did not attain remission. On an expanded brief psychiatric rating scale, both groups improved significantly, but without any significant differences between them. The average cost per remission was $3,300 for the ward and $565 for the special clinic. Although it is clear in this study that the special clinic patients did not do worse than the inpatient group, the Ns in each condition are so small as to prohibit adequate statistical analysis.

(8) Washburn, Vannicelli, Longabaugh, and Scheff (1976) randomly assigned patients to either an inpatient unit or a day-care unit following 2 to 6 weeks of inpatient evaluation (a conservative comparison given that all patients were hospitalized for some period of time prior to randomization). Both groups were treated at McLean Hospital in Massachusetts, a private nonprofit teaching hospital noted for exceptional service. However, if patients were homicidal, suicidal, or judged by their therapists as absolutely requiring hospitalization, they were not considered candidates for randomized assignment (58% of the total sample). In addition, 27% of the total sample refused or were unable to participate. This left 15% of the total sample, or 59 patients who were randomly assigned to either an inpatient unit (N = 30) or a day-care unit (N = 29). The data are very clear and indicate that "for the range of patients studied, day treatment is, on the whole, superior to inpatient treatment in five distinct areas: subjective distress; community functioning; family burden; total hospital costs; and days of attachment to the hospital program" (p. 665). The differences between conditions, however, lessened over an 18-month to 2-year period of time. The treatment costs for the two groups were quite different. The authors computed totals for 6-month periods across 18 months. Summing these figures, it appears that the average cost of inpatient care for each of the 30 H patients was about $22,000, or a total of over $650,000. The average cost for the day-care patient was less than $14,000, bringing the total for the 29 patients to about $400,000. The difference in cost of treatment between the two groups for the first 18 months of the study was, therefore, more than $250,000. The authors say that the AC group spent significantly fewer hospital days during the second 6 months of the study (and were otherwise similar).

(9) Zwerling and Wilder (1964), in an older but well-known study, attempted to ascertain whether psychiatric patients could be assigned in

an entirely random fashion from the admitting room of a general hospital to a day hospital. During a 4.5-month period, all patients admitted to the psychiatric service of the Bronx Municipal Hospital Center were randomly assigned either to inpatient treatment or to day care. A total of 189 patients were assigned to each treatment, but staff were allowed to treat the patients however they felt appropriate and the investigators made no attempt to keep the patients in the day hospital.

The principal problem with the study is that it is more an assessment of the attitudes of the staff in that particular hospital than it is a test of whether or not one can in fact treat all patients with day care. The staff were allowed to reject whomever they wished, and as noted, many staff are substantially opposed to treating a majority of the cases in day care.

Wilder, Levin, and Zwerling (1966) followed up on these patients and attempted to assess their status 24 months after their initial admission. One of the difficulties in assessing this follow-up is that the original day-care patients were considered as a statistical group, even though only 39% were treated solely in the day-care setting and another 34% of the "day-care" group were treated completely within the inpatient setting. No distinction was made between these subgroups. Most of the data came from an interview with the patient and a member of the patient's family in the home, part of which was conducted with the patient and the family member together.

The day group spent eight (five-day) weeks in the initial treatment, whereas the inpatient group had a median stay of about three (seven-day) weeks (the finding reported earlier as typical). However, the day-care group spent a somewhat smaller number of total days in the hospital over the two-year period than did the inpatient group. The proportion of AC patients hospitalized was slightly smaller (40%) than inpatients being readmitted (45%). The interview data revealed no significant differences between conditions in psychiatric stress. The authors conclude that "the day hospital was . . . generally as effective as the inpatient service in the treatment of acutely disturbed patients for most or all phases of their hospitalization" (p. 1101).

(10) In an unpublished study sponsored by Capital Blue Cross, Krowinski and Fitt (1978) compared a day-treatment center with inpatient care. Inpatient care included daily visits by a private psychiatrist for therapy and medication. The general inpatient approach was a mixture of medical and milieu models; staff included an occupational therapist, a clinical social worker, and a chief psychiatrist. The day-care center included several modular programs that emphasized helping the individual to function in the community. Staff consisted of three

MA-level psychologists, two clinical social workers, an occupational therapist, a registered nurse, and a part-time psychiatrist.

Patients were eligible if they demonstrated sufficient dysfunction to require inpatient care, but they were excluded prior to randomization if they were suicidal, violent, extremely agitated, disorganized, or drug or alcohol dependent (12%); not considered to require hospitalization (19%); or refused assignment to the unit (7%). Thus 38% of the total patient population considered initially were excluded prior to randomization, leaving a net sample of 101 patients.

The day-care patients improved more than the inpatient group on such scales of the psychiatric status schedule as subjective distress, lack of emotion, depressive anxiety, memory disorientation, and parent role (in all, 8 of 28 scales). The inpatient group improved more on one scale, agitation-excitement. Each sample improved on almost all of the 28 measures. On a "functional baseline system" with categories of impairment, 67% of the day-care group were considered to have improved, and 52% of the inpatient group also improved.

In a six-month follow up, differences between conditions had lessened somewhat. During the six-month period, 38% of the inpatient group had been readmitted to the hospital (for an average of 35 days), while 20% of the day-care group had been admitted (for an average of 26.5 days). The Krowinski and Fitt study is unique in its detailed discussion of costs. They compute actual costs of the original inpatient care to be $1,549 per patient and $1,414 for day care (including physician costs, but excluding research costs). Adding the cost of readmission, the total actual cost was $2,742 per inpatient and $1,933 per day-care patient, a difference of 38% over the six months.

(11) Polak and Kirby (1976; see also Brook, Cortes, March, & Sundberg-Stirling, 1976 for a different report of the same study) describe a study building upon the Fort Logan experience, described by Brook. The Southwest Denver Mental Health Services—a mental health center—and the Fort Logan Mental Health Center—a state hospital—have an intake process integrated into a single system. Their approach is called the Total Community Care System and has several distinguishing features: The preferred treatment site is the home; if either the family or the patient objects, then arrangements have been made with other families to accept the patient into their family home for a fee (base data of $7.50 per day for room, board, and client care); when constant observation is required (e.g., a suicidal patient), volunteers do it; home visits are carried out by staff, including four initial evaluations; a day-care teaching program for chronic patients is carried out in one of the homes; and a method of rapid tranquilization is used in acute crises. Hospitaliza-

tion is only seen as appropriate when there are significant side effects to medication; when important medical problems exist; when the patient's behavior is seen as uncontrollable; or to meet minimum legal requirements for involuntary hospitalization.

Polak and Kirby report a study, with random assignment, comparing treatment outcome in private homes with that in the mental hospital. The patients (N = 85) represented the total sample "requiring hospitalization" over an 18-month period,[3] so that no patients were excluded from the study.[4] Eighty percent of the patients had previously been inpatients.

Outcome measures included the Treatment Effectiveness Scale (TES), a goal attainment scale, a self-disclosure scale, and a community adjustment scale. Data were collected at admission, discharge and 4 months after discharge, from clients as well as from staff and family or friends.

On discharge, there were no statistical differences between groups as perceived by staff. However, clients in the AC group were more satisfied with treatment, perceived it to be more effective, and saw the staff as more concerned and competent, than did clients in the H group. In addition the families were more satisfied with treatment in the AC conditions. In addition, ignoring statistical significance, *all* mean differences favored the AC condition.

In the follow up, four months later, all scale means again favored the AC group, and client items that had been statistically significant continued to be so. In addition, greater treatment goal attainment and greater self-disclosure were found in the AC group.

(12) In a very brief report, Rittenhouse (1970) compared the effects of family unit therapy given in the home with therapeutic community treatment given in the hospital (N = 35 and 37, respectively). Patient assignment was random, but not otherwise described. There were no differences between the groups on "discharge." Rittenhouse's hypothesis was that the AC treatment would be more enduring; she took measurements at 3, 6, and 12 months. There were no differences in family pathology (some effects in favor of the H group) nor community functioning. Only a few differences were found in patient pathology (favoring the AC group). However, AC patients reported better functioning in the work area and reported seeking less psychiatric help than did H patients.

The major data reported are for readmission: In the first 3 months 1 AC patient and 16 H patients were readmitted.[5] Few admissions occurred for 6 and 12 months. The report is very brief and does not adequately describe patients, treatment, measures, exclusions, and so forth.

(13) Goodacre, Coles, MaCurdy, Coates, and Kendall (1975) carried out a flawed experiment in which patients were randomly assigned to conditions, but the treatment conditions were not implemented for the AC group. Patients were assigned to home treatment, hospital treatment, or hospital treatment followed by home treatment.[6]

Thirty-seven patients (43% of the home treatment condition) were admitted *within the first week, usually immediately after an initial assessment,* and an additional 21 patients were admitted at some time during the year, with a total of 10 readmissions. Eleven patients were admitted at least one week after the initial contact, and none of these eleven was subsequently readmitted during the study year. In these 11 admissions, the home treatment staff played an active role in planning with patients and relatives for the period of hospital stay and follow-up. By contrast, the 37 initial admissions were for the most part the result of suicidal or homicidal behavior, or such lack of support that the home treatment team were incapable of managing them out of hospital [p. 9].

This study appears to have serious flaws. In addition to a lack of implementation of the main condition, home treatment seems to have not received adequate attention and preparation (if 43% of the patients are judged incapable of receiving such treatment). Compare this study with the detailed and successful community treatment of Polak and Kirby (1976), for example.

Also, only 83% and 87% of the Hospital and Hospital plus Home patients were ever admitted. Further, ". . . on several occasions a rivalry between the hospital staff and the home treatment was observed, and patients going to home treatment for continuing care were kept in the hospital longer than similar patients being discharged to their own (and usually inadequate) resources" (p. 11). The only difference among conditions noted by the authors is that 33% of the home-treatment patients were never hospitalized during the year observed.

Considering the design and implementation flaws, very little can be concluded from this study. We include it only in the interest of thoroughness of coverage of studies with random assignment.

(14) Fenton, Tessier, and Struening (1979) compared home care with inpatient care in the psychiatric service unit at a Montreal teaching hospital. Their exclusion criteria are listed in Table 9.1: In all, these criteria would include only 55% of the total patient load there. Home care emphasized treatment within the family and use of community agencies, with psychotherapeutic intervention and drug treatment. Hospital care included short-term intensive treatment by the Department's regular

psychiatric and paramedical staff, with postdischarge follow up by a staff psychiatrist and a nurse. Outcome measures, taken at admission, and at 1, 3, 6, and 12 months, were carried out by a research team independently of either treatment group.

Both groups improved significantly during the year. No differences between groups were found for clinical symptoms, family burden, or role functioning. Some differences favoring the AC group, in role functioning and assumption of responsibility early in the study, decreased over time. Over time the two groups reversed patterns of use of outpatient care. During the first 90 days home care patients had significantly more outpatient visits than the H group (to be expected since therapy was an integrated part of their treatment). However, during the last 6 months the H group had significantly more outpatient visits than the AC group.

The use of inpatient facilities requires some detailed presentation. Fenton et al. say that 61.8% of AC patients had no inpatient care, another 30.3% had an average of 1.8 days of such care and that therefore, "hospitalization was prevented outright or minimized in 92.1% of the Home Care patients" (p. 1076). We can use these statistics to look more closely at their data. The average total number of inpatient days was reported as 14.5 for the AC group and 41.7 for the H group over the whole year. If the 30% (= 23 patients) who spent an "average of 1.8 days" are subtracted from the totals for the AC group, then we conclude that in that group were 6 patients (7.9%) who spent an average during the year of 177 days as an inpatient.

Why 30% of their AC patients were hospitalized for such a short period of time (mean of 1.8 days) is not explained. Further, how and why six AC patients spent an average of almost six months (177 days) of the study year in the hospital is similarly unexplained. Irrespective of these ambiguities, there is still a huge difference in average number of inpatient days between conditions (14.5 versus 41.7).

A Developing Consensus

We have mentioned that there have been several recent reviews of the literature comparing mental hospitalization with alternatives to hospitalization. We have concentrated here on studies with random assignment to condition, but there is significant overlap with the studies reviewed by others as well. It is instructive to look at the conclusions reached by the various authors in this area from their reviews. Kiesler (1982a) says, in no case were the outcomes of hospitalization more positive than alternative treatment. Typically alternative care was more effective regarding such outcome variables as psychiatric evaluation, probability of subsequent employment, independent living arrangement, and staying in school, as well as being decidedly less expensive. In aggregate, the studies provide clear evidence of the self-perpetuation of hospitalization of mental patients. Hospitalized patients were more likely to be readmitted to the hospital than were alternative care patients ever to be admitted [p. 349].

Greene and De La Cruz (1981) say,

a review of the comparative studies on day treatment as an alternative modality to traditional full-time hospitalization reveals impressive evidence of its superior effectiveness in facilitating the adjustment and reintegration of patients into the community. On other measures such as cost effectiveness, family stress, symptom alleviation, and relapse rate, day-treatment proves to be on a par with full-time hospitalization. [p. 191].

Braun et al. (1981) say, ". . . experimental alternatives to hospital care have led to psychiatric outcomes not different and occasionally superior to those patients in control groups. This conclusion is best supported for alternatives to admission and for modifications of conventional hospitalization" (p. 736). Mary Ann Test in her critical review of the literature (1981) says,

while we do not yet know how to cure chronic mental illness, much is known about how to improve the community tenure and quality of life of these persons. Specifically, if the full range of services outlined above is offered and if these services are delivered in the ways tested, the following results can be expected. . . . Hospitalization can be virtually eliminated for all but 15% to 25% of these individuals. Psychotic symptomatology can be dramatically reduced. Client satisfaction with life can be somewhat increased, social functioning can be maintained or restored to pre-morbid levels and in some cases improved. While many of these persons will be unable to sustain normal work and social roles, most will be able to participate in employment and social activities if on-going supportive or some semi-sheltered environments in these areas are provided [p. 82].

There is no reason for these reviewers to agree exactly, since they are not reviewing exactly the same batch of literature. On the other hand, even though the enthusiasm for potential conclusions from the literature and the degree of detailed criticisms of each study vary somewhat, there is a thread of a real consensus running through these summary comments. That is, across a wide variety of patient population and specific treatment strategies, alternative care is more effective than mental hospitalization.

All of these studies included patients who were seriously ill, certainly ill enough to have normally been treated in a hospital. The treatment modalities used seem to be applicable across a wide spectrum of patients. Only one study excluded a large proportion of patients prior to randomization, and three excluded essentially no one. It was typical, however, in these studies that excluded patients were either elderly or adolescent, had organic brain syndrome, or were alcohol or drug abusers. Given the array of studies here such exclusions seem reasonable, since none of the alternative treatments were designed for those populations. This issue is related to the more general case of consideration of alternative explanations for effects.

ARE THERE PLAUSIBLE ALTERNATIVE EXPLANATIONS FOR THESE EFFECTS?

To consider alternative explanations, one must ask what else could have produced the effect besides the alternative treatment per se. In looking for alternative explanations of these effects, one has to distinguish between an explanation for the aggregate effects across studies, and methodological deficiencies and design flaws within a particular study. One can easily criticize a majority of these studies on a variety of grounds. (Braun et al., 1981, in particular, criticize their specific studies in detail.) For example, a number of studies do not include a very detailed description of what the hospital treatment was. It is clear in most of the studies that the hospital treatment was of high quality, but the lack of detail makes it difficult to compare the efficacy of hospital treatment across studies. There is also a lack of detail on drugs used, with regard to type, amounts, follow through, side effects, and the like. There is often a lack of detail on previous psychiatric history of the patients. Mosher et al. (1975) emphasize that their two groups were young, first-admission schizophrenics. In most of the other studies it is unclear what the previous hospitalization history was, and whether the treatment was more or less effective as a function of that history. In some of the studies the ratings were not "blind," meaning that the raters knew which condition the patients were in, and therefore, could be criticized for the effects this knowledge might have on their judgmental processes. In some cases of alternative care treatment, there did not seem to be great effort to keep the patient out of the hospital (Zwerling

& Wilder, 1964, is the most extreme example). In some studies there is a lack of detail in describing the alternative treatment, including the number of home visits, the educational level of the mental health professional who made each home visit, and the relationship of all of these variables to outcome.

All these are reasonable criticisms of the individual studies reviewed in this chapter. However, none of them is a plausible alternative explanation for the aggregate of studies that we have described. If one wants to argue against the general conclusion of this aggregate of studies— namely that alternative care is more effective than mental hospitalization—then one has to explain the data across all the studies. The fact that some studies have flaws that others do not does not provide a consistent explanation across studies. If there were an important design or methodological flaw in each of the studies, then we would be justified in still having some doubts about the generalization to be drawn from them. Indeed the size of the difference between the impact of the alternative care and the hospital conditions does not seem to be a function of the type of methodological problem in any particular study.[7]

OTHER METHODOLOGICAL ISSUES

There are a number of *problems in measurement* in these studies. For example, a number of the measures included in even the better studies were scales designed to measure psychiatric symptomatology or family burden. While these scales often have very acceptable degrees of statistical reliability, one can point to questions of their validity, specifically as used in these settings. The critical element in these studies is not only to provide a reliable and valid measure of, say, psychiatric symptomatology, but to provide in addition a reliable measure of the change in that variable. Some scales in other areas of measurement that can be demonstrated to be reliable and valid on a given occasion are not very sensitive to change. Indeed some of the techniques used to increase reliability and validity of measurement in a given instance simultaneously decrease the sensitivity of the scaling instrument to detect change in the underlying variable (see Kiesler, 1983). Some of the studies to their credit have outcome measures at four or five different points in the assessment sequence. However, we are left hanging about how sensitive to change the instruments are when repeated so frequently.

THE LENGTH OF THE ASSESSMENT PERIOD

It seems quite clear from this array of studies that whatever differences exist between the AC and H conditions after treatment dissipate over time. Whatever differences exist somewhat later, say two years, still tend to favor the AC group, but certainly the number and the size of such differences generally have substantially decreased. Indeed Hogarty (1977) argues that the cessation of any kind of treatment results in reversal of initial treatment gains for a majority of patients. Test (1981) argues very strongly against what she calls the "time bound" treatment and argues for treatment tailored to individualized needs in a continuing involvement in an assessment and treatment of those needs. As yet, there has been little or no research related to techniques of maintaining the kinds of initial treatment gains shown in this aggregate of studies.

THE POWER OF THE EFFECT

Anthony (1979) argues that "the goal of the psychiatrically disabled client is to perform the physical, intellectual, and emotional skills needed to live, learn and work in his or her particular community given the least amount of support necessary from agents of the helping professions" (p. 30). Although alternative care is clearly more effective than mental hospitalization, there is still considerable doubt about whether or not the care described in these studies has a sufficiently powerful effect to meet the goals of the psychiatrically disabled client as defined by Anthony. Perhaps Anthony's goals are inappropriately severe and can never be met. On the other hand, several of the AC methods are sufficiently inexpensive and simple that they could be continued periodically almost indefinitely.

THE COMPLEXITIES OF TREATMENT

Most of the alternative care strategies used are fairly complex. For the most part they involve some drugs, some psychiatric therapy, some skills training, some lack of control over the patient's environment (in comparison with the hospitalized patient), some degree of nonprofessional contact, and the like. Subsequent research should try to assess the separate impact of these various components such that treatment might be enhanced through an appropriate aggregation of the more effective techniques. In some of the alternative care mechanisms, there is considerable emphasis on coping skills and independence training (e.g., Stein et al., 1975). Dellario and Anthony (1981, p. 26) argue that various reviews "all indicate that the effectiveness of skills training transcends setting and is a function of other considerations such as training technology and staff client interaction." They mean that although such training typically takes place in alternative care, there is no reason why it could not also take place in a hospital for hospitalized patients. To the extent it is a core element of the effectiveness of alternative care, it should also enhance the effectiveness of hospital treatment.

There is also a good deal of psychosocial contact in alternative care treatments of patients with people who are trained but not professionals. Paul and Lentz (1977) describe a hospital based form of care in which there is a great deal of emphasis in training everyone who comes into contact with patients, in a very detailed manner. One could enhance the effects of hospital care by specifically training lower-level or nonprofessional workers and increasing their contact with patients.

THE USE OF DRUGS

There is considerable variation among the alternative care treatments in the use of psychotropic drugs, ranging from the explicit lack of any use of drugs by Mosher and Menn to the rapid tranquilization technique of Polak and Kirby (1976). The use of drugs alone in alternative care treatments (without the other components of the treatment) does not seem very effective. More information about the use of psychotropic drugs in combinations with other treatment components is needed. Smith, Glass, and Miller (1980) review studies with random assignment comparing psychotherapy alone, psychotropic drugs alone, and drugs and therapy in combination. Their meta-analysis of such studies includes seriously ill patients, with about 50% of the total sample hospitalized. They find that the effects of drugs and the effects of psychotherapy in isolation are about equal. Further, and surprisingly, they found no statistical interaction of drugs and therapy. That is, the effects of psychotherapy plus drugs with seriously disturbed patients can be predicted very precisely from a simple addition of their effects alone. Whether this generalization can be specifically applied to alternative care is unknown. It is not clear from the Smith et al. meta-analysis whether one could reconstruct their data base in order to compare a quasi-alternative care treatment condition with a hospitalized treatment condition. If so, this could provide a partial answer to the question of the centrality or potential usefulness of drugs in alternative care. However, a more explicit test of the potential use of drugs in alternative care should be carried out with a very high priority.

THE INTERACTION OF DIAGNOSIS
WITH EFFICACY AND COST OF ALTERNATIVE CARE

As mentioned, most studies include several different types of diagnoses in the patients that they include. Except for Weisbrod's (1983) analysis of the data of Stein et al. (1975), we have noticed no analyses of the effectiveness of the alternative (and hospital) care as a function of the diagnosis of the patient. This is an especially important question because of the interaction found by Weisbrod in terms of the cost-effectiveness of the Stein et al. TCL program. Weisbrod found the TCL program to be much more cost-effective than hospitalization for schizophrenics and other psychotics. On the other hand, he found the alternative care to be substantially more costly than hospitalization for personality disorders.

Such interactions are not necessarily disturbing. Even if not planned, one might subconsciously structure one's alternative care program to be oriented toward the type of patient one most frequently sees (indeed that would be schizophrenics and other psychotics in this array of studies). In addition, Weisbrod did not find (nor assess) a difference in effectiveness of the two techniques for personality disorders, but did find rather substantial difference in costs. Personality disorders were discharged from the hospital much sooner. The inpatient costs for schizophrenics was $4276 per patient but only $1964 for personality disorders. For the H group, much less was spent for the treatment of personality disorders on the average than for schizophrenia, whereas the reverse was true in the AC condition. The net difference between the two conditions or the treatment of personality disorders favored the H group by $2577. Whether there was any difference in treatment effectiveness for the two diagnostic conditions as a function of treatment conditions is unknown.

There is no particular reason to expect a specific alternative treatment (or drug) to be uniformly effective across all disorders. Even though AC treatments are generally more effective (and less costly) than inpatient treatment in these studies, that generalization may not be true for all disorders, age groups, etc. Insufficient detail is provided in these studies to assess such questions even preliminarily.

THE ARRAY OF TYPES OF ALTERNATIVE TREATMENT

The type of alternative treatment varies considerably across studies in terms of professional involvement, supervision, and costs. However, the treatment alternatives typically, but not exclusively, involve social-systems intervention, basic support, and behavioral skill building. The variation in the type of treatment used adds some inferential power to the conclusions we can draw from the total array of studies. However, we cannot scientifically conclude therefore that the most effective alternative care treatment would emphasize social systems intervention, social support, and behavioral skills building. One simply cannot say if there are other forms of alternative care that would be as effective or perhaps more effective than the ones included in this array of studies.

READMISSION

The majority of the studies had some evidence related to the readmissions of the hospitalized patients, and eventual admissions of the AC patients. With one exception, in every case such differences were reported, they favored the AC condition. Fenton et al. (1979) provide one mild exception in the sense that 38% of the AC group were ultimately admitted within the first year of treatment, whereas 23.4% of the H group were readmitted to the hospital after initial discharge. A substantial exception is provided by Goodacre et al. (1975) in which only 33% of the AC group escaped hospitalization in the year of the study, a figure that is at substantial variance with other studies in this group. Indeed, in the Goodacre et al. study, 43% of the AC patients were hospitalized on the first day of treatment. Perhaps the patients in this study were more severely ill than those in other studies. Goodacre et al. say, "during the study period, staff shortages led to restricted admissions to the hospital, and consequently, the subjects of this study were drawn from a severely ill and highly pre-screened psychiatric hospital admission cohort" (p. 8). No patients were excluded. Whether or not a similar proportion of patients would have been immediately hospitalized and ultimately hospitalized in other experiments with a comparable population in severity of illness and no exclusions is unknown. The small difference in the Fenton et al. study and the large difference in the Goodacre et al. study provide the only exceptions to the generalization that Kiesler made in his original review, that "hospitalized patients were more likely to be readmitted to the hospital than alternative care patients were ever to be admitted" (p. 349).

Summary

Over all studies, H patients were much more likely to be readmitted to the hospital than AC patients were ever to be admitted. This empirical fact may be due to the factors described by sociologists in their studies of total institutions: increasing dependency, loss of social and behavioral skills, interruptions of positive social relationships and social support. It may also be due to inadequate inpatient treatment, such as described by Rosenhan (1973).

However, there is also another factor that could have the same effect: the central locus of treatment. All patients in all of these studies were treated by a physician who believed in the efficacy of hospital care for mental disorders. If not, then the patients would not have been sent to the mental hospital in the first place (in advance of random assignment). If, after treatment, the patient feels some recurrence of prior symptoms, whom do they see? It is rather likely that the H group might well return to the same physician (who already had shown a willingness to hospitalize). It also seems likely that the AC patient would see someone in the AC program—that is, someone who believed that effective care could be delivered outside a hospital.

Thus, the difference in the central locus of treatment (where decisions are made) may account for the difference in admissions and readmissions, rather than a long-term debilitating effect of the hospital treatment, per se. This alternative explanation suggests that it is the judgmental bias of the attending physician—and not the hospital itself—that produces the differences in readmission.

These two forces are not mutually exclusive. Both could have an independent influence. However, no data exist to sort between them as theoretical explanations.

The most general conclusion one can draw from this chapter is that alternative care is more effective and less costly than mental hospitalization. How much more effective is unknown. Whether even more effective alternative care programs could be developed is also unknown.

Research on ways to enhance the quality of care *within* a hospital (and afterward) is the topic of the next chapter.

Notes

1. Actually, one of the studies did not involve true random assignment but was sufficiently close to warrant inclusion. In that study, all of the patients in one five-month period were assigned to an inpatient crisis unit, and in the following five-month period all were assigned to the alternative treatment without hospitalization. Unless the patient population changed over time, nonrandom factors were unlikely to have influenced the results, and the study is included here.

2. In the Flomenhaft et al. report on half the 6-month data, these were reported to be 16 and 14, respectively.

3. Polak and Kirby (1976) say that, "the fact that only 85 clients required psychiatric hospitalization from a catchment area of 100,000 over an 18-month period reflects the impact of (these methods) so that the majority of clients who normally would be admitted were treated without separation from the real-life setting" (p. 18).

4. Actually 10 cases—mostly in the beginning months of the evaluation of the system, and the "vast majority" of whom were paranoid, could not be treated in the home setting because they were "overly violent or suicidal and posed management problems" (p. 18). Their exclusion actually made the hospital and home group more similar on various demographic measures.

5. Actually, only the mean readmissions are reported, and our numbers are extrapolated from them. Over a 3-month period, this is likely to be the same as the number of patients readmitted, but not necessarily.

6. The authors also present data from a second hospital plus home condition, but patients were not randomly assigned; we will discuss the three conditions with random assignment.

7. Straw (1982) is the exception. He argues that his coded variable "allegiance to the innovation" is correlated with the effect size. Allegiance was judged on the basis of the enthusiasm expressed about the data in the published article. However, Kiesler (1985) notes that one can conclude either bias or natural enthusiasm for a very impactful program. The use of the term "allegiance" implies the former, rather than the latter, whereas the two possible conclusions are equally plausible.

CHAPTER 10

DEINSTITUTIONALIZATION AND THE PROBLEMS OF SUBSEQUENT TREATMENT, CHRONICITY, AND THE HOMELESS

In Chapter 9, we described the only true experiments ever done,[1] comparing inpatient hospital care with systematic care outside a hospital. Those data are very clear: Within the limits tested, alternative care is more effective and less expensive. It also keeps people out of the hospital. In those studies, substantially more hospitalized patients were subsequently readmitted than alternative care patients ever admitted.

In spite of these data, the episodic rate of mental hospitalization has continued to rise. At the same time, with rare exceptions, alternative care as a treatment policy has not been fully implemented.

This chapter deals with some of the special issues that relate to policy development and change. We ask: Why do physicians continue to hospitalize people for mental disorders? What aspects of inpatient treatment or aftercare treatment are more effective? In what ways has the deinstitutionalization movement inadvertently worked against its own goals? What are the problems of treatment of the much discussed special populations of the chronic patient and the homeless?

Why Hospitalize Mental Patients?

At one level, the national data on inpatient episodes could be seen as simply the aggregate of a large number of physicians deciding to hospitalize mental patients rather than treating them outside a hospital. We ask here, what factors influence that decision to do so? Phrased a different way, what are the advantages of hospitalization for a mental patient? There are several.

(1) It is *easier*. Bachrach (1981), in a critique of deinstitutionalization, suggests that the full array of necessary services—psychiatric, medical, social, rehabilitative, and vocational services—is more easily arranged in a single setting. On the other hand, others (e.g., Bandura, 1978; Mosher, 1982) have argued that these services are more effective

when arranged outside an institutional setting. Everyone agrees, however, that for the attending professional, inpatient treatment is less complicated.

(2) *Insurance*—whether public or private—is easier to arrange for inpatient care. Indeed, public or private insurance coverage can typically only be arranged for inpatient care. It is possible—although awkward— for a state to arrange an exception in order that Medicaid and Medicare can be used to reimburse for community services. However, Mosher (1983) claims that private third-party payment has never been used to reimburse community care programs, except as an experiment (e.g., Krowinski & Fitt, 1978).[2]

(3) *Control and power*. In a mental hospital, the psychiatrist is in charge and everyone else does as instructed. When not otherwise instructed, the ward staff are in charge and the patient is told what to do and how to behave (with imperfect compliance, of course). We do not wish to demean any of the individuals involved, but nonetheless a mental hospital is an authoritarian environment, with a clear organizational structure. From organizational theory we know that such organizations are easier to run (for the people on top) but they do not promote independence.

Outside the hospital setting the patient has more power and independence. They may go to treatment or not, eat or not, take their medication or not. Effective treatment is much more complex outside a hospital. Stein and Test (1982) describe some of these problems well. Their staff often work alongside a patient in a new job until they are working effectively (and often return to do so again if problems arise or new learning is necessary). They sometimes work with store owners when patients overtly shoplift in order to be returned to the hospital (the hospital often being easier for the patient as well as the treatment provider). They develop special techniques to entice patients to take their medication.[3] Care outside a hospital is obviously more complex and difficult— probably for both patient and care provider.

(4) The patient is often very trying for the *family*. The frequency with which the family burden scale is used in studies described in Chapter 9 is evidence of the salience of this problem. Mental patients are difficult and trying to treat and to live with. Families can experience burnout as frequently as care providers do. However, Chapter 9 suggests that the family burden may be less with alternative care than hospitalization (in spite of the fact that families get a "vacation" when the patient is hospitalized).

(5) There has been an *ideological clash* over the deinstitutionalization movement. Etzioni (1976) called it a "policy fashion"; Dumont

(1982) . . . "a polite term for cutting mental health budgets." Bachrach (1983b) has criticized deinstitutionalization: "The shift to community settings did not, in general, lead to improved circumstances among the chronically mentally ill; despite their humane objectives and noble intentions, the initiatives of deinstitutionalization planners often resulted in patient neglect" (p. 9).

The ideological clash has been driven by philosophy and values, more than empirical data and theory. Perhaps as a result, the deinstitutionalization movement—both action and reaction—has interfered with, rather than promoted, the development of a plausible body of empirical data and theory.

We have experienced emotional reactions to the data presented in this book from both sides. From the proponents of deinstitutionalization, we have heard: Effectiveness of alternative care is irrelevant—it is basically a question of human rights and freedom; or alternatively, Why spend money carefully testing the effectiveness of alternative care, when it is obvious on a priori grounds that it must be more effective? From the opponents of deinstitutionalization, we have heard: Effectiveness of alternative care is irrelevent if programs of treatment do not exist; or, "My twenty-five years of clinical experience tell me hospital care is necessary for a mental patient" (irrespective of the data); or, Chronic patients require periodic care through their lives and the hospital is the only place to do that.

Our point is that debate on both sides of the deinstitutionalization movement has been more emotional than empirical. Both sides are supported by at least some data. We should get people out of mental hospitals—alternative treatment is more effective. On the other hand, the deinstitutionalized patient has typically not been in contact with effective treatment—if indeed, there has been any treatment at all. Deinstitutionalization became a social movement—with both idealistic and political overtones—rather than a well-planned national policy of more effective treatment of the mentally disorderd.

In addition, some have pointed out that there is an implicit professional clash as well. Alternative care tends to be psychosocial in approach, although usually with some medication. Grob (1983) has pointed to the cyclical "remedicalization" of psychiatry over the past 100 years. The current emphasis on the biological bases of mental illness is partly a function of the recent surge of feelings that psychiatry must develop closer ties with general medicine. Psychiatry is clearly in charge of hospital treatment; that is less clear in alternative care.

(6) *Treatment programs do not exist.* Mosher (1983) has pointed to the lack of third-party payment for alternative care. There has not been

much contact between CMHCs and state mental hospitals, although that was one intent of the original legislation (and the Joint Commission on Mental Illness and Health). Hansell (1978) has even suggested that CMHCs do not have the right organization to handle chronic patients; that they are more oriented toward the single episode user.

(7) *There are no real incentives for cost-effective care.* Money saved by a treatment center in handling a specific case is not retained by the center for other purposes. The treatment center typically gains nothing by being cost-effective (Kiesler, 1984).

The Community Support System was designed to facilitate alternative care (more specifically, care of chronic patients), but it has been inadequately financed, had only leverage funds, and has not been very successful (Love, 1984).

When programs do exist it takes special efforts to entice patients to use them. In Lamb's (1984a) study, almost half the patients in a board and care home would not use a psychosocial rehabilitation program when it was across the street. When a van ride was required only about a quarter would attend. When a public bus ride was required, 97% of the patients would not go! Obviously, special techniques and efforts are necessary to get patients to make use of existing programs (e.g., Stein & Test, 1982).

All of these factors work together to make it difficult to change existing patterns of mental hospitalization. We do not accuse anyone of bad faith or a lack of commitment to humane treatment. It is difficult to change public policy and perhaps equally difficult to change national professional practices, the roots of which go back a century and a half. In this case, these two factors work together to continue a national commitment to hospital care.

Are there effective forms of hospital care? Let's look at one.

Effective Hospital Care

Let us define what effective hospital care is. Effective hospital care, in our opinion, should be inpatient treatment that gets patients out of the hospital soon and keeps them out.

The most effective form of hospital treatment for severely disturbed patients that we have seen is the "social-learning" approach designed by Gordon Paul (see Paul & Lentz, 1977). Paul started with an especially difficult population, patients who on the average had been hospitalized for 17 years prior to his study. These patients had been continuously hospitalized despite repeated waves of deinstitutionalization efforts that had released the bulk of their fellow patients.

Paul randomly assigned patients to three forms of treatment: social-learning therapy; milieu therapy; or standard hospital treatment. All three were effective to some extent. Social-learning therapy, of Paul's devising, was based on a fairly extreme form of social learning theory (e.g., Bandura, 1978), which includes clear instructions ("do not act crazy!"), some aspects of a token economy system, some punishment (e.g., "time out"), explicit teaching of ordinary but forgotten skills, and a gradual elimination of drug treatment. The program deemphasized the clinical aspects of the environment: patients were called "residents"; staff dressed informally (and all staff, regardless of education and training, were called "change agents"); and patients were informed they would be leaving as soon as they relearned the forgotten skills of ordinary living.

The results are quite startling. The social-learning program was the most effective by far, followed by milieu therapy, and then standard hospital treatment. For example, the clinical frequency at release of "total appropriate" behavior was over 90% for the social-learning group; the increase of total appropriate behavior was over 250% and the increase in self-care behavior was almost 300%. Of the 40 social-learning patients, 36 were released to board and room homes and 3 others to self-supporting, independent living. Across all three treatment programs 74 patients were released and only two had returned at the end of an 18-month follow up (a 3% readmission rate).

Paul's treatment program involved total control over the patient's environment: 85% of each patient's waking hours were devoted to acquiring skills through social-learning procedures, continuing even during meals as well. Only 12% of the patient's time was not structured; 3% was given over to drug administration. By contrast, the hospital treatment condition involved 64% unstructured time, 19% for meals, 6.3% for administration of drugs, with only 5% devoted to classes, meetings, and focused activities.

The study was constructed so that the same level of staffing (FTEs) and the same professional-to-nonprofessional ratio was present for all three conditions. In addition, the same staff administered the social learning and milieu conditions, rotating every half day.

Paul's work demonstrates quite dramatically that even long-term chronic patients in the back wards in state hospitals can be treated, and effectively. Their bizarre and inappropriate behavior can be effectively reduced. They can live outside the institution at a fraction of what institutional care costs. All three conditions produced savings over custodial care but the savings produced by the social-learning approach was three times that of the hospital condition, and 30% more than the milieu condition.

The social-learning approach is highly organized: only 12% of the patient's time was unstructured (versus 64% in the hospital condition). It also demands training both professional and nonprofessional staff in the detailed aspects of treatment, but it does not demand more staff.

It is surprising that Paul's work has not had more impact on changing the treatment of chronic and seriously disturbed patients. For example, two recent and otherwise good books, *The Young Adult Chronic Patient* (Pepper & Ryglewicz, 1982) and *Deinstitutionalization* (Bachrach, 1983a) never even cite Paul's work. Indeed, Paul can be quite moving personally in describing the difficult time he has periodically in obtaining his research funds. There are probably several reasons for this. The social-learning approach is quite radical in nature, and does not blend easily with the training of psychiatrists or some clinical psychologists. It demands total control over the patients' environment, perhaps offending those especially concerned with the civil rights of patients. It is considered quite antidrug in perspective, contrary to the dominant theme in treatment of the mentally ill. Lastly, it demands detailed training of staff and extensive interaction with the patients, either of which might deter the average staff person. In any event, people who claim the chronically mentally ill cannot be treated should read Paul's research.

Paul has also argued in a personal communication against extreme views in favor of alternative care—meaning ours. The effectiveness of his approach depends on control over the patient's environment. Without extreme control (over 85% of the patients' time), appropriate and timely rewards and punishments cannot be given, and the theoretical impact of the social learning approach would be less. For Paul's approach to be effective, it needs to take place in a hospital (or other total institution). Our previous discussion of the mental hospital as a total institution becomes necessarily more complex.

The Chronic Mental Patient

In professional journals and the public media, the problems and prospects of the chronic mental patient have received considerable attention in recent years. The chronic patient was of central concern to the Joint Commission on Mental Illness and Health (*Action for Mental Health*, 1961). It was still a central concern for the President's Commission in 1978, which in turn precipitated a National Plan for the Chronically Mentally Ill in 1980 (see Department of Health and Human Services, 1981), and several more recent volumes (e.g., Bachrach, 1983a; Lamb, 1982; Pepper & Ryglewicz, 1982; Talbott, 1978, 1984). In particular, attention has been drawn to the new, younger and never-treated chronic patient (Pepper, Ryglewicz, & Kirshner, 1982; Bachrach, 1982).

Who are these people, how many of them are there, and how do they affect other issues raised in this volume?

These questions are not as straightforward as with counting inpatient episodes. National surveys are not regularly done, and the definitional issues are more complicated.

Two dimensions of *chronicity* and *disability* converge to define the group of "chronically mentally disabled" (President's Commission on Mental Health, 1978a; Minkoff, 1978). Minkoff (1978) includes a third dimension of institutionalization to describe a group with a history of several or prolonged hospitalizations, and it is these to whom he refers as the "deinstitutionalized." Therefore, people with mental disorders may or may not be "chronically mentally ill," may or may not be disabled in performance of important life tasks, and may or may not have a history of hospitalization.

The Group for the Advancement of Psychiatry's (GAP) report in 1978 used Bachrach's (1976) definition of "mental patient" to be "those individuals who are, have been or might have been, but for the deinstitutionalization movement, on the rolls of long term mental institutions, especially state hospitals."

Goldman, Gattozzi, and Taube (1981) encompass Minkoff's three dimensions of hospitalization in defining the "chronically mentally ill." Included are those who have certain mental disorders (usually psychotic disorders) that interfere with three or more areas of functioning in daily life (e.g., self-care, interpersonal relationships, learning) and that prevent economic self-sufficiency. A history of institutional stay is not a necessary criterion, but the authors note that "most" have been hospitalized or in nursing homes. They estimate 900,000 chronically mentally ill in institutions (psychiatric hospitals and nursing homes) and between 800,000 and 1.5 million in the community. Other community estimates of 800,000 severely mentally disabled come from surveys by the Urban Institute in 1973 and the Social Security Administration in 1966. An additional 700,000 are estimated to be "moderately" or "partially disabled," based on a Census Bureau survey in 1976.

It is difficult to capture the whereabouts of the deinstitutionalized and the chronically mentally ill in the community, as well as their flow in and out of institutions. The dynamics involve the probability of being hospitalized, the number at risk for rehospitalization, the length of stay if hospitalized, and the number discharged from various institutions each year.

The deinstitutionalized—many of whom will be rehospitalized and thereby earn the post hoc label of "chronic"—are an important issue in mental health policy. Much literature describes the unfortunate circumstances surrounding the deinstitutionalized, but studies vary in the extent to which actual data are reported. The Task Panel on "Deinstitutionalization, Rehabilitation, and Long-Term Care" (Platman, 1978) of the President's Commission on Mental Health argued that people with chronic mental disorders need high-quality services, regardless of whether the setting is institutional or some alternative. The Task Panel recommended removing financial disincentives to community care, providing funds for case management and staff training, and broadening vocational rehabilitation to include services appropriate to the chronically disabled. The GAP report briefly reviewed literature on the chronic population. They cited studies reporting several thousand ex-patients in various cities living in substandard housing surrounded by an unsavory population. Other studies, as well as the GAP report, note the inadequate aftercare ex-patients receive (e.g., Kirk & Therrien, 1975; Wolpert & Wolpert, 1976) mostly due to inadequate funding of aftercare services. Much publicity has depicted the deinstitutionalized as homeless, unemployed, and both victims and perpetrators of crime. They are also viewed as problematic, because they supposedly make "inappropriate" use of the existing mental health service system such as emergency rooms of general hospitals.

WHAT DOES "CHRONIC" MEAN: PROBLEMS OF CIRCULARITY

The basic problem in discussing the chronic mental patient is that the definition of the term is inherently circular and flawed. Both chronicity and disability are integral to defining the chronic mental patient. Neither is independent of treatment in general and treatment effectiveness in particular.

For example, consider the studies reviewed in the last chapter. Hospital care was less effective than alternative care; it was more expensive and led to repeated hospitalizations. In these studies one is more likely to be defined as a chronic mental patient if one is randomly assigned to treatment in a mental hospital! This is true of both dimensions of chronicity: disability (H patients were worse off clinically after treatment than were AC patients) and chronicity (H patients were more likely to be readmitted than AC patients were to ever be admitted).

The Community Support System defined chronic as a single episode of hospitalization of at least 6 months (in the previous 5 years) or two or more hospitalizations within a 12-month period. In one sense, all of Paul's patients were chronic patients for 17 years prior to treatment but essentially none were chronic after treatment (only 3% were readmitted within 18 months following treatment).

Disability itself is not independent of the type and effectiveness of treatment previously obtained. In its definition of chronicity, the *National Plan* emphasizes the erosion of such aspects of daily life as personal hygiene, self-care, interpersonal relationships, and social transitions, precisely the sorts of variables that Paul's social-learning approach had dramatic effects on for severely disabled people.

Our point is that the word "chronic" has a circular definition, and cannot be defined independently of the quality of treatment. Further, if a patient is chronic partly due to ineffective treatment, perhaps our collective attention should focus more on the treatment and less on the hapless patient. Finally, to define a patient as chronic is to imply a fatalistic expectation of future hospitalization—an expectation certain to increase the probability of hospitalization occurring.

Living Arrangements

Two types of studies attempt to document the living conditions of deinstitutionalized people with mental disorders. The first type occurs in the hospital reports and statistics on where the current patients are discharged to. The second takes place in the community and describes the status of former hospital patients. All studies we found were of state hospital populations and we emphasize the changing nature of that population over the last 3 decades. Although categories vary from study to study, the most commonly used categories of living arrangements are alone, with family and relatives, and in supervised living, such as board and care homes and halfway houses.

The GAP report concluded on the basis of studies done in the early 1960s that about 70% of discharged people returned to families (about half of those to spouses and half to other relatives) and the remaining lived alone or in community residences with equal frequency. Minkoff (1978) added that later studies showed a lower proportion of discharged patients returning home, probably the result of the changing demographics of discharged patients from state institutions over 15 years and the decreasing percentage of total patients treated there.

The largest data set on the chronically mentally ill is provided by the NIMH Community Support Program. This program funds demonstration sites, where a core service agency, via a case manager, coordinates 10 key service components. Tessler, Bernstein, Rosen, and Goldman (1982) and Goldstrom and Manderscheid (1982) report the results of a descriptive survey of 1,471 randomly selected clients from 18 sites. Their median age was 42 years, and 92% had been hospitalized for psychiatric care at some time; the median was 3 admissions per client, with a median of 23 total months in hospitals. Twenty-eight percent had spent a total of more than 10 years in institutions (and those presumably over 40 years old, given deinstitutionalization patterns). Almost a third had been psychiatrically hospitalized in the previous year for a median of 6 weeks. As for living arrangements, 32% lived with family members, 43% lived with other Community Support Program clients, and 15% lived alone.

Solomon, Davis, Gordon, Fishbein, & Mason (1983) found that at the time of admission, almost 70% of the 550 state hospital discharges lived with parents, spouses, or other relatives, and 20% lived alone. At discharge, living arrangements were similar, but 10% went to live in group homes as compared with 5% living there at admission.

Leaf (1977) and Strayer and Keith (1977) found similar distributions of living arrangements. Strayer and Keith's (1977) results cannot be directly compared with those of Solomon et al., but appear similar. The living arrangements of 87 long-term state hospital patients were assessed 4 days after their discharge. Two-thirds were in private residences, either alone or with parents, friends, or relatives. One-quarter were in transient hotels, and 7% in board and care facilities. A third lived alone, but the location was not specified.

Leaf (1977) reported that at discharge, 72% of state hospital patients went to live with family members, but only 3% lived alone, much lower than the approximately 20% in the previous studies. A difference in age may account for the difference in the percentage living alone. Leaf reports 19% discharged to nursing homes, while Solomon reported 10% discharged to all types of group homes, which presumably includes nursing homes. Twenty-seven percent of the Leaf group were discharged to parents, but the percentage of the Solomon group discharged to parents is not stated.

Leaf studied the same patients three years after discharge and found that 64% lived in nonsupervised settings (4% alone). The 37% in supervised facilities were composed of 19% in nursing homes, 14% in state hospitals or mental retardation facilities, and 4% in other supervised settings, such as group homes.

The living arrangements appear similar among the "young adult chronic patients," to be further described in the next section. Pepper et al. (1981) reported on a group of 294 people aged 18 to 30 categorized as "young adult chronics" because of their set of functional disabilities and needs for service. Sixty-eight percent lived with parents or other relatives or friends and 17% lived alone.

Baker and Intagliata (1984) describe a group of 844 chronically mentally ill people being served by community treatment and support services in New York State, excluding New York City. The median age was 56 years. Ten percent lived alone, and 31% lived with relatives or others. When dividing the sample into age groups, they found that 37% of clients aged 18 to 34 lived with parents, while only 17% of those 35 to 44 did, presumably the result of aging parents either dying or becoming incapacitated.

Goldman, Gattozzi, and Taube (1981) estimate that 300 to 400 thousand of the .8 to 1.5 million chronically disabled population live in board and care homes. This would be approximately 20% to 50%, somewhat more than that actually found in other studies.

Lamb and Goertzel (1972) followed up on all those who were in a California state hospital in 1965 and who had been hospitalized for at least half of the previous 2 years. The sample was limited to those 60 years and under. Five years later two-thirds were institutionalized—35% of those in a state hospital and 51% in boarding homes (Lamb and Goertzel consider boarding homes to function as institutions within a community). Only a third were living in noninstitutional settings—63% with a spouse or relatives, 27% alone, and 10% in satellite housing.

Lamb and Goertzel (1977) conducted an unusual study that surveyed the total population of long-term psychiatrically disabled patients in San Mateo, California, rather than tracking a cohort of discharges. They point out that only studying state hopitals misses a large proportion of psychiatrically disabled patients in the community, because many were never sent to a state hospital in the era of deinstitutionalization. In fact, over 60% did not have an inpatient episode anywhere in the previous two years (an unusually low rate). They defined their "long-term psychiatrically disabled population" as those between the ages of 18 and 64 years with a functional psychotic diagnosis and who had been receiving Supplemental Security Insurance (SSI) for psychiatric reasons for at least 18 months. A sample of 99 was obtained by randomly selecting names from all SSI recipients meeting the criteria. The median age of the women (N = 50) was 44 years and was 31 years for men (N = 49).

Of the sample, 60% had at least one state hospitalization at some time in their life—70% of those were over 30 years old.

At the time of the study the following living arrangements were present: 25% lived alone, 23% with parents, 18% with spouse, 10% with other relatives, 14% in board and care homes,[4] and the rest with friends or in other arrangements. The authors note that over two-thirds were living alone or with family members, contrary to the conception that most psychiatrically disabled people live in board and care homes or other segregated arrangements.

In general, discharged "chronic patients" live mostly with their families and group living arrangements. Only Strayer and Keith found any substantial number in transient hotels (SROs) and only Leaf found a substantial proportion (19%) discharged to nursing homes. Young chronics especially live with their families.

Characteristics of the Deinstitutionalized

Bachrach (1979) divides the "chronic population" needing help into five subgroups. In the community are those discharged from hospitals and those never hospitalized (although who presumably would have been before the deinstitutionalization movement). In the hospital are the old long-stay patients who never made it out despite deinstitutionalization, and recent admissions who will stay a brief time. The hospitals also house new long-stay patients—recent admissions who will not be discharged for a long time. Taube et al. (1983) report NIMH data showing that 41% (35,812) of the state hospital residents, who had been there for more than a year in 1979, were "new long-stay"; they had been continuously hospitalized from 1 to 5 years.

In a literature review, Bachrach (1982) focused on the "young adult chronic" patients, what Caton (1981) calls the "new chronic" patients. The postwar baby boom has created about 60 million people who are now between 18 and 36 years. This is the prime time for onset of schizophrenia, often a chronic condition. Coupled with the deinstitutionalization movement, a large number of "young adult chronics" have become visible to the public and service providers, because they are not confined to long-term institutions. Formal documentation of their situation has just begun.

Pepper et al. (1981) describe them as being extremely vulnerable to stress, having difficulty maintaining stable relationships, and having an apparent inability to learn from experience. Only 24% of their sample were self-supporting; 57% had some form of public assistance, and 19% were supported by parents.

Clinicians complain of their unwillingness to stay in outpatient programs, such as day hospitals and drug treatment programs. Young chronics simultaneously demand immediate help via emergency rooms while rejecting it and provoking an attitude of rejection from the staff (Pepper et al., 1981; Bassuk & Gerson, 1980; Schwartz & Goldfinger, 1981).

Of course, studies of people in contact with hospitals only reflect those who have come in for treatment. In their 1972 study, Lamb and Goertzel assessed the level of functioning of the boarding home and non-institutional residents on a 4-point scale ranging from self-care only to self-supporting. The boarding home residents (median age = 52) were functioning at a lower level than the other community residents (median age = 45). About half in boarding homes were functioning only at the level of self-care, while just a quarter of the other community residents were at this lowest level of functioning. Half of the noninstitutional population functioned at the highest level, while only 15% of the boarding home residents did. Lamb (1979) later did a more intensive study of 101 board and care home residents, aged 65 or younger in California. Their median age was 39 years, 65% were men, 60% were white, 64% never married, and 92% had psychotic symptoms. Most (86%) obtained SSI support and the median total of all previous hospitalization was 18 months. Almost all the residents (94%) had medication prescribed, and for 63% of the residents, the visiting psychiatrist was the only mental health professional seen. Sixty-one percent were either currently involved in vocational rehabilitation activities or had been at one time. Almost a third had been hospitalized during the previous year. Only 48% had goals, defined as the desire to change anything in their lives, such as their work or social situations. About 40% seemed content and the same number predominantly unhappy. The authors describe them as having found refuge in a facility that had taken over the functions of the state hospitals.

Intagliata and Baker (1984) compared "young chronics" with older chronically disabled people and found that those 18 to 34 did not significantly differ on several characteristics from those 35 to 44. These age groups could perform the same number of basic self-care skills (e.g., dressing) and the same number of community living skills (e.g., manage money) and had the same work involvement. These two age groups also performed similarly to the 45 to 54 age group.

However, more incidents of seriously maladaptive behavior (e.g., property damage, assault) were reported for the 18 to 34 group, even when controlling for the disproportionate number of males in this age group. Refusing needed services was also characteristic of "young adult chronic" clients. The youngest group did not refuse significantly more needed services than those 35 to 44, but both these groups refused more than the older groups. Some of the characteristics ascribed to young chronic patients applied to those up to 45 years.

Studies describing discharged psychiatric patients consistently show a large percentage unemployed and a minority involved in vocational rehabilitation services, in large part due to the scarcity of these services. Although direct evidence does not exist, we would expect unemployment to be both a cause and effect of disabling mental conditions.

Anthony et al. (1972) review several studies regarding the employment status of discharged people. The base line full-time employment rates at one year from discharge were 20% to 30%. This is a high rate of employment when compared with more recent studies, but a more select group was being discharged earlier.

Lamb and Goertzel's (1977) study of the current status of discharged patients found that 44% had some structured activity; however, only 15% were in paid employment and not necessarily full-time.

The large NIMH study of Community Support Program clients showed 26% employed at some point after discharge, with the weekly mean number of hours worked 24. Less than half (42%) of the employed held competitive jobs obtained on the open market. An additional 37% worked in sheltered workshops. The majority of employed (71%) held unskilled jobs.

Pepper et al. (1981) similarly found that 24% of the clients of a community mental health center were self-supporting.

As might be expected, employment rates at time of admission to an inpatient psychiatric facility were even lower. Schwartz and Goldfinger (1981) and Solomon et al. (1983) each found about 10% employed at admission.

Crime among deinstitutionalized mental patients has always been a concern, with community residents typically fearing a higher rate of crime committed by ex-patients than in a nonpatient population, and mental health professionals arguing against this stereotype. Rabkin (1979) concluded from her review of prospective studies of discharged patients that their crime rate depends on their prehospital arrest record. Ex-patients with arrest records had much higher arrest rates than the general population or other patients. As the number of people hospitalized with prior arrest records increases (due to a channeling of them from the criminal justice system to the mental health system) the aggregate postdischarge crime rates have increased. Ex-patients without prior arrest records continue to have postdischarge arrest rates equal to or less than the general population.

The public also fears other inappropriate behavior among former mental patients. In the NIMH study of Community Support Program clients, Goldstrom and Manderscheid (1982) report the percentages of clients reported to have the following problems to either a minor, moderate, or serious extent, in decreasing order of number of clients involved (judgments were made by case managers): caused complaints from neighbors (34%; 15% to a minor extent), engaged in bizarre behavior (25%; 13% to a minor extent), had trouble at work or school (24%; 10% to a minor extent), exhibited temper tantrums (19%; 9% to a minor extent), caused community complaints (15%; 7% to a minor extent). The remaining 10 behavioral problems were reported as problems for 6% to 14% of the clients. The mean number of behavioral problems was about 2.

It is quite possible that the same behaviors would not be reported by neighbors or case managers if the clients were not known to be "mental cases." Aside from this possible overestimation of the clients' problematic behavior, these reported statistics indicate a sizable proportion of people acting deviantly. Considering how rigid our expectations of appropriate behavior typically are, it is quite conceivable that these people quickly become rejected by the mainstream.

As for the general functioning of deinstitutionalized mental patients, some studies assess functioning in terms of amount of time spent in structured activities, the extent of social networks, involvement in community activities, and bizarre or inappropriate behavior. It would be expected that an individual's involvement in community activities would vary depending on his or her living situation, social network, state of health, and community acceptance. The general impression is that the deinstitutionalized are to some degree incompetent in accomplishing everyday living skills and live drab existences. The NIMH CSP data support this perception. Although at least half of the sample could independently do 9 of the 13 basic skills, it is still striking that, for example, 30% were judged either unable or unwilling to use available transportation on familiar routes without assistance, 31% did not maintain personal hygiene without assistance, and 40%–49% did not go shopping, prepare meals, maintain adequate diets, or verbalize needs without assistance. About 50% to 60% could not manage available funds, use transportation on unfamiliar routes, take prescribed medication or secure necessary support services. Of course, these are exactly some of the behaviors emphasized for change in many alternative treatment programs.

Caton's (1981) New York City sample was assessed at quarterly intervals during the year after discharge for psychiatric symptoms. Sixty-one percent had at least 1 psychiatric symptom during the year, but only 34% to 46% did at any single assessment. Unfortunately, we do not know the conditions of people who are not receiving services, because all of these studies draw samples from populations involved in treatment.

Use of Services

Availability of community mental health services is seen as essential for maintaining discharged mental patients in the community and generally delaying hospital readmissions of the chronically mentally ill. As we saw in Chapter 8 on readmissions, few experimental studies have been done, but the evidence suggests that participants in aftercare services are still eventually rehospitalized but at less frequent intervals and for shorter total stays. Again, the relationship of aftercare services to readmission must be a function of which services exist, the style of aftercare (persistent or not) and the quality of the original treatment.

However, chronic patients, most of whom have been hospitalized at some time, are seen as a drain on the existing health care system. They are perceived to use expensive emergency and crisis services but do not engage in continuous outpatient care. The attitude among some clinicians (e.g., Schwartz & Goldfinger, 1981) is that a mismatch exists between the current delivery system and the chronic patients' style of use.

Deinstitutionalized people typically need a wide range of social services, such as social-skills training, financial assistance, transportation, and housing. Although some data exist on the services given to different populations, data on the match between need and receipt of particular services are sparse.

The study of the participants in the Community Support Program, the largest chronic population under study, assessed what services clients received in the previous month. Almost a quarter had participated in community skills activities, and almost half participated in work-oriented activities, such as vocational rehabilitation and training and sheltered workshops. Half received SSI benefits, 40% received social security benefits, and almost half were given transportation or money for it. Twelve percent were assisted in finding housing.

As for health and mental health care, 60% received outpatient mental health services in the previous month, and almost half received medical and dental care under entitlement benefits.

Because the procurement of services by case managers is viewed as the most effective way of getting clients needed services, we would expect a high percentage to have been in contact with case managers. About 80% had either contact in person or were telephoned by the case manager. Psychotropic medication was being prescribed for 84% of the clients at the time of the study, yet only 60% received outpatient mental health services in the previous month, according to case managers' reports.

Solomon et al. (1983) also extensively studied use of aftercare services by discharged mental patients, although they counted whether services were used within a year after discharge rather than in the previous month. They did find that 79% of those who contacted community agencies did so within a month after discharge. Almost two-thirds of the cohort contacted the welfare department of the Social Security Administration (SSA) for financial assistance, and two-thirds contacted mental health agencies. Forty-four percent of the cohort contacted both types of agencies.

Contact with the welfare department or SSA does not guarantee benefits will be granted. However, if we assume most were granted, the total of 63% receiving financial assistance (or social services in a few cases) seems to correspond to the CSP results showing 48%, 35%, and 22% received SSI, social security, or state benefits, respectively.

The three most common forms of service received by the entire cohort of 550 was case management (57%), individual therapy (51%), and chemotherapy (36%, but an underestimate because it could often not be separated from individual therapy). Only 15% received social rehabilitation and 8% received vocational rehabilitation services.

The major difference between this group and the CSP group is that a higher percentage of the latter received vocational help (about 50%) and social skills training (about 25%). These "high-intensity" services have been a focus of the Community Support Program.

When we look at the percentage of the Solomon group receiving the services they were judged to need, the results show that half of the 85% needing individual therapy received it, and 40% of the 90% needing drug treatment received it (recall this is an underestimate). However, only 19% of the 79% needing socialization training received it, and 14% of the 50% needing vocational rehabilitation received it. Also, only 6% of the half needing group therapy received it. Therefore, the only type of service supplied to at least half who needed it was the financial assistance given to 60% of the 55% judged to need it.

In all cases, the intensity of contact was low. Two-thirds of service receivers had less than 2 hours of service a month, and the median number of hours of service received in the entire year after discharge was only 12 hours. The extremely low level of actual service received is even more striking when individual types of service are considered. Based on the subgroup of 363 people who received services, the median number of hours of case management received during their community tenure was 2.5, the median number of hours of individual therapy received during their entire community tenure was 5.5, 2 hours was the median for chemotherapy, 7.5 hours for group therapy. The median number of hours of social rehabilitation was 2.5 (mean = 20 hours) and 20 days was the median for day treatment.

The Solomon et al. report is one of the few studies that makes some assessment of clients' perception of needed services and barriers to obtaining them. A sample of 59 were selected from the cohort of 550 and interviewed about a year after discharge. Of note are the discrepancies between their reported needs and those assessed by the hospital social workers at the time of discharge. A higher percentage of clients were judged to need the following service than judged by the clients themselves: group counseling (48% versus 26%), self-help groups (52% versus 26%), homemaker (35% versus 12%).

Results of studies on use of aftercare services, such as the ones just presented, and those in Chapter 8 strongly suggest that the mere funding of traditional case management and aftercare services is not sufficient, if such services are not seen as desirable by potential clients. Patients will not use such services anyway, unless helped to do so (Lamb, 1982).

As Bachrach (1984a) says,

> The majority of the chronically mentally ill in the U.S. today have not been fortunate enough to experience deinstitutionalization under optimal conditions. Problems associated with deinstitutionalization include the need for highly diversified programming, difficulties in achieving both continuity and comprehension of care, the emergence of a population of system 'misfits,' and service systems' failure to designate the dimensions of their responsibility to the chronically mentally ill (pp. 26–27).

In general, findings regarding the deinstitutionalized are quite diverse. It is clear that certain populations at risk have increased in size through the increase in the 18–44 age group. It is clear that clinicians regard the "new young chronic" as more aggressive, less accepting of treatment, and more difficult to manage. There are no good data regarding the potential of alternative care programs with this age group. However, the group as a whole resists hospitalization and might respond better to alternative care than more typical treatment (as others do).

With the total array of data, it is difficult to make straightforward conclusions regarding national policy. The definition of the chronic patient and indeed the deinstitutionalized are confounded with quality of care. That they are rehospitalized can be predicted from existing research described in Chapter 9: hospitalization leads to rehospitalization. All available data suggest (Chapter 8) that the national readmissions rate has not increased, contrary to the usual claim. Perhaps people are in and out of hospitals as often claimed, but not any more frequently than before. Most of the basic premises of the national discussion of the deinstitution-alized are quite simply unfounded in fact.

Aftercare services and funding for them are lacking. The CSP program has tried to provide a model for such services and stimulate the funding for them, but has not provided direct funds, and other funds have not been forthcoming.

When such services are available, ex-patients do not use them much. Studies consistently find this, but it should not surprise us. Excellent work by Stein and Test (1980, 1982), for example, demonstrates both that such services need to be better integrated into overall treatment and how difficult and complex a matter that is. However, they also demonstrate how effectively it can be done.

Most discharged patients do not go to board and care homes, SROs, or nursing homes. Most live with family or spouse. There has been very little work seeing the family as playing a critical role in treatment. Recent work by Goldstein, Rodnick, Evans et al. (1978), Falloon, Boyd, McGill, et al. (1982), and others have shown that systematic work with families can reduce symptomatology, rehospitalization rates, and the like (see Heinrichs, 1984).

The Homeless

The plight of the nation's homeless population has received extraordi-nary publicity recently. The *Philadelphia Inquirer* and the *New York Times*, among many others, have published extensive series of articles analyzing and graphically describing these problems. Both the U.S. House and the Senate have held rather dramatic public hearings, and several bills have been introduced in Congress (e.g., the Homeless Emergency Relief Act of 1985, introduced by Congressman Weiss of New York).

The American Psychiatric Association reviewed the problem and published a generally excellent summary of the issues (Lamb, 1984b). The American Public Health Association has chaired an interorganiza-tional action group, which includes the national organizations of the major groups of mental health professionals.

The public seems to believe that the bulk of the homeless are the deinstitutionalized. That belief means any book on mental hospitalization must deal with this issue. In this brief section we ask, who are the homeless? How many have a major mental disorder? How many have previously been hospitalized for a mental disorder? What are their treatment needs? How do answers to these questions relate to other issues raised in this book?

Answers to all these questions are surprisingly sparse. Let's deal with the issue of numbers first. Estimates of the number of homeless range from 250,000 to 3 million. HUD in 1984 estimated the number of homeless on a given day to be between 192,000 and 586,000, but "most probably" 250,000–350,000. They suggest the cumulative annual total— people homeless at some time or another during the year—to be between 750,000 and one million. This report has been widely attacked and more common estimates in the press and research literature are 2–3 million.

There have always been homeless—the wanderers of colonial times, for example. Skid rows, however, began to develop in metropolitan areas with recurrent depressions of the late nineteenth and early twentieth century. By the 1950s skid rows began to shrink. By 1958, Chicago's skid row was one-fourth its original size 50 years before (in spite of a doubled total population). New York City Men's shelter served 20,000 in 1958 and 12,500 in 1965 (Arce & Vergare, 1984).

Bachrach (1984a) says that all agree on three recent changes in the homeless population: (1) the number is increasing steadily; (2) the average age is dropping sharply; and (3) the proportion of them who are mentally ill is increasing rapidly. Some add a fourth: The proportion of the homeless who are women (estimated now at 15%–25%) has also been increasing.

Most research on the homeless and the mentally ill among them has taken place at emergency shelters and hospital emergency rooms (particularly psychiatric ERs). Estimates of the proportion of those who have major psychiatric disorders range from 20%–90% (Bassuk, 1983), but cluster in the 40%–60% range. Estimates of the proportion of the homeless who have been previously hospitalized cluster around one-third (Basuk & Lauriat, 1984). The average age of the homeless is now in the low 30s.

Bassuk and Lauriat describe four frequently cited reasons for the increase in homelessness: unemployment (and other government economic policies); lack of low-cost housing; reduced disability benefits; and deinstitutionalization.

Unemployment has been a national problem for some time. SSI review procedures have become tougher recently and the mentally ill have disproportionately lost their benefits (by a factor of 3 to 1; Baxter and Hopper, 1984). Other benefits, such as social security and veterans' benefits, cannot be successfully applied for without a home address (40%–60% of the homeless are estimated to be veterans).

Low-cost housing has indeed decreased in recent years, particularly SROs. Between 1970 and 1982, 87% of the total SROs in New York City were eliminated—and 47% of the total supply nationally disappeared, a decrease of over 1 million rooms (Baxter & Hopper, 1984).

The report of the committee of the American Psychiatric Association (Lamb, 1984b) lays the problem squarely at the feet of the deinstitutionalization movement. On publication of the report, the *New York Times* (September 13, 1984) headline read "Failure is Found in the Discharge of Mentally Ill," and the lead read, "The American Psychiatric Association said today that the practice of discharging mentally ill patients from state hospitals into ill-prepared communities had been a failure and a 'major societal tragedy' " (p. 1). Indeed, the report calls for a loosening of the laws regarding involuntary commitment and establishment of laws for involuntary outpatient treatment.

Our review of the hospitalization literature would suggest neither of those recommendations is valid. It is also difficult to see deinstitutionalization at the root of the problems of the mentally ill homeless. As Bassuk (1983) points out, there are no data about the chronically mentally ill homeless spanning the years of deinstitutionalization. Basuk and Lauriat (1984, p. 303) conclude, "There is no doubt that a significant percentage of the population suffer from chronic mental illness; nevertheless, existing data continue to be used as a basis for argument on every side of the issue."

The data on chronicity among the homeless are not very good, and it is difficult to know what to conclude. The problem is obviously very salient to the country at large. The homeless have substantial problems of food, shelter, and medical care, all of which have become more difficult for marginal people to obtain in recent years. The need for the various services provided by typical alternative care (and aftercare) programs is also obvious. The need for coordination among service and programs is accepted by all.

The various national estimates do not fit well together. Goldman et al. (1981) and others have estimated the noninstitutionalized chronics to number around 800,000 as we have described. If 50% of the homeless are chronics, this would argue for two conclusions: (1) The total homeless number about 1.6 million (above the HUD estimate but below commonly accepted beliefs, so not unreasonable); (2) Every chronic is homeless.

The latter conclusion does not fit with data we reviewed earlier on deinstitutionalization. The majority of ex-patients live with families or friends. In follow-ups they live with families, in group homes, board and care, or alone. But they can be found and they are not homeless. Frankly, we are puzzled by the lack of fit among these national statistics.

It seems reasonable to conclude that the homeless are disproportionately the new young chronic patient as claimed by clinicians: The average age of the homeless is decreasing and the size of the general population at risk has dramatically increased (through the baby boom). However, this generation—and particularly the marginal ones among them—distrust institutions in general. The young chronics resist traditional treatment and do not respond well to it.

These statistics argue, for us at least, that loosening commitment laws would not solve or even lessen the problem (except by once again getting the mentally ill out of sight). We suggest that the problems of the homeless argue strongly for extensive alternative care programs with nontraditional treatment.

Notes

1. At least the only ones we have been able to find. We suspect, however, that the review articles cited in Chapter 9 have been sufficiently discussed and commented on that any additional true experiments would have come to light.

2. Even that study perhaps was unwitting. C. Kiesler testified before the U.S. Senate Committee on Appropriations in November, 1984 and mentioned the Krowinski and Fitt study in passing. The next day he received a phone call from a Vice President of Blue Cross in Chicago, asking about the study, its details, and where he could get a copy of it.

3. The lack of compliance with medicinal regimens is a major problem with normal people but especially so with mental patients.

4. Between 1966 and 1971 about half of the discharges from San Mateo state hospital judged in need of board and care homes were placed outside the county and were thus ineligible for this study. Otherwise, perhaps twice as many would have been there.

SECTION IV

PROBLEMS WITH THE OVERALL SYSTEM

In this section we look at some of the issues regarding an overall de facto system of mental hospitalization: what it now costs, what we need to know to develop effective and innovative public policy, and why we do not use what we already know.

Chapter 11 details the cost of mental hospitalization; what we now spend for those three million episodes we have described. Our best estimate is that we are now (1981 data) spending about $12 billion in direct expenditures for inpatient care for mental disorders. However, that number is rapidly increasing, not only well in excess of the general inflation rate, but also that part of it related to health expenditures. About one-third of the total—over $4 billion—funds state mental hospitals, although those hospitals now treat only a small minority of the patients.

We will also learn that the overall cost of an inpatient episode—cost per stay, we will call it—is much more driven by the length of the stay than it is by the cost per day of treatment. The places least expensive on a per diem basis (state mental hospitals, VA hospitals, residential treatment centers) are the most expensive by far when one looks at the total stay.

In Chapter 12, we outline the needs for new knowledge in the treatment of serious mental disorders: knowledge regarding treatment efficacy, regarding *systems* of care and which ones work best, and regarding comparisons of different sites of care. Some of the needed research is rather expensive but we argue that it can be cost-effective.

In Chapter 13, we describe how and why current knowledge has not been better used by both the public and professionals alike. For similar reasons we infer that the basic data described in the book will also be resisted, as part of a more general problem of incorporating new or even current knowledge into public policy.

Last, in Chapter 14, we summarize the basic conclusions of the book and inspect some of the potential implications for the future.

CHAPTER 11

NATIONAL EXPENDITURES FOR MENTAL HOSPITALIZATION

In this chapter we discuss the direct costs of mental hospitalization in the United States. There are several major reasons why this topic is of interest. First, it has a direct relationship to overall policy considerations. That is, we seriously want to consider what we do in the name of mental health, with what effect, and at what cost. In some sense, what we now spend overall can be considered a baseline—a pool of current monetary commitment that conceivably could be reallocated to a different overall approach without increased costs at the margin. Phrased a different way, if we now spend, say, $20 billion for mental health treatment in the United States, then we can pose the question of how $20 billion might be most efficaciously spent.

Phrasing the question this way forces us to consider and justify our current commitments to treatment in mental hospitals in terms of both efficacy and cost. These processes of reconsideration and justification at an overall policy level are pragmatically the most important outcomes of such a sequence. Thoroughly overhauling our mental health policy would not be a simple matter, however badly needed. The political constraints against massive policy change are enormous, even if one can demonstrate that the total cost would not be increased. There is ordinarily considerable resistance to any organizational change, a principle to which the U.S. Congress and state legislatures are no exception. The vested interest in mental health policy include various professional organizations, powerful drug companies, and unions of workers in institutional settings. These groups are politically powerful and have resisted change in the past. The AMA, for example, has opposed every major piece of social legislation affecting health delivery in the last 50 years, including Social Security, Medicaid, and Medicare (Mechanic, 1980). The people who would benefit from change—the current patients and potential future patients—are ineffective. Current patients are weak and distracted, and could not be expected to promote effective political pressure. The potential for future patients, which includes epidemiological estimates of a substantial proportion of the U.S. population, are somewhat paradoxically very suspicious of both mental health patients and treatment. As we shall discuss in Chapter 13, the general public is very apprehensive and distrustful of mental patients and that opinion, even though it is weakening over time, still serves to support some of the least efficacious methods of treatment.

Consequently, when we say that we should consider the overall costs of mental hospitalization in the United States and consider that cost as a baseline to view alternative policies and changes in our current policy, we do not mean to suggest that this is likely to be more than an academic exercise. Nonetheless, it is a very informative exercise, and one in which both professionals and the general public alike can participate.

For this exercise we certainly would wish to look at alternative subcategories of cost. We should consider the cost-effectiveness of institutionalization versus alternative modes of care, short-term therapy versus long-term therapy, drugs versus psychotherapy, and the like. We should consider the match-up of services to the needs of underserved populations, e.g., women, children, minorities, and the aged. In addition, we now have some information on the efficacy of particular treatments and it is useful to see whether our financial commitments follow our notions of treatment efficacy. For example, there is some evidence that short-term therapy is more beneficial than long-term therapy (e.g., Cummings, 1977). Assuming that is true, a question that itself needs further explication, we certainly should be distressed if most of our money went to long-term treatment. Further, from Chapter 9 we conclude that alternative care is more efficacious and costs less than hospitalization—even short-term hospitalization—and it should distress us if the vast majority of our money went to hospitalization.

In general, if treatments A and B are equally efficacious, or if treatment B is not demonstrably better, we do not want to throw all of our financial commitment into B. Consequently, it is important to note both total amounts spent in mental health treatment (and related costs) and how that total is distributed in various categories.

Research is also an aspect of our concern with total cost of mental health treatment. Much of the research that we will suggest in Chapter 12 is indeed expensive to tackle. As a society we certainly should know how much we spend on policy implementation, both de jure and de facto. One way of posing the research question is to look at what percentage of the total costs research accounts for. If one outcome of the research is improved treatment, we might overcome resistance to change of treatment techniques by calculating what savings change might bring to society.

Although all of these questions are of great interest, most are beyond the scope of this book. Here we will focus specifically on costs of mental hospitalization. In particular, we will compare costs per day and per episode in various sites and over time. We will also calculate an aggregate total direct cost of mental hospitalization and inspect that trend over recent years.

Unfortunately, there are very few data related to any of these questions. Indeed, there are a number of problems in calculating just the costs of mental treatment, in or out of a hospital, and it is these to which we now turn.

Issues in Calculating Cost

Personal distress. One of the great incalculables that is associated with mental health problems is the personal pain and distress that such problems bring for both the patient and significant others around the patient. If 35% of the U.S. population is demoralized or worse (Dohrenwend et al., 1980) then the human suffering those people experience themselves and that affects their families, their co-workers, their employers, and others who come into contact with them is enormous. Such a cost is not directly calculable, of course, but there are economic techniques that approximate it. For example, in health policy some economists and decision theorists have used the technique of asking people to subjectively attach costs to particular kinds of problems. They might ask, for example, "How much would you pay to avoid having cancer?" (e.g., Mushkin & Dunlop, 1979). Such approaches are interesting in theory and could easily be directly used in calculating public support for particular policy changes, including the insurance of mental health benefits.

However, these subjective utility methods are less easily applied to mental health than to health. People are more apt to deny any chance of mental health problems than health problems (it can't happen to me); they have less experience with severe mental health than health problems; and they are less familiar with effective treatment methods in mental health. With such little information, how much they would value avoiding such problems is probably moot. Consequently, we will concentrate on actual dollars in the discussion to follow, although we will calculate some indirect costs of mental health problems.

Direct and indirect costs. In most discussions of costs of mental health problems, a distinction is made between direct costs and indirect costs. Direct costs are actual charges against the system by the patient or the family as a function of mental illness. These costs are usually categorized by treatment site (e.g., state mental hospital, nursing home, office-based psychiatrists) and reflect the reported expenditures or charges at these sites.

Indirect costs emphasize lost dollars. Rubin (1978) describes some of the issues and problems in calculating indirect cost. For example, indirect costs include lost wages due to hospitalization, absenteeism, or lowered capacity to work. If a man becomes a chronic schizophrenic at age 24 and never works again, included in estimates of indirect cost would be the wages he had lost for the rest of his life.

If the patient dies prematurely, the family loses potential income. This is a real issue for mental patients. For example, Freedman (1978) reports that death rates for all types of death—homicide, suicide, and natural—are higher in psychiatric populations than in the general population. Indeed, 16,600 patients died in state hospitals in 1974 alone (Kramer, 1977). Minkoff (1978) reports that, at least until the mid-1970s, mental hospitalization terminated in death for the elderly about as often as in discharge.

On the other hand, such indirect costs are lessened by other payments the patient might receive. If a person receives Social Security supplemental income, the indirect cost is lower. However, pension payments are ignored, since such payments would be paid to the patient whether they were mentally ill or not. Rubin suggests that survivor payments paid when a death was the result of a mental illness should reduce indirect costs as well.

Indirect costs are not a trivial part of the national commitment. For example, Levine and Levine (1975) estimated the total cost of mental illness for 1971, including direct and indirect cost, as well as research and training and other costs. Of their total estimated cost of $25 billion, $14 billion or 56% were indirect costs.[1] Levine and Willner (1976) used the same method to estimate total costs of mental illness for 1974. Of the estimated $36.8 billion total costs, $19.8 billion was attributable to indirect costs.

Rubin also distinguishes between *program expenditures* and *economic costs*. Public and private program expenditures are direct outlays through public programs or by individuals. Economic costs are resources used up or productivity foregone. The importance in this distinction is the economic concept of transfer payments. Transfer payments are funds taken from some people and given to others. Social Security and the Social Security supplemental income are both forms of transfer payment. This concept is important because economists assume that transfer payments are not involved in productivity. Therefore a transfer payment is a program expenditure but not an economic cost.

These issues complicate detailed discussion of the costs of mental illness in the United States. Costs of such programs as Medicare, Medicaid, and Social Security are sometimes submerged in calculations as transfer payments, which is typical economic practice. However, these transfer payments are real policy costs to society. They represent income that presumably could be used for other purposes, such as changing incentives within Medicaid and Medicare; and they are real expenditures.

Expenditures for Mental Hospitalization

Our approach here will be similar to that used in Section II on institutionalization. That is, we will look at the official national estimates of the appropriate federal agencies. We will then look at the bases on which these estimates were derived and look at other estimates based on other data. For example, we used this method in Chapter 3 and estimated that instead of 1.7 million episodes of mental hospitalization yearly in the United States, it was more likely that about 3 million episodes occurred. We went on to discuss public policy in terms of these revised estimates. We will revive some of that discussion for the current analysis. Following is a presentation of expenditure data as reported by various agencies. After reviewing these data we will discuss estimates of total costs of mental illness and the effects of insurance policies on hospitalization.

Two major problems in comparing cost data from various sources exist. The first is deciding on a unit of measure. As Rubin and others (e.g., Binner & Nassimbene, 1980; May, 1970) point out, the commonly used measure of cost per inpatient day, or cost per diem, is a measure of a unit of care produced. It is affected by characteristics of the institution and program, e.g., staff-patient ratio or intensity of treatment. However, the cost of a hospital day provides little information about the cost of treating an entire episode, which is a function of the cost per inpatient day times the number of days stayed.

It is cost per stay[2] that is necessary for comparing costs either across institutions or within the same institution over time. A particular type of inpatient care may appear cheaper than another, because the per diem cost is less. However, the average length of stay may be shorter in the second, creating a less costly total stay (e.g., Sheehan & Atkinson, 1974). In fact, cost per day can be misleading even for comparing across the same type of institution, e.g., state hospitals. Morrissey, Burton, Castellani, and Melnick (1979) showed that the difference in cost per day between two groups of New York state hospitals with low versus high rates was almost totally accounted for (after adjusting for current capital costs) by the percentage of chronic versus acute case load served. In other words, the cost per day for acute care was about equal in high versus low rate hospitals. The discrepancy in their overall rates reflected the relative amount of active versus custodial treatment. Higher quality, or more intensive, treatment will cost more per day, but if it results in a shorter length of stay, then the cost per stay could be cheaper (Binner & Nassimbene, 1980; McCaffree, 1969).

The second problem concerns how a particular unit of cost should be measured (Frank, 1981; Rubin, 1982). The same unit may not be comparable given that "cost" may or may not include indirect costs, capital costs, lost opportunity costs, physicians' fees, etc.

These problems of comparability become critical for comparing costs of treatment in general (e.g., Cassell, Smith, Grundberg, Boan, & Thomas, 1972) and doing cost-benefit and cost-effectiveness analyses in particular (Frank, 1981). Not only must the units be comparable, but all costs must be included for accurate conclusions as to which course of treatment has a lower ratio.

It is striking how few national data exist on the cost of psychiatric care in various types of facilities. The summary of NIMH annual expenditure data provided by Thompson et al. (1982) has been extended by Taube and Barrett (1983, 1985). Rubin presents primarily data on cost per inpatient day (mostly current years only) but he includes estimates from sources additional to NIMH. He found that state psychiatric hospitals were the least expensive, while a day in a CMHC and a general hospital (averaged over all medical diagnoses) was the most expensive.

Our purpose is to extend our previous presentations to show trend data on both cost per inpatient day and cost per stay in all inpatient sites for psychiatric care. In addition to per diem cost figures from NIMH and other sources, we will use true average length of stay figures, based on total days of care per discharge, to calculate cost per total stay. We limit our presentation to inpatient care, since that is the theme of this book. However, we note that inpatient costs comprise the majority of mental health expenditures.

As will be further explained in the method section, we used various sources of data to calculate cost per day and per stay for both the same and different types of institutions. We also look at total national costs. The data are difficult to come by and should not be interpreted as precise values but rather as indicators of trends. The sources of the data are quite similar to those previously described. The nontechnical reader may wish to skip to the results section of this chapter.

Sources of Data

Various national surveys of hospitals differ substantially in the universe covered, the data collected, and the definitions of the variables. Therefore, several data sources were used for the various statistics presented here.

Our interest is in the annual expenditures and the number of inpatient days in each type of inpatient facility. The first is divided by the second to obtain expenditures or cost per inpatient day.[3] We also present the true average length of stay per discharge that we have previously discussed (Chapter 5). Multiplying the length of stay by the cost per day equals the cost per stay.

The annual expenditures and inpatient days for state and private psychiatric hospitals are those reported by Taube and Barrett (1983, 1985), based on the NIMH National Reporting Program. (These total expenditures include a small percentage for outpatient care.)

Expenditures for mental health care in VA medical centers and in general hospitals are more complex, because people can be treated both in separate psychiatric units (or bed sections) or in general medical units. However, the cost per day in a medical bed section is not reported by diagnosis. Therefore, expenditures for the days spent there must be estimated.

We used the same approach for VA medical centers as for estimating characteristics of discharges with mental disorder diagnoses from general hospitals without separate psychiatric units (Chapter 4). We subtracted the days spent in separate psychiatric bed sections from the total days of care accumulated by all people discharged with a principal diagnosis of mental disorder. Then each subset of days was multiplied by their respective cost per day. The cost per day of treating a psychiatric case in a general medical bed section is not known. Using the average cost per day in a medical section may slightly overestimate these psychiatric expenditures, but there is no better estimate available. All data used in these calculations came from various VA surveys.

Our calculations for general hospitals used data from the National Institute of Mental Health, the NCHS Hospital Discharge Survey, and the American Hospital Association. Inpatient days in psychiatric units, as reported by NIMH, were substracted from total days accumulated by all people discharged with a principal diagnosis of mental disorder from all general hospitals (with or without a separate unit), as reported by the HDS. Then each subset of days was multiplied by the respective cost per day. Again, cost per day of treating a psychiatric case in a general medical area is not known at the national level. We used the average cost per day across all general hospitals, as reported by AHA.

To summarize our sources of data, NIMH days and expenditures were used for state and private psychiatric hospitals. The VA data came from their cost surveys and their surveys of aggregate data and discharge records. NIMH expenditures and days were used for general hospitals with separate psychiatric units. Days for hospitals without units were derived from the Hospital Discharge Survey and expenditures per day from AHA were used to calculate cost there.

The medical care component of the Consumer Price Index was used to convert current dollars to constant dollars (U.S. Bureau of the Census, 1984).[4]

Results

State mental hospitals. Table 11.1 shows trends in annual expenditures in state mental hospitals from 1969 to 1981 in current and constant dollars. Total inpatient days and expenditures per inpatient day, derived by dividing annual expenditures by inpatient days are also shown. Expenditures per total stay in current and constant dollars were derived by multiplying expenditures per day by the true average length of stay.

In constant dollars, annual expenditures steadily rose until 1975 (but have since stabilized), while inpatient days steadily decreased. The result was to almost triple the cost per day from $14 in 1969 to $40 in 1981 (constant dollars). Length of stay continued to decrease between 1969 and 1981. The effect on cost per stay in constant dollars was an increase from 1969 to 1975, followed by an overall decrease. The cost per stay in 1981 was the same as in 1969 in constant dollars. In current dollars, the cost per stay in a state mental hospital was almost $15,000 in 1981, and the total national expenditure in state mental hospitals was about $4½ billion.

Private psychiatric hospitals. Table 11.2 shows comparable data for private psychiatric hospitals. The annual expenditures in constant dollars rose faster than in state hospitals, but the inpatient days also have been slowly increasing. The length of stay has decreased since 1969 but has been stable recently. The net result is that the cost per stay has also been stable recently after adjusting for inflation. In 1981, the cost per stay in

TABLE 11.1
Total Expenditures in State and County Mental Hospitals and Expenditures per Day and per Stay in Current and Constant (1969) Dollars, 1969-1981

Year	Total Expenditures (in thousands) Current	Total Expenditures (in thousands) Constant	Inpatient Days	Expenditures per Inpatient Day Current	Expenditures per Inpatient Day Constant	L of S per Dischg	Expenditures/ Stay Current	Expenditures/ Stay Constant
1969	1,814,101	1,814,101	134,185,000	14	14	421	5,894	5,894
1971	2,359,000	2,083,922	119,200,000	20	17	367	7,340	6,239
1973	2,574,803	2,120,925	92,210,000	28	23	312	8,736	7,176
1975	3,185,049	2,141,929	70,584,000	45	30	270	12,150	8,100
1977	3,330,249	1,865,686	57,206,000	58	33	210	12,180	6,930
1979	3,756,754	1,777,083	50,589,000	74	35	162	11,988	5,670
1981	4,492,606	1,762,497	44,558,000	101	40	147	14,847	5,880

SOURCES: Expenditures and inpatient days: *Mental Health United States 1983* and *1985*, NIMH. Length of stay/discharge: 1971 and 1973: NCHS Vital and Health Statistics, Series 14, Nos. 12, 16. Other years: unpublished data from NCHS and AHA.

NOTE: The number of inpatient days reported here are from NIMH surveys. Therefore, they are slightly different from those reported in Chapter 6, which are from NCHS and AHA. NIMH days are used here to correspond with NIMH expenditures.

TABLE 11.2

Total Expenditures in Private Psychiatric Hospitals and Expenditures per Day and per Stay, in Current and Constant Dollars, 1969-1981

| Year | Total Expenditures (in thousands) | | Inpatient Days | Expenditures per Day | | L of S per Dischg | Expenditures/ Stay | |
	Current	Constant		Current	Constant		Current	Constant
1969	220,026	220,026	4,237,000	52	52	65	3,380	3,380
1971	276,000	243,816	4,220,000	65	58	50	3,250	2,900
1973	328,463	270,563	4,108,000	80	66	39	3,120	2,574
1975	466,720	313,867	4,401,000	106	71	39	4,134	2,769
1977	563,294	315,571	4,792,000	118	66	38	4,484	2,508
1979	743,037	351,484	5,074,000	146	69	36	5,256	2,484
1981	1,113,764	436,942	5,578,000	200	78	37	7,400	2,886

SOURCES: Expenditures and inpatient days: *Mental Health U.S. 1983* and *1985*, NIMH. Length of stay/discharge: NCHS Vital and Health Statistics, Series 14, Nos. 12 and 16. Other years: unpublished data from NCHS and AHA.

NOTES: The number of inpatient days reported here are from NIMH surveys. Therefore, they are slightly different from those reported in Chapter 6, which are from NCHS and AHA. We use NIMH days here to correspond with NIMH expenditures.

a private psychiatric hospital was about $7,400. The total national bill was slightly over $1 billion.

Veterans' Administration. Table 11.3 shows VA annual expenditures for total days accumulated by all discharges with a principal diagnosis of mental disorder from all bed sections. This total was derived by calculating expenditures separately for days in psychiatric bed sections and days in general medical bed sections.

Days in medical sections were estimated by subtracting days in psychiatric bed sections from total days accumulated by discharges with principal diagnoses of mental disorders. Expenditures were calculated by multiplying days by the cost per day in their respective bed sections. This analysis assumes the cost per day of a psychiatric case in a medical section is equal to the average cost there. It is likely to be somewhat of an overestimate.

One can see that the total number of inpatient days for mental disorders in VA hospitals has decreased substantially, even more so in medical bed sections than in psychiatric bed sections. The costs per day have risen only slightly in excess of the inflation rate for both psychiatric and medical bed sections (the current dollar costs in 1983 were 142 and 217, respectively). The current (1983) total national expenditure for mental disorders in VA hospitals is about $1.8 billion.

For the VA, the cost per stay is not an easy calculation. Recall from Chapter 5 (Table 5.3) that the length of stay varies considerably between general and psychiatric hospitals, even with diagnosis constant. For example, in 1978 (the last year types of hospitals were distinguished) the length of stay for psychotics was 160.6 days in psychiatric hospitals and 74.1 in general hospitals. For nonpsychotics, the lengths of stay were 52.9 and 28 days, respectively.

However, the VA no longer distinguishes between general and psychiatric hospitals, and we do not know the distribution of psychotics and nonpsychotics by type of bed section. For purposes of discussion, let us assume that all discharges from general hospitals were treated in general medical bed sections and all those from psychiatric hospitals were treated in psychiatric bed sections. (Recall that both types of hospitals had both types of bed sections.)

If we apply the length of stay figures for 1978 to the 1983 per diem costs, the estimated cost per stay for psychotics would be $22,805 in a psychiatric bed section and $16,080 in a medical bed section. For nonpsychotics, these costs would be $7,512 and $6,076, respectively. Giving due weight to the relative proportion of psychotics and others, the overall average cost of stay in a psychiatric bed section would be slightly over $14,000, and a general medical section approximately $9,500.

TABLE 11.3

Estimates of Total Expenditures for Mental Disorders in VA Medical Centers in Current and Constant Dollars (1969), 1975-1983

Year	Days in All Bed Sections for Mental Disorders [a]	Days in Psych Bed Sect. [b]	Days in Medical Bed Sect. [c]	Avg. Cost/Day Psych Bed Sect. [b] Current	Constant	Avg. Cost/Day Medical Sect. [a] Current	Constant	Expenditure in Psych Sect. [b] (in thous.)	Expenditure Medical Sect. (in thous.)	Total Expenditures Psych & Medical Sect. (in thous.) Current	Constant
1975	16,851,574	9,531,536	7,320,038	55	37	82	55	519,400	600,243	1,119,643	752,954
1976	15,234,838	9,090,753	6,144,085	65	40	94	58	586,800	577,544	1,164,344	714,760
1977	14,056,477	8,571,213	5,485,264	75	42	110	62	643,673	603,379	1,247,052	698,629
1978	12,872,994	8,335,030	4,537,964	86	44	127	66	718,251	576,321	1,294,572	669,029
1979	12,167,771	7,892,452	4,275,319	97	46	147	70	762,355	628,472	1,390,827	657,912
1980	11,164,637	7,692,623	3,472,014	110	47	159	68	847,471	552,050	1,399,521	596,811
1981	10,872,464	7,478,889	3,393,575	121	47	181	70	903,015	614,237	1,517,252	584,233
1982	10,801,881	7,443,999	3,357,882	130	45	199	69	970,002	668,219	1,638,221	565,099
1983	10,676,310	7,382,025	3,294,285	142	45	217	69	1,045,060	714,860	1,759,920	558,527

[a] Total days for all discharges with principal diagnoses of mental disorder (VA *Annual Reports*).

[b] Inpatient days (VA *Summary of Medical Programs*). Expenditures in psychiatric sections do not exactly equal days times cost/day due to our rounding of the published cost/day figures.

[c] Derived by subtracting days in psychiatric bed sections from all days for mental disorders.

[d] VA *Summary of Medical Programs*.

Although we do not have these cost by diagnosis by length of stay break-downs for other sites, it appears that the cost of stay in a VA psychiatric bed section is similar to that of a state mental hospital.

General hospitals. Table 11.4 presents data from general hospitals, broken down into hospitals with and without units. Recall that two-thirds of the episodes in general hospitals occur in hospitals without units. In spite of that, the total number of days spent in nonunits is somewhat less than units. However, hospitals without units cost much more per day (currently $244 and $121), resulting in total expenditures almost twice that of hospitals with separate units. The total bill for inpatient care in general hospitals for 1980 was $3.5 billion.

For the three-year period, 1977–1980, cost per day of care in non-units increased 41% in current dollars. We have assumed a similar increase for units, although that may be a serious underestimate.[5] We do not have any data for units more recent than that in Table 11.4. However, we do know that the cost per day of (nonspecified) care in a general hospital increased 50% from 1980 to 1983 (AHA, 1984). Sup-pose we assume a similar increase for units. Suppose further the number of days of care remain the same, a conservative assumption. This would mean that total expenditures for inpatient care in general hospitals in 1983 was over $5 billion.

The cost per stay in 1980 was similar for units ($2035) and nonunits ($1950). In 1983 the cost for nonunits had risen to $2925. We have no data on units but the cost per stay there was surely over $3000 by 1983.

CMHCs. Expenditure data for CMHCs have not been collected separately for inpatient and outpatient care at the national level. Total expenditures increased from $73 million in 1967 to $1.5 billion in 1980. Although only 13% of all CMHC episodes were for inpatient care in 1977 (Witkin, 1980), an inpatient day is a much more expensive unit of care than an outpatient visit. NIMH reports a cost of $140 for a day of inpatient care in 1977 (based on a study by Sorenson and Hanbery reported in Vischi, et al., 1980). Rubin (1982) reports a reimbursement rate of $177 for an inpatient day in a New Jersey CMHC in 1979. From these limited data, it appears that CMHC inpatient care has a cost greater than that of psychiatric units but somewhat less than hospitals without separate units. If we use 14 days as the average length of stay per episode (see Chapter 5), and $180 per day (midway between units and nonunits), the cost per stay would be approximately $2520 in 1980. We have no way of ascertaining whether the per diem costs in CMHCs have been rising as fast as those in psychiatric units, however.

Residential treatment centers for emotionally disturbed children. These are an additional site of inpatient mental health care. Annual

TABLE 11.4
Estimates of Total Expenditures for Mental Disorders in General Hospitals with and without Separate Inpatient Psychiatric Units, 1969-1980

Year	Days in All General Hospitals for Mental Disorders [a]	Days in Separate Units [c]	Days Not in Units [d]	Avg. Cost/Day Separate Units Current	Constant	Avg. Cost/Day All Gen. Hosp. [e] Current	Constant	Expenditures in Units (in thous.)	Expenditures Not in Units (in thous.) [f]	Total Expenditures (in thous.) Current	Constant
1969	9,760,000 [b]	6,500,000	3,260,000	$46	$46	$64	$64	$298,000	$208,640	$506,640	$506,640
1971	12,341,000	6,826,000	5,515,000	55	49	83	73	373,000	457,745	830,745	733,874
1973	14,176,000	6,990,000	7,186,000	64	53	102	84	450,715	732,972	1,183,687	975,030
1975	16,496,000	8,349,000	8,147,000	74	50	133	89	621,284	1,083,551	1,704,835	1,146,493
1977	17,606,000	8,435,000	9,171,000	86	48	173	97	722,868	1,586,583	2,309,451	1,293,810
1980	19,578,000	10,727,000	8,851,000	121	51	244	104	1,297,967	2,159,644	3,457,611	1,474,461

NOTE: Total expenditures include an unknown amount for outpatient care. This amount is expected to be a small percentage except for 1980 data, which includes some former CMHCs. See text.

[a] Days of care (discharge days) for all discharges with a principal diagnosis of mental disorder (NCHS Hospital Discharge Survey).

[b] 1968 data.

[c] Inpatient days and expenditures as reported by NIMH in *Mental Health United States 1983* and *1985*. See text for 1980 calculation.

[d] Derived by subtracting inpatient days in units from total days.

[e] These are adjusted expenses per inpatient day according to AHA. They equal total expenses times the ratio of inpatient to total patient revenue, all divided by the number of inpatient days.

[f] Calculated by multiplying days in general hospitals without units times average cost/day in general hospitals.

218

expenditures rose from $123 million in 1969 to $530 million in 1981. (These figures are a slight overestimate of inpatient expenditures to the extent they include an unknown amount of outpatient costs.) Dividing this figure by the 6.5 million days spent in RTCs (Chapter 6) yields a per diem figure of $82. There are no good figures on length of stay in RTCs, but the average is assumed to be over a year. This suggests the cost per stay is over $30,000; perhaps even as high as $50,000.

Costs per Stay

Over a 10-year period, state hospital per diem costs almost tripled in constant dollars. However, a simultaneous sharp decrease in length of stay has held down the cost per total stay. Our estimated cost per stay in a state hospital is still very expensive, and in most recent data was about $15,000. Our estimated cost per stay in the VA psychiatric bed section was similar, around $14,000.[6] That VA mean conceals huge differences between treatment of psychotics and other patients ($22,800 versus $7500) given their difference in length of stay. A similar difference in LoS and therefore cost must be true in state hospitals as well, although we cannot document it. The treatment differences in costs presumably apply to the medical bed sections of the VA as well, yielding an overall average of about $9500 (composed of treatment costs of $16,100 for psychotics and $6100 for others).

These public sites cost much more per stay than any of the other sites. In 1980, the cost per stay in general hospitals was $2035 in psychiatric units and $1950 in nonunits. We estimate an inpatient stay in a CMHC at that time to have been $2520. The comparable figure for a private psychiatric hospital is about $7400. The most expensive site of all, of course, are the RTCs, which we estimate to have a cost of stay over $30,000. However the number of episodes in RTCs is very small (33,000), as the reader may recall.

It is clear from these figures that the cost per day of treatment is not a good clue to total cost of stay. Length of stay dominates the total figure much more than per diem costs. The three least expensive sites on a per diem basis—state hospitals, VA psychiatric bed sections, and RTCs—have by far the most expensive costs of stay. We are certain that those three sites also have the most custodial care and the least intensive treatment.

These data suggest a clear policy question: Would it be possible to intensify the treatment in these sites, thereby driving the per diem costs up, but perhaps driving the length of stay down sufficiently to produce

for over 30% of total costs. In other treatment sites, annual total costs and costs per stay have remained relatively level, at least in constant dollars. The exception is private mental hospitals. Total inpatient expenditures have doubled there in constant dollars, although they represent a small part of the total national expenditure (9%).

Effectiveness. To have a well-articulated national policy in mental health we would need data on treatment effectiveness at each of these sites, most particularly in general hospitals. Alas, such data simply do not exist. The data in Chapter 9 suggest that alternative care programs are more effective than all of these sites (although no comparisons have been conducted involving general hospitals without psychiatric units). We do know there is some systematic variation in diagnoses by site. At the same time there is considerable overlap among sites. That is, all sites treat some of all mental disorders. Systematic and complete specialization does not exist. For example, state hospitals treat disproportionately the poor, black, male, nonyoung psychotic patient without private insurance. However, there still are many in the nonpoor, white, female, nonpsychotic and younger categories (and probably even the occasional insured patient). State hospitals probably "specialize" (by default) more than do the other sites. There are no comparisons of the treatment effectiveness of one site versus another for a particular disorder (at least with random assignment). Anecdotal evidence and the data on per diem expenditures strongly suggest state hospitals must be the least effective site, but it is commonly acknowledged both that they receive the most disturbed and difficult-to-treat patient, and that they do have some successes. No data and probably no uniformity of opinion exist about the other sites. Consequently, although we can speak clearly of the *costs* of inpatient treatment, we can say very little about the cost-*effectiveness* of treatment.

PROPORTION OF TOTAL COSTS
THAT ARE FOR INPATIENT CARE

The Alcohol, Drug Abuse, and Mental Health Administration (ADAMHA) published some projections in 1979 for 1980 for estimated expenditures, including outpatient care. We can meld some of their figures with ours to estimate what proportion of total direct costs for mental health care that is attributable to inpatient care. First, we add their figures for children's inpatient treatment programs ($206 million), halfway/community residences ($43 million) and physician visits to inpatients ($750 million) to our totals in Table 11.5. ADAMHA includes them under inpatient care and, for the purposes of this discussion, so will we. For outpatient treatment ADAMHA estimates $3.3 billion for organized settings (such as CMHCs), $387 million for HMOs and the like, and $1.8 billion for private office-based providers.

If we take our total in Table 11.5 (which excludes nursing homes), and add in the three inpatient items above, we derive a total inpatient figure of $12.985 billion. Adding in ADAMHA's outpatient estimate, we come to a figure of $18.465 billion for total direct costs. Approximately 70% of these total expenditures for mental health care in the United States goes for inpatient care.

Frank and Kamlet (1985) provide us with an independent estimate of total expenditures. Leaving aside their estimates for expenditures in schools and the criminal justice system, they estimate a range of $18.4–$19 billion for total expenditures. Our 70% estimate fits well with their estimates of the total. However, they include approximately $1.6 billion for nursing home expenditures for mental disorders. If one includes these expenditures as part of our total, then we would conclude that about 72% of all expenditures are for inpatient care. We note that including nursing homes results in a national total of $14.6 billion in direct expenditures for inpatient mental health care in the United States.

There are a number of costs that are not included in these statistics. For example, these figures do not include a wide variety of traditional medical problems in which there is a strong psychological or mental health component. Rapid progress has been made recently in both the treatment and study of such medical problems as cardiovascular disease (particularly that related to Type-A behavior), hypertension, chronic pain, bronchial asthma, obesity, migraine headaches, and the like. Medical psychology and its closely allied field, behavioral medicine, are making rapid strides in both the investigation and treatment of such conditions. However, such mental health-like activities are not included in national statistics about the cost of mental health treatment, inpatient or other.

Also not included in these statistics is a potentially important problem, misdiagnosis of mental health problems as medical. To some extent the probability of misdiagnosis varies as a function of both the attending professional and the site in which the service is delivered. Nonpsychiatric physicians, with little background in psychology and psychiatry, still see an enormous number of mental patients. They are much less likely to recognize mental health problems than are psychiatric physicians, and more likely to use drugs in their treatment of such problems. The unrecognized cases in this large sample have costs in treatment that are not represented in a summary of national figures.

The statistics do not include the indirect costs of mental health problems, such as alcoholism, in related medical diagnoses, such as the treatment of renal conditions. The extent to which the overall cost of treatment of liver conditions is a function of alcoholism of the patients involved is unknown. The cost of treating the condition in a more advanced state as long as the specific treatment refers to something physical, would be lumped under medical costs and not mental health.

Also not included are certain costs of patients being untreated or inappropriately treated. Untreated mental health problems may lead to such conditions as divorce, dropping out of school, absenteeism, and the like. Such costs are difficult to track and there are no appropriate national statistics for the untreated. The estimated cost for the untreated patient, which must be substantial, is not included in the national statistics. Inappropriately treated refers to the mental patients being treated by nonpsychiatric physicians. There is a good deal of inappropriate medication or unnecessary surgery that goes on for the treatment of conditions that are mental and not physical (Mechanic, 1980). An understanding of the cost of mental illness in context requires an analysis of how it is insured, to which we now turn.

THE EFFECTS OF INSURANCE PRACTICES ON HOSPITALIZATION RATES

Insurance programs, both public and private, dramatically affect the quality and type of mental health care. Because these programs offer incentives in favor of inpatient care, and inpatient care accounts for over 70% of the mental health dollar, insurance in essence drives de facto national mental health policy. NIMH has little to do with Medicaid policy, but Medicaid is the nation's largest single mental health program.[7]

The bias results from barriers erected against outpatient care. Medicare and most private insurance programs have copayments (often 50%) for outpatient care but would pay the full bill for inpatient care. We note parenthetically that this is also true for alcoholism treatment for which inpatient care is demonstratively less effective than outpatient care (see Vischi et al., 1980). The imbalance in the incentive structure produces a bias toward hospitalization and is inconsistent with the data on treatment effectiveness that we saw in Chapter 9. The reasoning behind the insurance policy is to handle the most serious mental health cases, but to inhibit seeking professional care for "ordinary problems of living." However, as David Mechanic (1980) says:

the present insurance structure that includes broader insurance coverage for inpatient care for mental illness provides incentives for *unnecessary* hospital care and encourages a medical approach to mental health problems in contrast to community alternatives in education and rehabilitative models . . . [these] programs . . . effectively limit total expenditures for psychiatric services, but also reinforce traditional, ineffective and inefficient patterns of mental health care, inhibit innovation and use of less expensive mental health personnel, and reinforce a medical as compared with a social or educational approach to patients' psychological problems [p. 141].

To some extent this attitude toward hospitalization depends on an overly developed analogy of mental health with medicine, i.e., that the most serious cases—physical or mental—should go to a "hospital." Politicians and insurance executives intuitively accept that and have been supportive in developing funds for hospitalization of mental patients. Indeed, hospitalizing serious mental cases has some face validity, even to the very best trained professionals. However, the acceptance of the face validity of institutionalization has helped produce the environmental press on the overall system. That is, we have not to any extent applied the same tough-minded evaluative critique of the basic premise of hospitalization as we have with, say, psychotherapy. People have argued for years over the effects of psychotherapy, while at the same time implicitly accepting the premises behind hospitalizing mental patients.

To be more explicit, suppose a family were considering the mental problems of one of the parents. They might consult with their friends to decide which options were open to them. What they are likely to find is that if they take the parent for psychotherapy that they will have to pay 50% of the cost of psychotherapy. Thus, if they consider that the case is serious enough to warrant, say, 20 sessions of psychotherapy at $50 an hour (a total of a $1,000 bill), then they would have to anticipate paying $500 for that treatment. If, on the other hand, they hospitalize the parent they are very likely to receive no bills for those services, in spite of the fact that the total cost for hospitalizing the patient for even 3 days is probably very similar to 20 therapy visits.

This bias in the system of insuring mental health treatment—providing free (or inexpensive) hospital care but erecting financial barriers against outpatient care—is most explicit in private insurance programs. In a university we know well, for example, the overall insurance program provides all the costs of going to a general MD for any physical problem, and all of the cost of going to a mental hospital for up to

120 days. However, the program until recently has provided only 50% of the cost for going to a psychotherapist, and none of the first $200 of such costs.

We note also that this bias in insurance incentives carries an unintended message to the consumers of services (or their relatives) when contemplating alternative forms of care. In the process of offering different incentives, differential credibility of the services is inadvertently communicated as well. If an insurance company (or the government) says it will pay all of treatment A and only half of treatment B, then the message is inescapable that the company feels that treatment A is more effective and preferred. In this example, A is hospitalization and B is outpatient or other alternative care. It is true that outpatient care is not preferred by insurance companies. However, other data suggest that it is more effective. In many cases, perhaps all, cost and perceived effectiveness work together in the patient's mind to lead him or her to choose the objectively less efficacious treatment alternative. For example, Zook, Moore, and Zeckhauser (1981) cite a California Medicaid study in which a charge of only $1.00 per physician visit decreased those visits and increased hospital services which remained free. If $1 can have that sort of effect, consider what the $500 difference in our example above could produce in the behavior of potential patients or their custodial relatives.

Summary

The cost of a day of inpatient care for a mental patient continues to rise in all sites. The rise has been quite sharp even in constant dollars. However, in all sites but one, the length of stay has decreased sufficiently so that the cost of an episode has remained relatively constant.

This is not the case in the general hospital where length of stay has been constant, but the cost per day has increased very sharply, well in excess of the cost of living, or the cost of other health services.

The general hospital also has had a dramatic effect on total direct costs. From a fairly trivial program in 1965, the general hospital now accounts for over 30% of total inpatient direct costs for the country as a whole, and we project that a rise to over 50% is possible.

Notes

1. Three and a half billion dollars due to death, $7.4 billion to disability and $3.2 billion due to "patient-care activities."

2. We use the term "cost per stay" rather than "cost per episode," because the latter is often used by others to mean the cost of all inpatient days divided by the number of episodes.

3. We use the terms "cost" and "expenditures" interchangeably, for purposes of this presentation.

4. This technique probably overestimates the inflation rate somewhat. Frank and Kamlet (1985) report a real growth rate (over inflation) of 1.7% per year for mental health costs, compared to 3.6% for health care.

5. We really do not know the cost per day in a separate psychiatric unit in 1980. In previous years we calculated it by dividing total expenditures by the number of inpatient days. (This is a slight overestimate given that total expenditures include some outpatient services.) However, between 1977 and 1980 the reported inpatient days increased 27%, while the expenditures almost tripled. Dividing expenditures by days would result in a cost/day that was about 70% higher in constant dollars, while the nonspecific cost/day in general hospitals only increased 7% in constant dollars. We suspect that the reclassification of former CMHCs with general hospital services substantially increased the outpatient component of total expenditures. Therefore, we assumed the same increase in cost per day for inpatient units as nonunits (7% in constant dollars).

6. Recall that these estimates are based on differences in LoS between psychiatric and general VA hospitals, rather than bed sections. However, they are probably not far off.

7. Medicaid and Medicare are substantial supporters of inpatient mental health care. They are also very complicated programs and we have included some detailed description of them in Appendix 11-A, page 228.

APPENDIX 11-A

THE MEDICARE AND MEDICAID PROGRAMS

The purpose of this appendix is to give a more detailed description of the relevant aspects of the two largest public health insurance programs—Medicare and Medicaid.[1]

The Social Security Act

An array of programs designed to assist the aged, poor, and disabled were created under the Social Security Act, which was enacted in 1935. It has been periodically amended; Medicare and Medicaid were major amendments in 1965. Medicare is Title XVIII of the Social Security Act, titled "Health Insurance for the Aged and Disabled." Medicaid is Title XIX, "Grants to States for Medical Assistance Programs."

These programs, administered by the Health Care Financing Administration (HCFA), are quite different from each other. All those aged 65 and over who are entitled to monthly Social Security checks are eligible for Medicare coverage, as are those who meet the Social Security criteria for disability (which includes psychiatric disability). In 1980 90% of Medicare enrollees were age 65 or over and 10% were disabled. The aged enrollees received 87% of the reimbursements, and the disabled received 13%. Medicare is not the only health insurance held by the majority of the elderly; 65% also have private insurance, and 10% have both Medicare and Medicaid coverage, but no other insurance.

Medicaid is actually 54 different programs; 49 states, Washington, DC, and four territories have a program.[2] The federal government shares the cost with the states of providing medical care for certain categories of poor people. The federal share varies according to the states' per capita income and ranges from 50% to 78%. The states are required by statute to provide certain services under Medicaid; other services are optional. States also have some discretion in setting copayments and deductibles. This state by state variation makes it difficult to summarize any particular kind of coverage, as we will attempt to do for mental health benefits.

Medicare and Medicaid differ in terms of the types and amounts of health care reimbursed. Medicare funds primarily acute care; inpatient short-stay hospital care accounted for almost two-thirds of its reimbursements in 1980. However, Medicaid payments for inpatient hospital services accounted for only 28%, while payments for long-term care in nursing homes (both skilled and intermediate) absorbed 43% of Medicaid payments in 1980 (Health Care Financing Administration, 1983). Medicaid's support of long-term care is primarily for the aged: 72% of skilled nursing facility service recipients were aged, and 80% of intermediate care facility service recipients were aged in 1980. The expense of such long-term care is reflected in the distribution showing that only 15% of Medicaid recipients were aged in 1984, but they received 37% of the payments. In contrast, children and adults eligible for Medicaid under Aid to Families with Dependent Children (AFDC) comprised 72% of recipients in 1984 but accounted for only 25% of the total payments. A more detailed description of these programs follows.

Medicare

COVERAGE AND LIMITATIONS

Medicare consists of two parts: Hospital Insurance (Part A) and Supplementary Medical Insurance (Part B). Part A is an entitlement program; all persons over the age of 65 may receive these benefits. Part B is an optional program in which beneficiaries may enroll by paying a monthly premium. The distinction between Parts A and B is essentially between services provided as part of an inpatient stay in a hospital or skilled nursing home (Part A) and those provided by a physician or providers authorized by the physician (Part B). The difference between Part A and Part B is not simply inpatient versus outpatient categories used in the mental health literature, because physicians are reimbursed for their services under Part B whether provided in the hospital or not. There are four parts to Part A: (1) inpatient hospital services, which cover all services typically received while an inpatient, such as room and board, nursing services, drugs, and supplies; a 190-day lifetime limit for psychiatric hospital stays is also included; (2) limited coverage for stays in skilled nursing homes; (3) certain home health services; and (4) a hospice benefit option. The first two are described below.

Coverage for *inpatient hospital* care is 90 days during any benefit period. A benefit period begins on the first day of hospitalization and ends 60 consecutive days after discharge. Therefore, a benefit period can consist of more than one hospitalization, but there must be at least 60 days without hospitalization between benefit periods.

Hospital coverage is not without cost to the beneficiary, who must pay an "inpatient hospital deductible" (IHD) at the beginning of each benefit period. The deductible is about the cost of one day in a hospital; the IHD was $304 in 1983, 83% of the $368 average cost per day in non-federal general hospitals (American Hospital Association, 1984). In 1986 the deductible was $492 (unpublished data from HCFA), meaning the beneficiary must pay all charges up to $492, and Medicare pays the balance of the bill. In addition, the beneficiary must pay coinsurance for each day in the hospital after the 60th day. The inpatient daily coinsurance is one quarter the deductible, or $123 in 1986.[3]

When the beneficiary uses up the 90 hospital days in a benefit period, he or she can use up to 60 more lifetime reserve days. The coinsurance for each reserve day is one-half the inpatient hospital deductible, or $246 in 1986.

The psychiatric hospital benefit limitation (a lifetime limit of 190 days) does not apply to psychiatric care in general hospitals, regardless of whether or not the care is in a psychiatric unit. This limitation could act as an incentive for beneficiaries to seek care in general hospitals rather than psychiatric hospitals.[4] Medicare can pay for all services in *skilled nursing facilities* (SNF) for up to 100 days in a benefit period, if the patient meets skilled level of care criteria. The beneficiary must have been hospitalized for 3 consecutive days and the transfer to a SNF must be within 30 days of discharge. Costs for the first 20 days are fully reimbursable, after which the beneficiary pays daily coinsurance equal to one-eighth the hospital deductible, or $61.50 in 1986.

Covered services under Supplementary Medical Insurance (Part B) are those provided by a physician and those "incident to" or furnished in conjunction with his or her services. Services performed directly by a physician can be provided in any setting, e.g., as part of a hospital stay, in a nursing home, through the outpatient department of a hospital, as a home visit, in a private office, or community health center. However, services furnished "incident to" a physician, and not in an institutional setting, must be authorized and supervised by the physician. The physician must essentially employ any nonphysicians who provide services to Medicare beneficiaries. This arrangement seriously limits the coverage for mental health services, given that services such as psychotherapy can be supplied by nonphysicians, such as psychologists and clinical social workers. Nonphysician suppliers cannot bill Medicare directly for nearly all outpatient services, and can only be paid for them through the physician's direct billing. The only exception for mental health care is for diagnostic testing by a psychologist. These services must also be authorized by a physician, but the psychologist may bill Medicare directly for them.

Part B services are reimbursed at 80%; the beneficiary pays 20% of all charges after a deductible. The annual deductible has been $75 since 1982; the beneficiary pays all charges up to $75 each year and 20% of all charges thereafter. The Supplementary Medical Insurance program also has a monthly premium of $15.50 in 1986.

Before the change to a prospective payment system in 1983,[5] ancillary services could be reimbursed under Part B whether the beneficiary was in a hospital or not. Now, all services provided to hospitalized patients must be included under Part A, except those personally provided by a physician. Therefore, services "incident to" a physician, and other medical services provided by any nonphysician professional, are now "bundled" into Part A coverage if the person is hospitalized (Uyeda & Moldawsky, 1986). Although the physician must still authorize and supervise these services, the Medicare patient no longer pays the 20% copayment generally required for Part B services.

Nonphysician providers of services to hospitalized patients must now arrange to be paid by the hospital. This also applies to those who could formerly bill Medicare directly for certain services, such as psychologists doing diagnostic testing. Services incident to a physician (and other medical services) remain subject to applicable Part B deductibles and copayments when delivered outside a hospital, as before prospective reimbursement.

Reimbursement for outpatient mental health services is limited to $250 a year and, in effect, requires 50% coinsurance. After the deductible of $75, a person could purchase up to $500 of outpatient care and have half of it paid for.[6]

The $250 limit applies to outpatient mental health services, regardless of what type of physician provides them. Therefore, general practitioners treating, for example, depression with psychotropic drugs, would be subject to the $250 limit, if they billed for the services appropriately. This creates an incentive for nonpsychiatrist physicians to mislabel mental disorder diagnoses so as to avoid the $250 limit.

It is not clear how the respective inpatient and outpatient deductibles, coinsurance, and limits influence the decision to hospitalize. Although mental-health services are subject to less cost sharing when provided in a hospital, the patient is faced with a large deductible. Empirical evidence is not available on the impact that "bundling" Part B services has on the provision of mental health services to hospitalized patients. Anecdotal information suggests that hospitals are reluctant to provide any service that is not considered essential for patient care or does not show a clear cost saving.

As we saw from Chapter 9 on alternative care, ambulatory care is only one form of nonhospital care. Someone who is a typical candidate for hospital admission, but is not admitted in favor of appropriate and available alternative care, would presumably receive a range of services, such as those in a halfway house or a day hospital program. Medicare creates an incentive for hospitalization to the extent that alternative services, such as these, are not covered under Part B as "medically necessary" services. Services provided by nonphysicians are not themselves subject to the $250 annual limit, but physician charges, which are subject to the $250 limit, would have to be billed at some point, in order to show active involvement of the physician. Once the limit is met for physician charges, the "incident to" services are no longer covered. As part of a cost containment effort, HCFA is closely scrutinizing the use of Medicare payments for certain psychosocial rehabilitation services, including day treatment (Mental Health Reports, July 31, 1985). This effort will likely make Medicare coverage for any form of alternative care more difficult.

Medicaid

COVERAGE AND LIMITATIONS

Medicaid provides medical care to the "categorically needy," those who are low income as well as being aged, blind, disabled, or children in families with only one parent capable of support (i.e., the other parent is absent, dead, or incapacitated). The federal government shares the cost for these programs with the states. A person's eligibility for Aid to Families with Dependent Children (AFDC) and Supplemental Security Income (SSI),[7] two cash welfare programs under the Social Security Act, includes automatic eligibility for Medicaid.[8] In addition, the states can offer Medicaid to the "medically needy," those who cannot afford large medical bills, but whose income is too high to qualify for cash benefits.

The Social Security Act requires the states to offer the following mandatory services:

- inpatient hospital services (except in institutions for mental disease)[9]
- outpatient hospital services
- laboratory and X-ray services

- skilled nursing facilities for those 21 and over (except in institutions for mental disease)
- home health care (for those eligible for skilled nursing facility services)
- physician services
- family planning services
- rural health clinic services
- early and periodic screening, diagnosis, and treatment (EPSDT) services for children (under 21)
- services by a nurse-midwife where legally authorized

However, the states may limit the scope of coverage for any of these required services.

The states may also provide a number of optional services, which the federal government will share the cost of; those relevant to mental health care are listed below:[10]

- clinic services: services furnished to outpatients by or under the direction of a physician or dentist in a facility that is not part of a hospital
- prescribed drugs

and various services in different types of institutions, as follows:

- services for those aged 65 or older in institutions for mental disease: inpatient hospital, skilled nursing facility, and intermediate care facility services
- intermediate care facility (ICF) services (except in institutions for mental disease)
- ICF services in institutions for the mentally retarded
- inpatient psychiatric service for those age 21 and under
- skilled nursing facility (SNF) services for under age 21

The major optional and mandatory services that apply to mental health care are physician services, outpatient hospital services, clinic services, and all of the institutional services. The categories of institutional services are confusing, because hospital, skilled nursing, and intermediate care services can all be provided in institutions for mental disease (IMDs), as well as in general care hospitals, SNFs, and ICFs. However, services provided in IMDs are classified as IMD services, and an IMD is typically reimbursed at either the hospital, SNF, or ICF level of care. In other words, SNF services provided in a general care SNF are SNF services, but they are IMD services when provided in a SNF-level IMD.

In summarizing the institutional services reimbursed by Medicaid, the age of recipient is a critical factor. Services in institutions for mental disease are reimbursed only for people under age 21 and age 65 and over. However, services in general hospitals, skilled nursing facilities, and intermediate care facilities may be reimbursed for all ages.

In addition to limits on the amount or duration of services, states can impose restrictions by requiring prior authorization or other kinds of review procedures to assure that the service is "medically necessary." This is a state-level determination, and varies accordingly.

We saw that Medicare limits long-term mental health care by imposing a 190-day lifetime limit on psychiatric specialty hospitals, by not funding intermediate care facilities, and by limiting skilled nursing facilities to 100 days per benefit period (with coinsurance of one-eighth the hospital deductible beginning on the 21st day). However, these are precisely the long-term care services that Medicaid can choose to pay for within applicable limits.

In 1984, 44% of Medicaid funds were spent on SNF and ICF services and an additional 29% paid for inpatient hospital services, for both general and mental health care. The expense of institutional care is illustrated by the fact that the 44% of payments for SNF and ICF services were spent on only 7% of the recipients. When inpatient hospital services are included, 26% of the recipients accounted for 73% of Medicaid expenditures. As we saw in Chapter 1, about 80% of Medicaid mental health expenditures were spent on institutional care.

STATE VARIATION IN MENTAL HEALTH COVERAGE

It is not unexpected that expenditures for inpatient care would be disproportionately high, relative to the number of recipients, given the high cost of institutional care and long nursing home stays. However, it is possible that the structure of Medicaid reimbursement encourages institutionalizaton, and to some extent, contributes to these disproportionate expenditures.

Unlike private insurance plans and Medicare, the copayments in Medicaid are almost exclusively for drug prescriptions and are nominal amounts of about $1.00. In 1983, 16 states had copayments for prescriptions (Clinkscale, McCue, Fisher, & Hyatt, 1983) and only 7 states had copayments for clinic or outpatient hospital services.[11] Therefore, copayments are unlikely to operate as an incentive for hospitalization by requiring more out-of-pocket payment for outpatient care.

Toff (1984) studied state variation in mental health services covered under Medicaid, by asking state offices to describe their programs as of

January 1984. A comparison of inpatient and outpatient benefits for both general health and mental health care would be necessary for a full analysis of whether certain categories had more generous benefits than others. Although the Toff study did not systematically report the limits in each of these categories, it provides the best available evidence on Medicaid funded mental health service provision. The limits on reimbursed services for the following categories were observed: IMDs, general hospital inpatient, hospital outpatient, physician, and clinic services.

Limitations on services were not usually specific to mental health treatment, but applied to all diagnoses. For example, only 8 states specifically limited outpatient hospital services for mental health care in some way. However, about 30 states had some type of limit on hospital outpatient services in general. Likewise, more states limited physician services in general than specifically limited physician visits for mental health care.

All but 6 states reimbursed IMDs at some level in 1984.[12] Of the 42 that did, 39 reimbursed at the hospital level of care and 23 of these also reimbursed at the ICF or SNF level of care. Of the 39 states providing hospital services in IMDs, slightly more than half had no limit. The most common type of limit was prior authorization or a requirement for some kind of utilization review. Twenty-seven states and Washington, D.C. provided inpatient psychiatric services for individuals under 21, either with or without some type of limitation or review requirement.

The most frequent limits on general hospital, outpatient, physician, and clinic services were on the number of days in a general hospital and the number of physician, outpatient, or clinic visits. (Limits include those specific to mental health, as well as those that apply to all diagnoses.) The frequency distributions of the number of states having these limits were similar for general hospital, outpatient, and physician services. About 30%–40% indicated a limit; about 20%–25% limited the service, providing more subject to review; about 15% required some kind of review before providing the service; and about 25%–35% had no limit indicated. For clinic services, about 40% of the states indicated no limit, and about 25% of the states had a limit.[13]

A problem with inferring availability of services from stated limits is that limits and guidelines do not necessarily indicate actual service provision. Two states with the same stated limits may in fact fund different amounts of services by applying prior authorization or utilization review differently. For example, two states may have the same limit on the number of physician visits but may differ in how liberally prior authorization is granted. Similarly, mental health services may not be deemed "medically necessary" as frequently as general health services are.

Expenditures for hospitalization might be related to allowable coverage for outpatient care; the proportion that a state spends on mental hospitalization might be inversely related to the availability of outpatient services. However, analysis of this hypothesis is hampered by lack of data on actual availability and utilization of services. Also, national Medicaid expenditure data, collected by HCFA, do not separate mental health payments from general health, except for payments made to IMDs. Therefore, estimates for mental health care in general hospitals and in outpatient settings would be needed.

With the provision of Section 2176 waivers, under the Omnibus Budget Reconciliation Act of 1981, empirical data could be forthcoming to explore the relationship between expenditures on institutional care and the availability of alternative care for the treatment of mental disorders. These waivers allow Medicaid reimbursement for a variety of nonmedical services (e.g., case management, respite care, homemaker services) that could be used as cost-effective alternatives to institutional care.

Notes

1. The discussions on Medicare and Medicaid in this Appendix are based on the following sources: Code of Federal Regulations, Title 42, 1984, *Social Security Bulletin Annual Statistical Supplement 1983* (Social Security Administration, 1984a), *Social Security Handbook* (Social Security Administration, 1984b), *The Medicare and Medicaid Data Book 1983* (Health Care Financing Administration, 1983), Wilson and Neuhauser, 1982. Health Care Financing Administration staff members were very helpful in clarifying the facts on which this discussion is based. We also thank Gail Toff and Mary Uyeda for their comments.

2. Arizona's program is unique and is not included in this discussion.

3. See the *Social Security Bulletin Annual Statistical Supplement, 1983,* for a trend table showing cost sharing since the beginning of the program.

4. In fact, a study (Cooper, 1969) comparing the number of discharges and days of care for psychiatric diagnoses in general hospitals (both with and without psychiatric units) during the 18 months before and after Medicare took effect showed that discharges increased for both those under and over age 65, but the percentage change was much higher for those over 65 (29% versus 1%).

5. As part of the Social Security Amendments (P.L. 28–91), hospitals are now paid at predetermined rates for each Medicare patient. The rate received is

based on the average cost of treating a patient in a particular diagnosis-related group (DRG).

6. Medicare payment for noninpatient mental health services is limited to 62.5% of reasonable charges, up to a maximum of $500; 62.5% of $500 is $312.50, and $312.50 minus 20% coinsurance leaves $250.

7. AFDC provides income to families with incomes below a certain level, as determined by state standards. SSI provides cash assistance to the aged, blind, and disabled, and states can supplement the basic federal SSI payment (Social Security Administration, 1984a).

8. However, 14 states choose the option allowing them to use more restrictive eligibility requirements for the aged, blind, and disabled.

9. Most institutions for mental disease (IMDs) are psychiatric hospitals. Some nursing homes are classified as IMDs, because their overall character is that of a facility that primarily provides mental health treatment.

10. See the Code of Federal Regulations (Title 42) or the *Medicare and Medicaid Data Book* for a complete list of optional services.

11. A few more had copayments for inpatient care.

12. The analysis of IMDs excludes Connecticut and West Virginia, the data of which were ambiguous.

13. Coverage of clinic services is particularly difficult to code validly, because one state may offer a broad range of services and limit a few, while another state may offer an unlimited amount of fewer services. In our rough coding scheme, states with limits on any service were grouped together.

CHAPTER 12

NEEDS FOR NEW KNOWLEDGE

In the previous chapters we have presented, discussed, and reanalyzed the national data regarding mental hospitalization and our de facto mental health policy. We began by reviewing the trends in statistics on hospitalization and then considered the effectiveness of alternative forms of treatment and aftercare. The last Chapter (11) analyzed the direct expenditures for mental hospitalization. The purpose of this chapter is to crystalize some policy issues surrounding hospitalization by exploring policy-relevant research areas.

Our discussion here is limited to policy issues in mental hospitalization, rather than the more general area of mental health. We specifically focus on the gaps in knowledge which, if filled, would immediately allow us to design a better overall system of service delivery—to develop better mental health policy. We also look at existing data that have been insufficiently integrated into national policy.

Alternative Services and Volunteer Groups

In addition to hospitalization and the fee-for-service system of outpatient care, a huge, largely informal and unconnected network of services exists. Assuming that noninstitutionalization could be implemented on a larger scale, tracking and evaluating this network becomes very important.

Although terms and definitions vary considerably in the literature, one might categorize these services, in decreasing order of formality, as the community support system,[1] alternative services, and volunteer programs.

The community support system includes formal and funded mechanisms to expand culturally sensitive services, to multiply effects of professional and institutional services, to help bridge public and private systems of care across such areas as justice, health, and social services, and to lessen the impact of deinstitutionalizing patients (e.g., Johnson, 1983). It would include such service-oriented projects as the consultation and education services delivered by CMHCs; the work of professionals in the care of the chronic patient in the community (Budson, 1978); and such special projects as, for example, the discharge patient advocacy project of the Mental Health Association of Essex County, New Jersey, which actively links persons discharged into the community to other resources and services (Christmas, 1978). In this definition, the major intent of such programs is to expand the existing care of individuals in the community and to link up systems of care. They tend to be federally funded.

The Community Support Program (CSP) is the major federal effort in this area (Love, 1984). For the CSP, NIMH awarded contracts to states to stimulate the development of local sytems of community support. The CSP has always been modestly funded: Between 1978–1984, only $42 million was provided from federal funds. For several years, the Reagan Administration reduced this budget to zero, and only a concentrated effort by an interorganizational group of citizens and professionals has saved it. The intent of the CSP has always been to use a small amount of federal funds to leverage a larger commitment by the states.

Consistent with the amount of funds invested, the outcomes of the Program have been modest. Some states have increased support funding substantially, along with some better integration with other federal agencies (e.g., HUD); a few states have integrated the community support model into state mental health plans, and about a third have made the chronically mentally ill a priority group. However, for the most part this Program—originally a good idea, we think—had the worst of timing. It got underway just about as the Reagan Administration implemented its austerity views of social programs (see Love, 1984, for a recent review).

One of the reasons we define community support systems more formally than most writers in this area is that they then are part and parcel of the national mental health policy. As such, the descriptive parameters of the system should be thoroughly outlined; its epidemiological aspects studied in detail; and its psychological impact studied in the comparative sense (versus other services), in the absolute sense (whether any impact at all), with due attention to cost efficiency.

There are frequently evaluations of specific demonstration projects in the more general community support system. However, there is seldom any detailed look at the policy potential of a project in the sense of attempting to evaluate the project for widespread national use. "Middle-level testing," research in that large area between demonstration and national projection, is almost nonexistent. Nor is there any comparative evaluation (the impact of one set of services versus another, including what Kiesler [1973] once referred to as the "bargain basement alternative,") or evaluation of the cost efficiency of such projects. There is a great deal of research regarding bits and pieces of the community support system, but only a very small proportion, if any, is directly related to policy issues.

Alternative services are substitutes for other services that might otherwise be expected or delivered. Several of these alternatives, which were experimentally tested, were reviewed in Chapter 9. Care after hospitalization, depending exactly on how it is conducted, could fit the definition of either alternative services or community support systems (e.g., Budson, 1978). Careful scientific investigation of either group of services is sparse (but see Rose, 1979; and Taber, 1980 for reviews). There are evaluations of particular sets of services, but they tend to be demonstrations rather than fulfillments of careful scientific criteria. Evaluation research in this area has been underfunded and most evaluations do not meet minimal scientific criteria for either (1) assessing the absolute impact of a particular service (compared to no treatment), or (2) comparing one instance of service delivery with other ones (a comparative assessment).

Community support systems and alternative care are two primary mechanisms for expanding the potential of service delivery to large populations. As such, they need to be investigated very carefully, not only with an eye to their absolute efficacy, but also comparing alternative strategies of delivering such services. In particular, cost-benefit analyses of these services are needed that specifically address the question of developing such services for a national system of service delivery (Schulberg, 1979).

Volunteer groups providing services to people with mental problems are a potentially great national resource, but relatively uninvestigated (but see Silverman, 1978; Lieberman & Borman, 1976; Christmas, 1978). These volunteer groups are often composed of ex-patients and, for a variety of reasons, unsympathetic to more traditional modes of care. We include here both self-help groups and volunteers who devote time to helping others. Some of the groups include what might be called mutual aid; that is, people with the same problem attempting to help each other. Others might be called sequential aid; a person who had a particular mental problem but who is much improved, now attempts to help others with the same problem.

The PCMH estimates that there are 500,000 self-help groups in the country. They specifically draw attention to the National Association for Retarded Citizens, with 1,300 local units and more than 130,000 members, and Alcoholics Anonymous, with over 750,000 members worldwide. Indeed, there is a self-help group for almost every imaginable mental health problem. These groups treat a variety of people who might otherwise come under a more formal system of care, such as parents who abuse their children, drug and alcohol abusers, the suicide prone, discharged patients, and parents of schizophrenic patients. Other groups include people with perhaps equally important problems who might not as often come under a formal mental health system of care, such as some veterans, families of prisoners, widows, old people, and women who have had mastectomies. Many of these groups are very action oriented, focusing on changing public attitudes and policies. The groups are often very uncooperative, and view outsiders in general as being unsympathetic to their goals. Their cooperation in research is, therefore, difficult to obtain. Observational research is one obvious method to use. Such research, however, is highly technical in nature, and not at all easy to do.

We need to know more about the demographic and sociological characteristics of such groups, even as a preliminary step. On the other hand, our ultimate interest is in learning about the effectiveness of such groups in ameliorating mental health problems. Consequently, outcome research is needed, but the careful detail needed in such research is typically difficult to come by when the organization being studied is loosely organized. Such groups need to be evaluated both as a substitute for other services and as a potential expansion of such services. For example, one would like to know whether psychotherapeutic intervention interferes with or facilitates the impact of such groups (and if it facilitates, whether the effect is additive or multiplicative). This implies a detailed personal history of people involved in the group, which frequently would be nearly impossible to obtain. Further, these groups are indeed volunteer groups, which raises some basic scientific problems in studying them. Typically, an individual who is a member of a voluntary self-help group is a person who acknowledges the problem, is seeking help from others, and views himself or herself as being helped. Of course, acknowledging one has a particular mental problem is often a significant step in ameliorating the problem.

The major scientific issue in studying such groups is self-selection. A person who does not believe that the group will be at least somewhat helpful, will not join. A person who joins a group and feels that the group is not effective, will drop out. There are few barriers to dropping out of such groups, surely less than the barriers against dropping out of psychotherapy, for example, or a mental institution. Knowledge of the degree of such self-selection is an important ingredient in assessing the effectiveness of a voluntary self-help group. At minimum, this means studying the group over time so that the dropout rate could be estimated, and its potential impact on outcome data assessed.

Aside from self-help groups, there is enormous potential in volunteer groups. Sainer (1976) has described the RSVP program (Retired Senior Volunteer Program) begun 20 years ago by a private social agency. Today more than 700 RSVP programs exist, with 165,000 volunteers. A similar program, the federally funded foster grandparents program, included at last estimate 16,000 older people, each of whom was willing to spend 20 hours a week working with deinstitutionalized younger patients. The potential of such programs is enormous, although relatively unexplored. Evaluation research oriented toward outcome effectiveness in these programs would be very valuable. In addition, the potential of such individuals for further practical training and handling of mental health problems is also relatively unexplored. That is, one must distinguish between the current effectiveness of such groups (which surely must be substantial), and the potential effectiveness of such groups were public policy to place emphasis on them as potential service providers.

Issues in Alternative Care

We have previously indicated that the best studies done show that alternative care is more effective and less expensive than hospitalization. That general conclusion seems warranted by the scientific evidence available, but there are a host of questions unanswered and unaddressed by that scientific evidence that are important for responsible public policy. Some of them relate more generally to the care of the mentally disabled. For example, consider the question of appropriate training of nonprofessional personnel. Alternative care models and the work of Gordon Paul suggest that nonprofessionals in traditional inpatient settings are typically not well trained and their efforts are not coordinated toward overall treatment goals. Recall, in Paul and Lentz (1977) that there was extensive and detailed training given the nonprofessionals both in how to treat those back ward patients and how to monitor their own behavior in the treatment process. Recall, from the work of Stein and Test, (1980, 1982), that they employ extensive training procedures for their nonprofessional personnel. Those personnel often work along with the patient in a new job, or will come into the job setting when the patient experiences problems or has difficulty coping with changes. Their nonprofessional personnel are out in the community helping the patient, teaching them how to make change, take buses, get to care centers, and the like. One wonders how effective traditional hospital care might be if there were such extensive and detailed training during the course of hospitalization and after. One further wonders what the appropriate mix of professional and nonprofessional personnel is in any care of the seriously mentally disabled. The degree and type of mix has not been an independent variable in research. However, one is struck by the critical importance and centrality of nonprofessional personnel to effective care of the mentally disordered.

Some of the resistance to alternative care and its proper funding is related to potential abuses in the system. In essence, one can have custodial care in a halfway house or in an alternative care program, in theory at least, as well as one can have it in a state hospital. The question is how to ensure that third-party payment is being used for a specific and effective care. A recent review by the Health Care Financing Administration of Medicare payments for mental health care alleged that Medicare was "paying for clients playing Trivial Pursuit" (Mental Health Reports, July 31, 1985). It is true that any public program must have oversight of expenditures and their propriety. That oversight is more difficult to accomplish outside a hospital than inside. Effective programmatic means of doing so could play an important role in the implementation of alternative care mechanisms.

Components of successful alternative care programs. Bachrach (1983c) has reviewed the alternative care literature and the model programs for the care of the chronically mentally ill. From this literature she has extracted what she feels are the main planning principles that run through successful programs. First, she feels that precision in goals and objectives is necessary, including defining carefully the target population in any particular program. Second, she mentions interagency cooperation and linkage. "Resource linkage is essential for integrating service delivery, for avoiding duplication of services, for controlling or reducing service delivery cost and for attacking turf-related opposition to specific program initiatives" (p. 96). Third, she stresses that individual treatment is necessary, enhancing the patients' skill development and emphasizing the patients' potential and capabilities. Last, she decribes information needs as a planning principle. These needs relate to the characteristics and service requirements of individual patients; data assessing program effectiveness; and data on the assessment of the impact of the treatment.

Bachrach has extracted these from her reading of the literature on successful model programs for the alternative treatment of the seriously mentally ill. On the other hand, as we have noted in Chapter 9, there has not been extensive variation in the types of model programs that have been attempted. That is, the existing literature is heavily tilted toward social rehabilitation and competence building. While there is theoretical justification for such programs being effective, these do not exhaust the possibilities for alternative programs. Thus, Bachrach's principles are extrapolations from a biased subset of programs. They help us build upon those programs, but they should not be taken to mean that those are the only principles possible for effective alternative care programs. Indeed, much research is needed on the components of effective alternative programs in order to enhance the effectiveness of the existing ones.

Effectiveness of Psychotherapy

At least two major reviews of the effectiveness of psychotherapy have appeared. One is the paper on efficacy and cost-effectiveness of psychotherapy prepared by Leonard Saxe (1980) for the Office of Technology Assessment (see also Yates & Newman, 1981). This paper is recommended to the reader and includes a bibliography of over 300 entries. It concludes (p. 5) that,

> in summary, OTA finds that psychotherapy is a complex—yet scientifically assessable—set of technologies. It also finds good evidence of psychotherapy's positive effects. Although therapy may not be generalizable to the wide range of problems for which therapy is employed, it suggests that additional research may provide data useful for the development of mental health policy. Given the potential net benefits of psychotherapy, this effort would seem to be justified.

The other major review of psychotherapy outcomes is the meta-analysis provided by Smith and Glass (1977), and later expanded in book form by Smith, et al. (1980). Meta-analysis is an extremely useful technique for psychological studies related to public policy.[2] It derives quantitative measures in a manner that can be aggregated across studies. Specific measures are referred to as effect sizes, which are derived by calculating the difference between the mean of an experimental group and the mean of a control group for each measure in a given study, divided by the standard deviation of the control group. In this manner, the effect of the experimental manipulation for a specific study is represented as the number of standard deviations separating the means of the two groups. Their meta-analysis of 475 controlled studies of psychotherapy (with 766 effect-size measures), led to an average finding of effect size of 0.85. This means that in the typical experimental study comparing psychotherapy with no treatment, the average patient after therapy had responses sufficiently positive to be at the 80th percentile of the control group. Thus, a consistent, clear effect of psychotherapy was noted. Exactly what this means for public policy is unclear since it is difficult to state clearly how desirable it is to be at the 80 percentile of the control group (Kiesler, 1981a). We note that the effect sizes themselves are considered as if they were independent in this analysis. However, when each study is considered to have only one effect size, similar but slightly stronger results were found (Landman & Dawes, 1982; see also Glass et al., 1981).

There are major policy questions regarding psychotherapy, even if acknowledged to be effective as demonstrated by Smith et al., or cost-effective as discussed by Saxe. These include: the marginal utility of psychotherapy, when added to a system of existing services (Kiesler, 1980); comparative or summative effects of psychotherapy compared to drug therapy (Smith et al., 1980); the effects of adding psychotherapy to the existing system of health care (Jones & Vischi, 1980); the cost-effectiveness of psychotherapy when compared to such things as prevention (Albee & Joffe, 1977); the moral hazard of insuring psychotherapy, since many fear that, if insured, almost everyone will undertake therapy (McGuire, 1981); and the question of how best to integrate psycho-therapy into an organized system of mental health care (Budman, 1981; Cummings & VandenBos, 1979; Albee & Kessler, 1977). Each of these issues will be raised later in this chapter.

The Effectiveness of Drugs

In policy considerations, drugs as an integral component of mental health services are a tantalizing alternative. When considering potential public policy in mental health it is conceptually easier to consider giving millions of drug dosages than to consider either, say, a community mental health center within the reach of everyone needing the service, or 16 hours of traditional psychotherapy per patient. Given the number of general physicians in the country, there are more people trained to give drugs than there are people to give therapy, and it does not require the consideration of the training of a great new cadre of service providers. As one hears this policy alternative discussed at a national level, one presumably only has to train physicians to recognize symptoms specific to diagnostic categories, with instructions of which drugs to use for which categories. To some extent this describes what we do now nation-ally. Indeed one national survey found 31% of Americans admitted using a psychotherapeutic drug in the previous year (Mellinger, Balter, Parry, Manheimer, & Cisin, 1974; also see Hingson, Matthews, & Scotch, 1979).

The average general practitioner in the United States sees more patients with mental disorders than does the average psychiatrist (Regier et al., 1978), although the time spent with each patient is dramatically different. Nonpsychiatric physicians are four times as likely as psychiatrists to use drugs in treatment of psychiatric cases. There is considerable variation among general physicians with respect to prescribing drugs. Some use them with almost everybody with a mental disorder, while others are very sparing in their usage (Gillis & Moran, 1981). In a study of antipsychotic drug use in nursing homes, the size of the physician's nursing home practice had a powerful effect on prescriptive practices. The 14% of physicians with the largest practices prescribed 81% of the antipsychotic medication, and were disproportionately family practitioners (Ray, Federspiel, & Schaffner, 1980). Drug prescriptions apparently allowed those physicians to expand their practices.

Effectiveness equal, the policy advantages of drugs in the treatment of mental disorders are: simplicity of the policy itself and the ease with which it can be communicated to decision makers and the public; the ease of access of people needing treatment to service providers, since potentially the whole network of nonpsychiatric physicians could be utilized; training of service providers is simplified since diagnosis could be emphasized rather than detailed treatment methods; more people could be treated, since the time necessary to treat each one would be sharply reduced if other treatment were not necessary; the cyclical valleys in the long-term progression of a mental disorder could presumably be reduced by occasional reinstatement of a drug regimen; and patients do not have to be monitored as closely, perhaps, as with more traditional psychotherapeutic treatment.

One can see why policymakers are so enthusiastic about the potential for drugs and why federal agencies often tout them. Policy questions directly relate to whether or not the advantages listed above are in fact empirically valid. Further, in the implementation of such a policy, one would have to be very concerned about typical conditions under which the drug may be used rather than the optimal conditions. Indeed, there is a lively controversy in the literature in reviews of outcome studies of drugs in mental health services, about which studies should be included in the review and which not. People can review essentially the same literature but have quite different arrays of studies from which conclusions are drawn. An interesting exception to this is the meta-analysis carried out by Smith et al. (1980) on drug research, which includes studies of drugs versus controls or comparison treatments, and a separate group of studies in which both drugs and psychotherapy were included in the experimental design. In all, they included 151 papers in their meta-analysis. Overall, they found the effect size for studies of drugs-only was approximately equal to psychotherapy-only. Considerable caution must be applied since the studies may be qualitatively different, particularly with respect to the use of placebos in the drug studies (as Smith et al., 1980, point out).

Of specific interest to us are the studies that included both drug therapy and psychotherapy separately or in combinations, with a proper experimental design. These results are really quite startling. In looking only at studies that include such conditions, the effects of drugs alone are approximately equal to the effects of psychotherapy alone. The two treatments, moreover, do not interact. That is, the effects of drugs and psychotherapy used in combination are equal to the additive effects of them used in isolation. The notion, for example, that drugs can be used for psychotics in order to get them to the point where psychotherapy would be more effective is not supported by these data. If that were the case then a clear interaction would be obtained: The effects of drugs plus psychotherapy would be more than the sum of their effects alone. Smith et al. do a very detailed and convincing analysis that demonstrates, at least for these studies, that such an interaction simply does not exist.

Smith et al. further analyze their data with respect to individual drugs within the categories of antipsychotics, antidepressants, and antianxiety agents. Within categories of disorders they did not find great variation in effect *among* the types of drugs, although there is some considerable variation *within* type of drug. Take antipsychotic drugs for example. On the basis of these data, one could not say that chlorpromazine was more effective in the studies in which it was used than, say, reserpine or lithium, irrespective of category of mental disorder.

The Smith et al. meta-analysis of drug studies and drug plus psychotherapy studies are probably the best evidence regarding the policy implications of drug use with mental disorders. The results suggest very clearly that more caution should be used about drug therapy in general, and specific drugs in particular, than has been the case. For example, there is no evidence in these studies that lithium is anything like the magic cure it is often touted to be (although the number of effect sizes in this study for lithium is very small).

On the other hand, although Smith et al. provide a fairly comprehensive review of the studies in which drugs and psychotherapy were used alone or in combination, their analysis of the drug-alone studies is but a sampling of the existing literature (of studies including both control conditions and random assignment). Needed is an exhaustive review of the literature of those studies, even though such an effort might be almost beyond the capacity of individual investigators to carry out. Meta-analysis of studies with only a particular drug appears to be less promising than one might otherwise think. Judging by the results of the effect sizes across drugs, there is some considerable danger in looking only at a specific drug used with a specific mental condition. It appears that one must look at all of the conditions for which a drug is used plus all of the other drugs that are used for those conditions as well.

Further, the more exhaustive number of studies is needed partly to obtain a more stable number of effect sizes with particular drugs in specific situations than the results of Smith et al. allow. Needed are detailed breakdowns of patient populations, including demographic characteristics that control a good deal of the variance in specific mental disorders, as well as institutions versus outpatient care, the specific institutional site, and the characteristics of the service provider (e.g., psychiatrist versus nonpsychiatric physician). Further, there is considerable evidence regarding relatively permanent negative side-effects of prolonged antipsychotic medication (e.g., Berger, 1978; American Psychiatric Association, 1980b). Measures of such side effects need to be included in evaluative studies of drug therapy. Use of meta-analysis has opened a new door to the assessment of drug effectiveness for mental disorders.

Relationship Between Physical and Mental Health

Goplerud (1981) reviews the literature indicating the coincidence of physical and mental health problems. He suggests (p. 59) that 30%–60% of medical patients in general hospitals and 50%–80% of medical patients treated by general practitioners have emotional problems sufficient "to pose problems in medical management." At the same time, psychiatric patients tend to have concurrent medical problems (we have already noted in Chapter 10 their elevated death rate). Goplerud estimates that 30%–50% of psychiatric inpatients and outpatients have significant physical disorders.[3]

Schwab et al. (1979) conducted a survey of a stratified community sample in one county in Florida. Based on self-report, they estimated 28% had emotional problems that could benefit from treatment, 39% had at least one physical illness, and 26% had psychosomatic conditions (e.g., hypertension, peptic ulcer, colitis, headaches). Interestingly, 10% of the sample reported all three types of disorders.

Koranyi (1972, 1979) twice studied consecutive admissions to a psychiatric clinic. About half the patients had major physical illnesses, and about half of these had not been detected by the referring source. Physicians—both psychiatric and nonpsychiatric—missed about one-third of physical illnesses in their referred patients. In both studies Koranyi found that for about 10% of the patients, a physical disorder was the sole cause of the patients' problem (most typically, diabetes).

A psychiatric disorder increased the chances of hospitalization for nonpsychiatric reasons. Browning, Miller, and Tyson (1974) followed up on patients receiving psychiatric emergency-room treatment. Six months later, their hospitalization rate for *nonpsychiatric* diagnoses was double than otherwise was expected. This confirms our point in other chapters that our data on costs and rates of mental hospitalization must be taken as conservative national estimates.

A substantial proportion of the patients psychiatrists and other mental health professionals see have fairly serious physical disorders, which go undetected. A substantial proportion of patients nonpsychiatric physicians see have fairly serious mental disorders, which go undetected.

This suggests a number of policy issues. The interrelationships between physical and mental disorders is not well understood and deserves considerable national attention. How their relationship affects cost of care, hospitalization (and readmission) rates, treatment efficacy and related programmatic needs is not well understood—for both somatic and psychological conditions. Yet rational national policies depend on such knowledge for both physical and mental health policy.

Consider, for example, the national reduction in total hospital inpatient days that we discussed in Chapter 6. We found that 98% of the total reduction in inpatient days for all disorders was specifically a reduction in inpatient days for mental disorders. Consider then another fact: The cost of health care nationally has risen far in excess of the inflation rate for decades. How much of that increase is due to untreated and undiagnosed mental disorders? Would that surprise us as much as the 98% above surprised us?

We do know some related facts. The majority of patients with mental disorders are treated by nonpsychiatric physicians (only about 20% of them by mental health professionals: Regier, Goldberg, & Taube, 1978). Nonpsychiatric physicians do not reliably detect mental disorders (e.g., Eastwood, 1975); and when detected, nonpsychiatric physicians are much more likely to treat a mental disorder with drugs than are psychiatrists or psychologists (e.g., World Health Organization, 1973). If they try therapy, it only lasts 3 minutes longer than the average of 13 minutes for all primary care visits (Burns, Orso, Jacobson, Leet, & Goldner, 1977). If a psychiatric disorder is not diagnosed, it may lead to the unnecessary tests, exploratory surgery, and nonpsychotropic drug treatments actually found with these patients (Goplerud, 1981).

All of these issues can seriously distort national statistics, our sense of what we understand about physical and mental disorders, and a rational understanding of what the public policy alternatives are for the future. These are serious public policy problems that only policy research can solve for us.

Medical Utilization

As implied above, people with various mental disorders are very high users of the physical health system. They are frequent complainers of physical symptoms, users of emergency rooms, and they receive unnecessary tests and surgery. Does mental health treatment reduce utilization of the physical health system?

Jones and Vischi (1980) reviewed 13 studies in which mental health services were introduced into an organized system of medical care. In 12 of the 13 studies, there was a fairly sharp reduction in the use of medical resources, for those patients who utilized the mental health services. Across the thousands of patients in the studies the median reduction was 20%. As one of the more dramatic examples, the Kaiser-Permanente plan (Cummings & Follette, 1976) found that those patients engaged in short-term psychotherapy of 8 hours or less reduced their use of medical resources as much as 70% over the following five years. Interestingly, they found a similar reduction in absenteeism from the work place for the same time period.

We now spend well over $200 billion per year on medical care in the United States, with the number increasing yearly well in excess of the inflation rate. Productivity is a national problem and absenteeism from work is a costly national expense. If it is generally true that psychotherapy (or other mental health care) decreases medical utilization and absenteeism, then it is a tool of considerable national importance.

The effect of mental health services on medical utilization has recently played a central role in policy discussions of various national insurance plans. However, it is a point that needs to be accepted with some caution. For example, we still do not know why the effect occurs, at any reasonable level of theoretical understanding. We do not know if it generalizes across practitioners and sites. The studies reviewed by Jones and Vischi were all conducted in health maintenance organizations (HMOs) or other organized systems of care. There are several reasons why such an effect might occur at an HMO, but not in CMHCs, or in private practice (Kiesler, 1981a). However, Schlesinger, Mumford, Glass, Patrick, and Sharfstein (1983) reported a similar medical offset in a large national fee-for-service plan. Differences in medical offset as a function of patient characteristics, service setting, and the like remain to be investigated (e.g., Mumford, Schlesinger, & Glass, 1981).

At one level, we don't know whether the effect is due more to the success of the mental health services than the failure of the physical health services system. That is, we need to consider which changes in current medical practice could also reduce medical utilization, and whether such changes overlap with or are distinct from the reductions produced by mental health services. Given there are not many doctoral-level mental health service providers in the country, it would be important to ascertain whether other mental health professionals such as psychiatric social workers and psychiatric nurses could produce a similar effect (Kiesler, 1983). We have no sense of whether these effects are general across people or specific to particular types of patients with specific sorts of problems. Generally, the sorts of patients who are seeking out psychotherapy in an organized system of care tend to have already been very high utilizers of the medical system (Tessler, Mechanic, & Dimond, 1976). Whether specific intervention techniques or changes in medical practice could reduce medical utilization even more when applied earlier in the course of help-seeking is unknown. In sum, this is a critical national area with a generally robust empirical finding. Why medical utilization decreases following psychotherapy is not now well understood, however (see Kiesler, 1981b for further discussion). That understanding is critical to developing rational public policy.

Insuring Mental Health Care

In discussions of insurance in mental health, the following questions typically come up (see McGuire & Weisbrod, 1981; Davis, 1975; Califano, 1979). Does psychotherapy work, and can it be insured by the typical methods? If insured, will everyone use psychotherapy and thereby "break the bank"? If one adds mental health services to an existing system of insured medical care, will medical utilization drop? What are the factors that might enhance or reduce the effect on medical utilization? What is the moral hazard in insuring mental health services? That is, how many more people (and with which problems) would use mental health services if they were free under an insurance plan? Specifically, what is the "income-price cross-elasticity of demand," a term economists use to refer to the changes in use patterns among groups of different income as a function of cost of the services. Insurance companies are also worried about adverse selection: that only people who need the services elect that insurance plan, which, as described later, starts a cycle that ensures the ultimate failure of the plan.

Insurance companies are very reluctant to offer a total plan for mental health care. In particular, the concepts of moral hazard, adverse selection, and price elasticity dominate their thinking. There is evidence to suggest that such fears are unjustified. For example, Dorken (1977) studied the civilian health and medical program of the uniform services (CHAMPUS), with a total insured population of over 6 million across the country. He found that less than 2% of the beneficiaries used mental health services when they were insured and that the average cost per person covered was approximately $1.75 a month. NIMH has found similar data for the federal employees health benefit plan (FEHBA), with an average cost per covered person of approximately $1.00 per month (NIMH, 1976). Utilization rates in other plans have been fairly similar to these. Liptzin, Regier, and Goldberg (1980) analyzed the 1975 data for the 2.3 million people covered by Michigan Blue Cross/Blue Shield. They found 2.6% of the covered population used psychiatric services for a specific disorder; 4.6% if one includes those with an unspecified diagnosis. The cost per person covered was $1.75 a month.

The plans that work best are those that do not offer a choice to the beneficiary. McGuire (1981) describes this issue very effectively. If the election of mental health benefits is voluntary for each participant in an insurance plan, the following sequence of adverse selection is not at all unusual. People who initially elect to have the benefits are those who think they need them soon. Thus in the initial experiences of the plan, an "unexpectedly" large number of people will seek mental health care. As a result of the large cost of such care, the following year the actuaries will increase the cost of that set of services in the insurance plan. As a result of the increased premium, people who have already been treated or those who are less certain of the need will drop the optional plan. The remaining insurees must be confident that they will need the care, since they are willing to pay an increased amount for it. This leaves a smaller number, but an even greater density of people electing the plan who need care, thus increasing the rate of utilization, and increasing the cost of the plan the following year. The sequence across years is one of increasing density of utilization and rapidly escalating costs per person covered. Under these conditions, the plan will ultimately either break the bank or prove so costly that nobody will choose it.

Mental health is not the only area in which adverse selection occurs, of course. Dental plans have much the same sorts of problems: People do sense how much they need dental treatment, and those who need the service disproportionately join the plans. Insurance companies understand this, and typically refuse to insure an organization without all employees being part of the plan. Further, to avoid some of the density of initial use, people often must demonstrate no immediate need. Thus patients must pay for any needed dental care prior to entering the plan. The plan is then composed of people with little need, it insures only future occurrences of need, and the fiscal underpinnings are quite different.

McGuire emphasizes that utilization rates are only part of the total picture, particularly regarding mental health services. Increased rates of utilization may be seriously misleading. That is, one must inspect the alternative costs when such benefits are not part of a plan. If people are using inappropriate services, such as general physicians and nursing homes when mental health benefits are not available, then those costs should decrease when such benefits are available. Further, the lack of mental health benefits has other costs, such as medical utilization and general physical costs of stress, which mental health care might reduce.

When mental health services are insured, and use of such services thereby increases, it does not necessarily follow that the services are being overly utilized. Indeed, the increased services may reflect more adequate and needed utilization, which could provide substantial savings elsewhere—such savings perhaps even exceeding the increased direct charges. The various contingencies affecting utilization and outcome of insured mental health services are in great need of investigation (see Broskowski, Marks, & Budman, 1981).

One logical policy alternative is to attempt to develop systems that prevent or inhibit hospitalization of mental patients. One way is to erect barriers against hospitalization, by insisting on certain forms of care being delivered in advance of a hospitalization. A partial form of this exists in the county surrounding Pittsburgh. One cannot be committed to a state mental hospital in that county without first having spent a maximum of 20 days in one of the short-stay hospitals in the area. Initial hospitalization in one of the short-stay hospitals is for 72 hours for observation. A special order must be obtained in order to commit the patient beyond that; the patients are unable to stay in these hospitals legally beyond a 20-day limit. The whole notion is to erect strong barriers against putting people in state mental hospitals, and also weak barriers to hospitalizing them at all. The effect of such programs on the practice of professionals is illustrated by the fact that although patients can stay in these hospitals only a maximun of 20 days legally, the average stay for all patients for mental health disorders is approximately 19 days.

Thus the average patient tends to be kept about as long as he or she legally can be. In any event one could erect other barriers against the initial hospitalization by insisting on certain forms of alternative care or intensive outpatient treatment before allowing hospitalization to be free.

The same bias in design of insurance programs can be seen in discussions of mental health benefits in national health insurance. At last report, the leading bills (none very actively considered) were all catastrophic bills—those that would insure only the "most serious" and expensive cases. Although well-meaning and superficially reasonable, the immediate effect would be to increase dramatically mental hospitalization and associated expenses. Because such programs reinforce traditional practice and because they encourage hospitalization, the total cost of the system is not necessarily less. Zook et al. (1981) deduced that catastrophic insurance costs more than noncatastrophic insurance in physical health *and* mental health. We do have the knowledge, we believe, to design a cost-beneficial and cost-effective insurance plan, incorporating more appropriate incentives for desired outcomes. What we do not have is a zeitgeist that allows such knowledge to be effectively used.

Decisions to Hospitalize

We have discussed mental hospitalization as if each instance were a rational, objective, informed human judgment by the physician. We have assumed that the physician making the decision has been trained to do so (although some unspecifiable number of hospitalizations are by nonpsychiatric physicians); that he or she looks dispassionately at the case, obtains the relevant information, and makes the right decision.

However, other data already indicate that even such well-informed decisions are fraught with systematic error (e.g., Fiske & Taylor, 1984). People—even scientists and physicians—consistently make certain kinds of errors in complex human judgments. For example, infrequent events are judged even more rare; very frequent events are judged near constant—both making the end points of a distribution seem more distinctive than they really are. Events that stand out in the perceptual field (hallucinations or other bizarre behavior could be such) are given disproportionate weight in a judgment. Decision alternatives that have risk associated with them tend to be made very conservatively, substantially in excess of the objective level of risk. Prior, often hidden, assumptions (statisticians call them "priors") affect a final judgment far beyond their mathematical predictiveness.

Further, people making a complex judgment involving a number of factors are unable to say correctly how they weighted the various factors. For example, consider admitting students into college where high-school grades, principal and teacher evaluations, outside activities, sports skills, the quality of the high school, leadership qualities, and SAT scores all have to be taken into account. There is a good deal of research on just this type of decision. One first asks the evaluators how much weight they give each factor after making a number of decisions. One then compares that with the mathematically derived actual weights that the person used. People are unable to assess with any accuracy the implicit weights that they used.

These same psychological distortions of the decision-making process must be equally true of the decision to put any given patient in a hospital for mental health treatment.

Factors to be taken into account are such things as: the seriousness of the disorder (itself a complex judgment); financial resources open to the patient (e.g., insurance); hospitals available to receive the patient and whether or not the physician has staff privileges; pressures from hospital administrators to fill beds; how disruptive the patient is to others; how dangerous the patient is (another complex and risky judgment); whether or not the family wants the patient to be admitted; whether or not the family could care for the patient, if not admitted; whether or not the last decision(s) could be judged as a "successful" decision; and so forth.

There is also a number of "priors," hidden assumptions not easily verbalized or assessed by the individual making a complex decision. These would include here: the training of the psychiatrist (are they socially or biologically oriented?); the belief in the hospital syllogism (the seriously mentally ill get treated in hospitals); whether or not the physician already is treating someone in that hospital, making it much easier to treat another patient there (at the margin); that complex history called "clinical experience" (which for all the reasons previously discribed could lead to systematic and serious errors of judgment); and so forth.

One can argue that the diagnosis and the severity of the disorder should rationally dominate the decision to commit. However, when one considers that the reliability of diagnosis of mental disorders is not high, the potential for these other factors and priors to affect the decision to commit is extreme and substantial. Add to that the increasing influence of the police and the courts in commitment decisions and one could have a situation in which the preponderance of variables statistically determining the decision to commit or not has little to do with the professional and personal needs of the patients.

This is a fascinating and very important area for policy-related research. As we have discussed there is considerable public and psychiatric resistance to alternative care—which the evidence suggests is more effective and less expensive. Research on the judgmental processes underlying each decision to hospitalize might well elucidate the current professional resistance to change.

Sites of Mental Health Service Delivery

Whether analyzing current policy, developing alternative policies for the future, or considering the potential research questions in mental health policy, one must consider the total system and the elements within it. One aspect of the overall system that has not received sufficient attention is the sites or places where services are actually delivered. There have been insufficient attempts to analyze each of these, as well as inappropriate application of data obtained at one site to another. Consider briefly four general sites in which services are delivered: community mental health centers; HMOs; private practice; and the various sites of hospitalization.

Most research on CMHCs is not evaluative (Cook & Shadish, 1982). It describes the number of CMHCs, the practitioners, patients, funding, and the like. This descriptive research is oriented toward ascertaining whether or not national policies regarding CMHCs have been successfully implemented. While this is a reasonable form of research, it does not assess the effectiveness of CMHCs in terms of treatment outcome, nor does it often assess the interrelationship of CMHCs with other sites of service delivery. There is some controversy about cost-effectiveness of CMHCs, as well as some question of whether they simply replaced existing outpatient clinics (Buck, 1984). Most professionals feel very positive about CMHCs, and do not think there is a reasonable alternative for the kinds of services that they are legislated to deliver. The original Joint Commission on Mental Illness and Health (*Action for Mental Health*, 1961), when proposing what eventually turned out to be the CMHC system, thought them to be a critical element in the treatment and transition of patients deinstitutionalized from state and county mental hospitals. This is less clear in the subsequent enabling legislation, and certainly has not been a central component of the history of the CMHC system. CMHCs have been more effective as alternatives to hospitalization, and most have active day care services. Less well known are the increasing inpatient services utilized by CMHCs. In 1980, the CMHC system had 250,000 clinical inpatient episodes across the country, with a total of 4 million inpatient days. Thus, CMHCs had more inpatient episodes and days than either private for-profit or not-for-profit mental hospitals.

One critical issue is the effect of the changes in funding CMHCs by President Reagan. NIMH has been the funder and initiator of the CMHC system, even though it provided only about 20% of the total funds for the system just prior to the election of Reagan. Reagan eliminated NIMH as a funder of the system, cut the total federal dollars by 25%, and gave the remainder as block grants to the individual states. Even if the states pass all of these dollars on to the CMHCs within their borders, the budgets for individual centers will be reduced. Some of them will not survive (survival was a frequent issue before the budget cuts). One policy issue is how the others can survive. Preliminary evidence suggests that the first few years after the change had a less negative impact than expected (Kiesler et al., 1983). However, little is known about more recent events.

One outcome is that the CMHCs must look for other funds to ensure their future. One possibility is to increase funds from third-party payers. However, third-party payment plans favor inpatient care. Although no data exist it seems very likely that CMHCs will increase their inpatient care both in frequency of inpatient episodes and perhaps even length of stay. It would be ironic if the system designed to be the national centerpiece in developing easily accessible outpatient care becomes a central proponent of inpatient care in order to survive.

The popularity of adding mental health services to HMOs is a relatively recent phenomenon even though examples of it go back at least 20 years (e.g., Kaiser-Permanente). Descriptive research is needed indicating more clearly the problems handled in HMOs, at what cost (particularly related to other services offered), and with what outcome. Comparative research is also needed, contrasting HMOs with other sites, regarding array of patients, diagnoses, costs, and outcomes. Most of the data on HMOs is aggregate data in which it is difficult to track individual patients. Although it is possible to look at outcome effectiveness in aggregate data, it is difficult to inspect the theoretical underpinnings of that effectiveness (patient by patient), and to theorize how the effectiveness might be enhanced. Particularly with the financial crippling of CMHCs, the inclusion of mental health services in HMOs could well be the wave of the future. A good deal of the data on the effectiveness of mental health services in an organized system of care has been accumulated in HMOs. Data on the effect of psychotherapy on the utilization of medical services have been disproportionately gathered in HMOs. We literally do not know whether or not such services in other sites will produce the same effect (although see Schlesinger et al., 1983). There is at least some reason to suspect that the specific organization of an HMO to some degree enhances the effect on medical utilization (Kiesler, 1981a; Mechanic, 1979). Whether this is true or not remains to be investigated. In short, we need outcome data specific to HMOs, but also data comparing outcomes to other methods and sites of delivering services.

The details of private practice as a site of mental health service delivery are least well known. There have been some surveys of psychiatrists in private practice (Marmor et al., 1975) and private practice psychologists (Gottfredson & Dyer, 1978) but these barely scratch the surface. Some state and county psychiatric registers attempt to track the patients who are treated in private practice settings, but they depend on the cooperation of the private practitioner and in all cases are limited to psychiatrists. They do not attempt to track other mental health professionals such as psychologists and clinical social workers. The large-scale study of private practice psychiatrists was methodologically flawed (Albee, 1976), although McGuire (1980) has demonstrated that regression techniques could overcome most of the survey flaws. There are some data on utilization of services when private practice is insured (Liptzin et al., 1980), but there are very few data on the outcomes of such services. Note also that in Liptzin et al.'s study of the Michigan experience, almost 50% "of those individuals who submitted a claim for physician services for a specific mental disorder received at least some of those services from nonpsychiatric physicians" (p. 556). Outcome data could be extremely informative. One also needs to ask such policy questions as the relative cost-effectiveness of insuring services from private practitioners compared to insuring services within the HMO concept.

The changing sites of mental hospitalization have been relatively uninvestigated. The traditional sites—at least from the public's point of view—now account for a rather small percentage of the total clinical episodes. We know very little indeed about what occurs in the site where most clinical episodes occur—the general hospital without a psychiatric unit.

We can outline some basic policy questions regarding alternative sites of service delivery. Where shall we put our public money for the greatest effectiveness and cost benefit? What should we ask the private sector—through legislation and other incentives—to do? In what ways could the public and private sectors cooperate/coordinate better to have a more effective system of service delivery? Does each site play a unique role, thereby being worthy of public support? Where should we put the most money so as to have the greatest overall effect? If all are uniquely worthwhile and to be supported, what mix of services nationally would make the best public policy? If we design insurance schemes or quasi-insurance schemes, how should we array the incentives and disincentives? Should we have a system in which it is easier and cheaper for the patient to be treated in a CMHC or an HMO, with disincentives for being treated in private practice? Should we erect insurance barriers against mental hospitalization, and incentives favoring outpatient care? If so, should the system be intentionally biased toward a particular form of outpatient care? Which national mix of service delivery systems and sites would have the largest effect on outcomes such as medical utilization and absenteeism? These questions deal very basically with the overall design of a national mental health system. As such, they are central to any discussion of our public policy, as well as consideration of alternative policies for the future. As a whole, however, these policy questions have been relatively uninvestigated.

Notes

1. Note that the term *community support system* is often defined to include both alternative services and volunteer programs.

2. Meta-analysis as a technique is not without its critics and there are some lively controversies (Bandura, 1978; Cook & Leviton, 1980; Paul & Licht, 1978). See Kiesler (1985) for discussion of ways to enhance the usefulness of meta-analysis for policy research.

3. Unfortunately, evidence indicates that psychiatrists, the real bridge between the fields of physical and mental health, recognize only about 50% of the physical disorders present in these patients.

CHAPTER 13

BARRIERS TO EFFECTIVE KNOWLEDGE ACQUISITION AND USE[1]

We have reanalyzed the national data base in mental hospitalization. Many of these data shatter currently held views of the "facts"; and many of our collective assumptions about mental hospitalization turn out to be myths. They are myths in the sense that they are commonly held beliefs that turn out to be inaccurate.

Not all the information we have presented is new. Some of it had been noted before. For example, the large number of inpatient episodes in general hospitals had been recently noted (Taube & Barrett, 1983). But no one tried to investigate it further, and it was not tracked over time (and indeed it was the change in episodic rate over time that made this datum especially intriguing). In some cases part of the information was well known, but overly generalized. For example, the decrease in length of stay in state hospitals was widely publicized. However, the small proportion of episodes handled there and the lack of decrease in length of stay in other sites were not.

However, some things were not known because no one had asked the question. For example, we discovered we could derive total inpatient days for mental disorders from NCHS surveys. We realized with that information, we could calculate total national hospital inpatient days for mental disorders as a percentage of all hospital days. That datum had been the big missing piece. Since a national discussion was ensuing regarding hospital cost containment, other people had noted that the total number of inpatient days had decreased. However, because the question had never been asked, no one knew that 98% of the decrease in total inpatient days in the United States was accounted for by mental disorders.

All of these data were there to be analyzed. Every time we looked for data relevant to questions regarding hospitalization, the data surprised us by disconfirming or seriously qualifying commonly held professional views. Our experience has been that the data—partly because they disconfirm commonly held assumptions—initially provoked a strong reaction from others—negative, in the case of some, such as many psychiatrists; positive in the case of others such as citizens' groups and many psychologists.

This chapter addresses the questions of why people didn't look at the whole system with a detached view before, and which problems and issues will inhibit or facilitate the use of these data in public policy formation in the future. We submit that there are barriers to both gathering and using the data—issues of knowledge acquisition and use.

Knowledge acquisition and use is a field of research in itself, perhaps epitomized by the journal *Knowledge: Creation, Diffusion, Utilization,* begun in 1979. The roots of these questions, of course, date to pre-Christian times and are historically linked to philosophy and history of science. More recently, however, there has been a developing focus on the creation and use of knowledge for public policy. It is interesting to recall how recent some of these emphases are.

As Rich (1979, p. 11) says, "Although the applicability of science to national goals was recognized early in the United States by Thomas Jefferson and Benjamin Franklin (among others), the idea that government should actively intervene in the private economy to support systematic research and development (R&D) on 'nationally significant technologies' was never forcefully advocated until after the Manhattan Project," which was completed in 1945. Indeed, both the National Science Foundation and National Institute of Mental Health were not begun until after World War II, in the late 1940s.

The more recent history of research in public policy has been a checkered one. The great burgeoning of social programs regarding health, welfare, and mental health in the 1960s was based less on scientific research than on values and conviction. The major changes in the 1970s in the area of mental health were based more on major court decisions, than on either research or public policy development.

People working in the research area of knowledge use and utilization regard it as naive to assume that public policy ought to be rational and based on systematic knowledge, scientifically produced and accumulated. Many (e.g., Rich, 1981) see public policymakers as relatively immune to the findings of social research. Others (Weiss, 1977) are quite upbeat about the degree to which research findings can be used to develop and implement public policy. In the 1980s the Reagan Administration has been quite hostile toward the use of social policy research in public policy and indeed insisted that NIMH discontinue research support for social policy research.

In short, there have been significant barriers in the past inhibiting knowledge acquisition in the area of mental hospitalization. In addition, there is good reason to believe that similar barriers will exist against use of these data for public policy in the future.

Health Policy Domination of Mental Health Policy

One might consider that health policy and mental health policy nationally could be considered coequal in importance and economic support. In the survey data previously reviewed, the frequency of mental health problems among people surveyed was substantial and approached the frequency of health problems. The interrelationship and coincidence of these problems was substantial (although not well understood). We noted the substantial proportion of patients who visit general practitioners, who in fact have no documentable medical problem, but presumably have psychological problems. Psychological knowledge and mental health treatment practices have recently demonstrated usefulness in the treatment of such quasi-medical problems as hypertension and peptic ulcers. Mental health treatment has also been quite promising in such areas as medical offset and absenteeism.

In general health, dramatically increasing the financial commitment to health practice will not change the physical health of the nation much at the margin. Indeed, it has often been argued that it is the change of certain behaviors and habits related to health that can have the most dramatic impact on health of the average citizen in the United States (e.g., Bandura, 1978, Fuchs, 1974). A recent report by the National Academy of Medicine concluded that of the top ten causes of death, seven were environmentally or behaviorally related. In short, what we know about human psychology and mental health treatment practices could have a substantial effect on the physical health of the average citizen. In this sense, one could imagine that these two sets of policies would be coequal and receive similar levels of support.

In fact, health policy has totally dominated mental health policy both financially and in practice. It is not unfair to characterize mental health policy as the current poor cousin of physical health policy. For example, consider research funds. The National Institute of Health currently spends about $6 billion a year for research that is biomedical in nature, and less than 1% of it goes for behavioral research. Contrast that with the amount spent at NIMH (FY 1981) of about $145 million dollars. The federal spending on physical health research is at least 20 times that of the spending on research for mental health. This is approximately the same ratio as the country spends on treatment. Physical health treatment accounts for about 20 times the money spent on mental health treatment.

To some extent, this affects how scientists think about their research, and where they can get it funded. To many psychiatrists and some psychologists, being part of the physical health system implies a less uncertain future. Within the physical health funding picture, they feel that the problems of seeking federal support are eased. They feel that the general medical credibility and prestige can enhance the field of mental health. Further, there is a great potential in mental health for financial "fallout" from physical health, partly because of the large discrepancy in dollars available. With the huge discrepancy between research funds available at NIH and NIMH, even a 1% NIH fallout for research of interest to NIMH would result in the equivalent of over 20% increase in NIMH research funds. A research crumb to one agency is a cake to another.

The political groups interested in physical health are also much more powerful than those interested in mental health, through both professional associations (e.g., the American Medical Association) and various citizens' associations (e.g., American Heart Association). Mental health also gets the crumbs of public policy. Medicare is perhaps the largest public program in creating funds for mental health. However, it is not a mental health program per se; it is a program for physical health of the elderly, and the mental health aspects of that legislation are fairly trivial. The major programs for mental health in the United States, both public and private, are actually programs for physical health, in which mental health is merely an add-on. As such, the style of delivering treatment, the methods for reimbursement, the review mechanisms, and the like, are dictated for mental health practitioners by physical health practitioners. That these may not be the most advantageous ways to deliver mental health services is frankly seldom raised. This is a serious disadvantage for mental health practitioners. On the other hand, the economic security from third-party payments for service is a major advantage.

However, there are also many disadvantages to mental health policy being driven by physical health policy. For one, a *zeitgeist* is developed that is a traditional medical one in nature. As such, mental health gets pulled toward traditional medical solutions, such as hospitalization, and questioning such practices is actively discouraged. Second, the typical "doctor—sees—patient" relationship in physical health could not be successfully extrapolated to mental health, partly because of the mismatch between providers available and services needed. We have also seen that the typical reactive method of service delivery for physical health, in which a doctor sits in an office waiting for the patient to come to him or her, is not the best way to deliver mental health services, particularly to the seriously disordered. Most of the successful alternative care programs involve very nontraditional service delivery, with various staff out in the field with the patient.

Yet another disadvantage is that with a power differential between two groups (health and mental health), certain kinds of questions tend to be closed off. If, for example, it is indeed true that 50%–70% of the visits at general practitioners' offices are for problems that are largely psychological in nature, then it seems wise not to have the people in charge who are the least knowledgeable about that set of problems. Yet there has been considerable resistance in medicine to having psychiatrists or psychologists actively involved in the delivery of primary care.

The national research portfolio also changes as a function of such denomination. Even prior to Reagan's election, ADAMHA moved to increase research funds in the biomedical area and decrease them in the behavioral area. Given the current state of knowledge and science's inability to state what is knowable, it is difficult to argue that decreasing the nation's investment in behavioral research is in the long-term national interest. Clearly, a balanced portfolio of research involvement is the wisest long-term strategy for science in general and mental health in particular.

The backgound of psychiatrists should not be discounted here. They receive a traditional medical training and a generic medical licence. Their internship and residency differs from other MDs, and there are some data suggesting that psychiatrists in general are much more "people oriented" (along with pediatricians) than are the typical MDs. However, the practice of psychiatry is not limited to formally trained psychiatrists. The medical license is generic, and anyone with an MD can practice psychiatry, although they may not necessarily be allowed hospital staff privileges and they cannot join the American Psychiatric Association without a three-year psychiatric residency. However, psychiatrists were the first professionals to be involved in mental health service, and they have dominated the other mental health professionals in terms of impact on public policy. Although there have cyclical "remedicalization" movements in psychiatry over the last 100 years, and cyclical debate between social psychiatrists and those who regard themselves as neuroscientists for almost the same period of time, psychiatry has never deviated very far in training and outlook from traditional medicine.

The influence of medicine on mental health policy and mental health treatment over the decades has been very substantial. For example, since its inception the NIMH has always had a psychiatrist as its director. All of these things work together to pull mental health policy under the general umbrella of health policy and, implicitly and explicitly, tilt the treatment of mental disorders toward the traditional medical model.

Bandura (1978) refers to this as "the sickness ideology" and is articulate in his rejection of the medical domination over mental health (and clinical psychology indirectly). "In virtually every respect—the nomenclature, the preoccupation with pathology and the structure of administrations—psychological services mimic traditional medical practices" (p. 98). He goes on to say, "We have the knowledge and the means to bring benefits to many. We have the experimental methodology with which to advance psychological knowledge and practice. But to accomplish this calls for . . . a fundamental change in the uses to which our knowledge is put" (p. 96). "The sickness ideology undermines valued research strategies for advancing knowledge" (p. 79).

There are two aspects of the "sickness ideology" that inhibit effective policy analysis. First it leads to a focus on diagnostic categories that surface in professional offices and mental institutions and disregards the underlying theme of social failure in mental disorders. Bandura points out that what most people see in mental health treatment are the failures with such disorders, rather than a random assortment of people with such disorders. He points to Lincoln as being an example of a successful depressive.

Further, one must keep in mind that changes or innovations in public policy are typically implemented at the margin. That is, they are implemented in addition to existing systems rather than instead of them (Kiesler, 1980). Thus, increasing the number of physicians would probably not affect the health of the nation much (Fuchs, 1974), nor might additional traditional psychotherapists affect the mental health of the nation much. Bandura (1978) suggests that the most substantial marginal utilities are in changing health threatening personal habits and environmental conditions. We do know a great deal about changing habits, but it is seldom included in mental health policy discussions.

Part of this issue is the question of what a mental health problem is assumed to be. Discussion focuses on the extent to which the basic issues are strictly medical in nature, or psychosocial in nature (and further whether those are discrete categories or a continuum). As Mechanic (1980) says,

> If mental illnesses are fundamentally different from ordinary problems of living and are defined not by social standards but by medical diagnosis of disease, public health policy should give the highest priority to those patients who are clearly sick in a traditional psychiatric sense . . . . Then public policy must give greatest emphasis to retarding and alleviating the

disability of the chronically ill patient. In contrast, if chronic mental illness and the psychoses are part of the same continuum as are other problems, we can treat all such conditions in fundamentally the same way—chronic disability is simply a manifestation of untreated neglected illnesses. Indeed, early intervention may prevent chronic and severe mental illness . . . [and] . . . it is reasonable to devote considerable resources to preventive work and to treating mild and moderate psychological disabilities [p. 37].

Academic disciplines have different views on the underlying issues in both the causes and treatment of mental disorders. Psychiatry is obviously driven more by a medical model, and psychology by a behavioral one. Wise public policy, given the lack of definitive scientific evidence, should not assume that either one or the other is valid. There is exciting work going on in neuroscience on basic questions of the brain's function, which may shed much light on the underlying problems in mental disorders. At the same time there is also exciting research, some of which is described in Chapter 9, regarding effective treatment for the mentally disordered. A public policy based on a more balanced view of the scientific literature is surely wiser than one that presupposes that one point of view or the other is the only accurate one. It is interesting to note that the President's Commission on Mental Health did not use the term "mental illness," and never defined the term "mental health" (Levine & Levine, 1981). In any event, the kind of posture one takes on these issues has a substantial effect on how one views the effectiveness of current public policy and the wisest course for future public policy.

Reliance on Drugs

Part of the salvation that led to deinstitutionalization is also part of the current problem—drugs. Over $100 million in drugs for mental health care is funded annually by Medicaid alone. Today at any given time, one in every seven Americans is regularly taking a psychotropic drug prescribed by a physician (Cummings, 1979). This practice is not limited to inpatient treatment in mental institutions. Ray et al. (1980), in a recent study of 5,900 Medicaid patients in 173 Tennessee nursing homes found that 43% of the patients received antipsychotic drugs, and 9% received an average of at least one dose per day. There were large differences among physicians. Physicians with large nursing home practices (10 or more patients) prescribed 81% of the total antipsychotic medication. Continued use of such medication can have serious long-term and irreversible neurological implications.

In social psychology we talk often about the attribution of causality. Two aspects of this phenomenon relate here. One is patients' attributions for changes in their own behavior. Davison and Valins (1969) found that drug-induced changes tend not to persist in individuals, since the person attributes the mood changes, even positive ones, to external causes. This might suggest that one can produce short-term change with drugs but any long-term change for the patient might well have to depend on other modes of treatment, including psychotherapy and the development of social support networks and social competencies. A different aspect of how attributions can work in this situation relates to interpretations by therapists and policymakers. If one interprets the success of the deinstitutionalization movement to be due to drugs, one is going to invest in the development of more and better drugs, and one is going to worry very little about the general system of delivery of mental health services. We mentioned in Chapter 2 that there is some controversy over the relative contributions of psychotropic drugs versus changes in administrative practices, in affecting deinstitutionalization. If one is convinced that drugs are the main reason, then one is not going to look very closely at administrative practices, nor attempt to do further research on refining them, nor perhaps indeed be terribly interested in keeping people out of hospitals.

It is not that psychotropic drugs do not have a positive effect. They do, although there is considerable variation in treatment response (see Kane, 1984, for a recent review). Recent evidence suggests that in schizophrenia, for example, neuroleptics may affect acute symptoms, such as hallucinations and delusions, in as many as 80% of the patients, but are relatively ineffective in longer-term symptoms such as lack of goal directed activity, blunting of affect and verbal paucity (see Keith & Matthews, 1984). In spite of an apparent 20% rate of tardive dyskinesia (Kane & Smith, 1982), the effectiveness of drugs in mental illness is widely accepted.

We do not review this literature in detail any more than we review the literature on psychotherapy in detail. Our point here is twofold: (1) It is not clear that drug therapy is any more effective than psychotherapy; and (2) therefore, a public policy that puts disproportionate weight on drug therapy is imbalanced. As we have described, an imbalanced policy inhibits certain kinds of questions being asked of science and service delivery, keeps some data from being gathered, inhibits self-criticism, and is a very high scientific risk for the long-run. We are open to drug therapy ultimately proving extremely effective and the treatment of choice for all patients. However, we question a public policy based on the *assumption* that this will ultimately be the case.

Public Attitudes toward Mental Illness

The stigma of mental illness has frequently been discussed in the literature. The public tends to characterize the mentally ill as dangerous and unpredictable: Tringo (1970) found that out of 21 different categories of disability groups, the least preferred were the mentally ill. Hazelton, Mandrill, and Stern (1975) found in a California survey that only 17% of the respondents agreed that "mental patients are not dangerous" (see also Rabkin, 1980). The perception of the mental patient as dangerous can interfere quite seriously with the public's concern with quality of care. For example, the economist Rubin (1978) hypothesizes that the main reason we institutionalize the mentally disturbed is because they make us uncomfortable and fearful. Looking at this issue from a cost-benefit analysis, Rubin suggests that if this out-of-sight phenomenon is sufficiently rewarding by itself, there would be no need to be concerned with the quality of care after institutionalization. That is, in this view the public's benefit would be served by hiding the patient, and no further substantial benefit would be derived from quality care.

Rabkin (1984) reviews more recent work and concludes that public attitudes have changed; changed to the point that the word "stigma" is no longer appropriate. She suggests much of the change toward ex-patients might be attributed to the community mental health center movement. It is clear, however, that patients still worry about their acceptance by family, friends, and employees after discharge.

The chronically mentally ill are rejected but the data suggest not simply because they are chronics, but at least equally important for their lack of social status and social graces, their appearance and their bizarre public behavior. As Rabkin (p. 328) says, "Desire for social distance, then, is not necessarily equivalent to rejection of the mentally ill."

Attitudes do not necessarily predict behavior, and opposition to group homes in one's neighborhood is extremely frequent. Wealthier, better educated people proclaim greater tolerance for the mentally ill but are more successful in avoiding having them nearby. It is frequently noted that people may object to a group home nearby, but are unlikely to have noticed the patients (as patients) if they were unaware of the home (see Rabkin, 1984 for a description of several studies).

Rabkin also notes that public attitudes vary about sites for treatment. More negatively viewed are inpatient facilities (versus outpatient), public facilities (versus private) and specialized psychiatric hospitals (versus general hospitals). Indeed, those sites viewed more positively are also those whose treatment episodes have been increasing.

There are several points worth making in reference to the relationship of public attitudes to public policy. To the extent the public sees the mentally disordered as dangerous and unpredictable, they may actively support long-term incarceration and more involvement by the judicial system. To the extent that people are defensive about its personal relevance they may not wish to discuss the topic at all.

Mental health problems of all types can produce defensive reactions in the discussant. Although we can all conceive of ourselves as possibly getting cancer, it is apparently more difficult to believe that we might become psychotic. Intelligent discussion of public policy alternatives, even with members of Congress, is inhibited by the defensive reactions to the potential prevalence of the problem.

The Total System

Perhaps the most important barrier to effective mental health policy is our collective failure to consider the whole mental health system, both de facto and de jure, at one time. As we have described, much of the national discussion among professionals and the public alike has really focused on public mental hospitals, a very small part of the overall mental hospitalization picture. As a result of only looking at slices of the de facto and de jure public policies, we can get serious distortions in alternative public policies.

For example, our overall public policies do not follow our national priorities. Our national priorities are deinstitutionalization and outpatient care. Our commitment nationally is to inpatient care. The major barrier to effective knowledge use in public policy in mental health is that we fail to consider all components at the same time. The narrow view implies a quite different set of needs for both knowledge and consequent research priorities, as well as current public policy problems.

Summary and Conclusions

Clearly, our national mental health policy should receive a substantial overhaul and change. In any organization, resistance to change is a quite natural phenomenon, partly due to the uncertainty of the future and partly to do with the comfort of the present. In mental health, this natural resistance to change is heightened in several ways. First, traditional modes of thought and the subsuming of mental health under health policy keep us to a very narrow view of mental health. Second, we have existing large federal and state bureaucracies, which are awkward themselves, but do not coordinate well with each other. Issues of coordinating with the state and federal governments are probably as critical for mental health as any other public policy. The traditionally perceived failure of CMHCs to care for the deinstitutionalized represents a failure of coordination between the federal and state governments. Third, there are other large, significant social policies such as social security, health, and education, which have more influence on mental health, typically indirectly and often unintentionally, than does national mental health policy itself. All of these influences inhibit self-criticism, undercut a broader perspective that would promote alternative points of view and alternative research strategies, and keep us in a public policy stance that many would consider to be outmoded and ineffective.

Note

1. This chapter leans heavily on the following article by Kiesler: "Barriers to Effective Knowledge Use and Acquisition" (1981a).

CHAPTER 14

SUMMARY AND CONCLUSIONS

As we described in the beginning of this book, this is really a research monograph. We have taken as our task a major reanalysis of the empirical data regarding mental hospitalization. Some issues raised during our investigation led us into related areas such as nursing homes and the homeless.

We have found these data startling. Time after time we found a priori expectations disconfirmed by the data. There is a current zeitgeist that is built upon an interrelated set of beliefs about mental hospitalization. These beliefs, held about as often by professionals as the lay public, are almost invariably wrong. When not, they have to be so seriously qualified as to change their real meaning.

Kiesler (1982b) has referred to these beliefs as the "myths" of mental hospitalization. They are myths in the sense that they are commonly held beliefs with little empirical basis.

We have often found that people, when presented with the data contradicting a myth, will metaphorically leap to another.

"You say that inpatient episodes are increasing rapidly in general hospitals without units. I wouldn't have expected that, but they are probably just being held for referral."

"Alternative care is more effective than inpatient care. I wouldn't have expected that, but it can't be true of serious cases."

"People with mental disorders have increased in nursing homes? That's because they've been dumped there from state mental hospitals. They haven't? Then they probably would have been there before deinstitutionalization."

When discussing mental hospitalization, it is very important to keep a number of findings in mind at the same time. To simplify that task, let us review the major findings and conclusions from each chapter.

Summary

Chapter 1. Our national de jure mental health policy rests on outpatient care and deinstitutionalization. Our de facto policy, however, is inpatient care.

There are many more outpatient episodes than inpatient episodes. However, over twice as much money is spent on inpatient care.

The lack of precise data has seriously interfered with discussions of national alternatives for mental health policy.

Chapter 2. Mental hospitalization has been a dominant medical practice in the United States for over 150 years.

The effectiveness of mental hospitalization has fluctuated rather widely over those years. It is not the case that there has been steady scientific progress in treatment effectiveness, culminating in a current, effective treatment of choice.

Chapter 3. The total number of inpatient episodes is currently almost 3 million, about 60% more than that typically reported in the literature. The difference is entirely due to general hospitals without separate psychiatric units.

The most frequent inpatient site for mental hospitalization is the general hospital. Within that category, more episodes occur in those without separate psychiatric units.

Chapter 4. The episodic rate of mental hospitalization has been increasing in recent years. Over a 15-year period, the absolute number of inpatient episodes increased about 60% (or 1 million cases).

The increase in the rate is totally due to the patients being treated in general hospitals without psychiatric units. These patients have the shortest length of stay of any site. From Friedman's (1985) data, we conclude that patients are actively treated in general hospitals without psychiatric units, and not simply held for referral as commonly believed.

Chapter 5. In most hospital sites, the average length of stay has been fairly stable in recent years. In only two sites, the state mental hospital and the VA, has the length of stay decreased recently. However, these two sites have always involved the longest lengths of stay and still do. However, they have improved. For example, "a person diagnosed psychotic in a state hospital in 1950 would stay there for an average of 20 years, a neurotic for 9 years" (Brown, 1985, p. 2).

Chapter 6. About 25% of all inpatient days in all hospitals in the United States are for diagnosed mental disorders. This percentage has decreased from over 50% 35 years ago.

This decrease affects our conclusions about general hospital practices for nonpsychiatric disorders. Total inpatient days for all disorders has decreased substantially in recent years, but 98% of the decrease in total days for all disorders is accounted for by the decrease in psychiatric days.

Chapter 7. State mental hospitals are not a haven of the elderly. The proportion of *residents* who are elderly is not large (25%–30%), and has not changed since 1964 (at least). The proportion of net *releases* who are elderly is tiny, only about 5%. The number of elderly releases has been fairly constant for years.

Nursing homes are the next step for many elderly who are released from state mental hospitals. This proportion may be substantial, and it may be a majority.

Nursing homes do not play a role in the care of the nonelderly mental patient (less than age 65) who is released from a state hospital. The number of younger patients in nursing homes has increased, but still is a small fraction of the total. Probably less than 2% of nonelderly patients released from state hospitals go to nursing homes.

The number of patients with chronic mental disorders in nursing homes is increasing very rapidly. A substantial majority of all nursing home patients are chronic mental patients (although they average 3.5 physical problems as well).

Only a small fraction of the increase of the mentally ill in nursing homes is due to the increase in the number of the elderly in the general population; most of the increase represents a change in *rate* of institutionalization at each age level.

Of the change in the rate for the elderly, only half or less can be accounted for by releases from state hospitals or a change in institutionalization practices. The remainder represent a new phenomenon in the United States. However, the change in national practices could, at least numerically, account for the increase in younger nursing home residents with mental disorders.

Deinstitutionalization *did not* cause the current increase in patients in nursing homes, nor even that subpart with mental disorders. It did not cause it either in the sense of patients released from mental hospitals or in the sense of changed hospitalization practices from the deinstitutionalization movement. Neither source accounts for even a majority of the increased number of mental patients in nursing homes.

Chapter 8. If one takes proper account of the increasing number of ex-patients at risk, then the best evidence is that the revolving door does not exist. That is, the national readmission rate to hospitals has not changed over the last 15 years or so. Indeed, there is some evidence that the readmission rate, properly calculated, has decreased somewhat. About the only thing that predicts readmission for an individual patient is the number of previous admissions.

Chapter 9. The most reasonable conclusion to be drawn from the best studies clearly indicates that alternative care outside of a hospital is more effective and less costly than mental hospitalization at its best. How much more effective is unknown.

An effective technology now exists for the treatment of serious mental disorders outside a hospital.

Chapter 10. The psychology of the attending physician has a greater effect on a decision to hospitalize someone with a mental disorder than do such patient variables as the severity of the disorder, the specific diagnosis, and the demographic characteristics of the patient. We assume that the same "physician variables" affect the length of stay of the patient in a mental hospital, as well.

There are treatment methods, such as Gordon Paul's, that are very effective inpatient treatment methods. Such treatment methods, however, have not become standard practice.

The definition of "chronic mental patient" is circular. A patient is as likely to be defined as chronic because of ineffective treatment methods as anything due to the disorder itself.

Demographically, the number of people at risk for certain types of mental disorders such as schizophrenia has increased dramatically in our population in the last 15 years. Although we know of no data, the increase in the population at risk may well account for the increase in the number of people and the rate of people hospitalized.

The homeless are disproportionately the new young chronic patients. The average age of the homeless population is decreasing, and the size of the general population at risk for certain mental disorders has increased through the baby boom. This generation, and particularly the marginal ones among them, distrust institutions in general, resist traditional treatment, and do not respond well to it.

Chapter 11. The cost of a day of inpatient care for a mental patient continues to rise in all sites. The rise has been quite sharp even in constant dollars. However, in all sites but one, the length of stay has decreased sufficiently so that the cost of an episode has remained relatively constant in deflated dollars.

In the general hospital, where the length of stay has been constant, the cost per day has increased sharply, well in excess of the cost of living or the cost of other health services. The general hospital now accounts for over 30% of total mental inpatient direct cost for the country as a whole, and we project that a rise to over 50% is likely.

Chapter 12. We argue that an effective and rational public policy is being held back through a lack of research specific to major questions for policy. Specifically, we advocate research dealing with: alternative services; community support systems; the effectiveness of both psychotherapy and drugs within a larger context of treatment; the relationship between physical and mental health; the best system mix of services for ensuring effective care; the effect of hospital site, overall service system, and training of attending professionals on quality of care; and the cognitive processes related to the individual attending physician's decision to hospitalize people.

Better national policies could be described now, but even more effective policy could be developed with research on these issues.

Chapter 13. Resistance to change is a natural human phenomenon, and is partly due to the uncertainty of the future and partly to do with the comfort of the present. However, there are a number of ways in which this natural resistance to change in mental health policy is heightened.

Traditional modes of thought and subsuming mental health under health policy keep the nation to a very narrow view of mental health.

We have large federal and state bureaucracies that are difficult to coordinate and often are at odds in policy development.

There are other large significant social policies regarding social security, health, and education that have more influence on mental health than does national mental health policy itself.

All of these inhibit a broader perspective that would promote alternative points of view and alternative research strategies; and they keep us in a public policy stance that many would consider to be outmoded and ineffective.

Conclusions

We feel these data speak for themselves. They argue quite forcefully for some changes in mental health policy. However, as is the wont of data, they do not argue for any particular change.

We do know that simply committing additional resources alone has not been the answer in the past. For example, Frank and Kamlet (1986) found that when revenues for mental health care were increased in a state, the quality of the care did not increase accordingly. Rather, the number of people treated increased.

We also know that legislation, at least in recent years, has not had the greatest impact in mental health services. Frank and Kamlet, among others, argue effectively that the most successful changes in mental health policy have recently occurred in the courts, in such cases as Wyatt versus Stickney. Many of these legal issues continue to percolate in our court systems, particularly regarding civil commitment, the right to treatment, competency to stand trial, and the insanity defense (Mechanic, 1980).

Even small programmatic changes in mental health policy have been difficult to implement. "Once particular approaches have been found to be superior to conventional services, it has often been difficult to achieve their widespread adoption because of reimbursement rules, conflicting interest between traditional programs and new innovations, and the pattern of traditionally organized professional relationships. Innovation requires more than having a good idea. It necessitates understanding of financial aspects of care and the political organization of service agencies and professional relationships. It also requires the leadership to attract people in new roles and tasks and to stimulate their motivation and commitment" (Mechanic, 1980; p. 182–183). Dain (1980) in his biography of Clifford Beers makes a similar point but grounded in history:

What he [Beers] and most others seem not to understand was that every reform effort in the field of mental illness had floundered on the inability to sustain in therapeutic or humane care of the mentally ill for which its leaders originally fought. This was true of reform movements in the 18th century, the 19th century, and the 20th. There is an initial strong push for reform, some improvements are made, then backsliding begins, and finally retrogression sets in [pp. 329–330].

Part of the difficulty in change is that institutionalizing patients serves a purpose for the public that is independent of care per se. "Much of the benefit of public provision of institutional mental health care is due to the perceived protection of society from the dangerously mentally ill and the capacity of institutions to 'protect' society from those whose behavior is particularly unsettling but not necessarily physically harmful. *These benefits arise out of institutionalization of a mentally disabled person and not the delivery of adequate care*" (Rubin, 1978, p. 112, his italics).

We believe the technology exists to treat people more effectively, probably even less expensively, outside of a hospital setting. That statement, at minimum, applies to the vast majority of patients. In the work of Test and Stein, for example, very few patients are ever hospitalized. A few are, but even then not for very long.

A major issue underlying the success of Test and Stein is that of proper financial incentives. Mental hospitals, by and large, have no incentive for cost-effective care. If they treat (or lead others to treat) a patient outside the hospital setting they don't reap any savings involved. Indeed, an unoccupied bed would cost, not save.

Programs like Test and Stein, however, receive monies for needed treatments for a population within a specified geographical area. If they can treat a particular patient as well and less expensively outside the hospital setting, it is to their economic advantage to do so.

When Kiesler testified before the U.S. Senate Appropriations Committee in November, 1984, he suggested "three major approaches to changes in federal policy which should enhance both the effectiveness and cost effectiveness of mental health care in the United States."

(1) Develop a better national data base, particularly regarding the outcomes of treatments. This demands research in which individual patients are tracked across time.
(2) We need to better understand the effects of different *systems* of service delivery, and the effects of health insurance coverage (both public and private) on utilization of services.
(3) Promote the use of the Wisconsin experience, and that of other places, testing the effects of channeling all public funds to a single administrative unit such as the county. Organize demonstration projects, research and conferences promoting cooperation between the public and private sectors.

There has been a great deal of public outcry in recent years about treatment of people with mental disorders, including the homeless and those in nursing homes. I have suggested several factors underlying the public crisis and for taking immediate action. We need to better understand why hospital inpatient rates have increased, why the problems of the homeless remain unsolved, and why the number of people in nursing homes with diagnosed mental disorders has increased so sharply. For a group which accounts for 25% of all inpatient hospital days in the United States, the problems of the mentally disturbed have remarkably been kept in the closet. The time for serious national discussion and the consideration of dramatic changes in public policy has arrived [pp. 7–8].

References

Action for Mental Health. (1961). Joint Commission on Mental Illness and Health. New York: Basic Books.

Albee, G. (1976). Into the valley of therapy rode the six thousand. *Contemporary Psychology, 21*, 525–527.

Albee, G. W. & Joffe, J. M. (Eds.). (1977). *The issues: An overview of primary prevention.* Hanover, NH: University Press of New England.

Albee, G. W., & Kessler, M. (1977). Evaluating individual deliverers: Private practice and professional standards review organizations. *Professional Psychology, 8*, 502–515.

Altman, H., Sletten, I. W., & Nebel, M. E. (1973). Length-of-stay and readmission rates in Missouri state hospitals. *Hospital and Community Psychiatry, 24*, 773–776.

American Hospital Association. (1978). *Hospital Statistics.* Chicago: Author.

American Hospital Association. (1981). *Guide to the health care field.* Chicago: Author.

American Psychiatric Association. (1968). *Diagnostic and statistical manual of mental disorders, second edition.* Washington, DC: Author.

American Psychiatric Association. (1980a). *Diagnostic and statistical manual of mental disorders, 3rd edition.* Washington, DC: Author.

American Psychiatric Association. (1980b). *Tardive dyskinesia.* Washington, DC: Author.

Anthony, W. A. (1979). *Principles of psychiatric rehabilitation.* Baltimore, MD: University Park Press.

Anthony, W. A., & Buell, G. J. (1974). Predicting psychiatric rehabilitation outcome using demographic characteristics: A replication. *Journal of Counseling Psychology, 21*, 421–422.

Anthony, W. A., Buell, G. J., Sharratt, S., & Althoff, M. E. (1972). Efficacy of psychiatric rehabilitation. *Psychological Bulletin, 78*, 447–456.

Anthony, W. A., Cohen, M. R., & Vitalo, R. (1978). The measurement of rehabilitation outcome. *Schizophrenia Bulletin, 4*, 365-383.

Arce, A., & Vergare, M. (1984). Identifying and characterizing the mentally ill among the homeless. In H. R. Lamb (Ed.), *The homeless mentally ill.* Washington, DC: American Psychiatric Association.

Babigian, H. M. (1977). The impact of community mental health centers on the utilization of services. *Archives of General Psychiatry, 34*, 385–394.

Bachrach, L. L. (1976). Deinstitutionalization: An analytical review and sociological perspective. (Mental Health Statistics Series D, No. 4) DHEW No. (ADM) 79–351. Washington, DC: U.S. Government Printing Office.

Bachrach, L. L. (1979). Planning mental health services for chronic patients. *Hospital and Community Psychiatry, 30*, 387–393.

Bachrach, L. L. (1981). Continuity of care for chronic mental patients: A conceptual analysis. *American Journal of Psychiatry, 138*, 1449–1456.

Bachrach, L. L. (1982). Young adult chronic patients: An analytical review of the literature. *Hospital and Community Psychiatry, 33*, 189–197.

Bachrach, L. L. (Ed.). (1983a). *Deinstitutionalization* San Francisco: Jossey-Bass.

Bachrach, L. L. (1983b). An overview of deinstitutionalization. In L. Bachrach (Ed.), *Deinstitutionalization* San Francisco: Jossey-Bass.

Bachrach, L. L. (1983c). New directions in deinstitutionalization planning. In L. Bachrach (Ed.), *Deinstitutionalization* San Francisco: Jossey-Bass.

Bachrach, L. L. (1984a). The homeless mentally ill and mental health services: An analytical review of the literature. In H. R. Lamb (Ed.), *The homeless mentally ill*. Washington, DC: American Psychiatric Association.

Bachrach, L. L. (1984b). Principles of planning for chronic psychiatric patients: A synthesis. In J. Talbott (Ed.), *The chronic mental patient five years later*. New York: Grune & Stratton.

Bahn, A. K., Gorwitz, K., Klee, G. D., Kramer, M., & Tuerk, I. (1965). Services received by Maryland residents in facilities directed by a psychiatrist. *Public Health Reports, 80*, 405–416.

Baker, F., & Intagliata, J. (1984). The New York State community support system: A profile of clients. *Hospital and Community Psychiatry, 35*, 39–44.

Bandura, A. (1978). On paradigms and recycled ideologies. *Cognitive Therapy and Research, 2*, 79–103.

Barnes, R. H., & Adams, R. L. (1974). The impact of a mental health center on admissions to a state hospital system. *Hospital and Community Psychiatry, 25*, 402–407.

Bassuk, E. L. (1983). *Homelessness/review of the literature*. Boston: Harvard Medical School.

Bassuk, E. L., & Gerson, S. (1978). Deinstitutionalization and mental health services. *Scientific American, 238*, 46–53.

Bassuk, E., & Gerson, S. (1980). Chronic crisis patients: A discrete clinical group. *American Journal of Psychiatry, 137*, 1513–1517.

Bassuk, E. L., & Lauriat, A. S. (1984). The politics of homelessness. In H. R. Lamb (Ed.), *The homeless mentally ill*. Washington, DC: American Psychiatric Association.

Baxter, E. & Hopper, K. (1984). Troubled on the streets: The mentally disabled homeless poor. In J. Talbott (Ed.), *The chronic mental patient five years later*. New York: Grune & Stratton.

Beard, J. H., Malamud, T. J., & Rossman, E. (1978). Psychiatric rehabilitation and long-term rehospitalization rates: The findings of two research studies. *Schizophrenia Bulletin, 4*, 622–635.

Beers, C. W. (1908). *A mind that found itself*. New York: Longmans, Green and Company.

Berger, P. A. (1978). Medical treatment of mental illness. *Science, 200*, 974–981.

Billings, A. (1978). The impact of a community screening program on psychiatric hospital admissions. *American Journal of Community Psychology, 6*, 599–605.

Binner, P. R., & Nassimbene, R. (1980). Mental hospital costs since the 1960s. *Administration in Mental Health, 8*, 83–102.

Bockoven, J. S. (1972). *Moral treatment in community mental health.* New York: Springer.

Bockoven, J. S. (1956). Moral treatment in American psychiatry. *Journal of Nervous and Mental Disease, 124*, 167–194, 292–321.

Bond, E. D. (1954). Results of treatment in psychoses with a control series. II. Involutional psychotic reaction. *American Journal of Psychiatry, 110*, 881–883.

Braff, J., & Lefkowitz, M. M. (1979). Community mental health treatment: What works for whom? *Psychiatric Quarterly, 51*, 119–134.

Braun, P., Kochansky, G., Shapiro, R., Greenberg, S., Gudeman, J. E., Johnson, S., & Shore, M. F. (1981). Overview: Deinstitutionalization of psychiatric patients, a critical review of outcome studies. *American Journal of Psychiatry, 138*, 736–749.

Brenner, M. H. (1973). *Mental illness and the economy.* Cambridge, MA: Harvard University Press.

Brill, H. R., & Patton, R. E. (1957). Analysis of 1955–1956 population fall in New York State mental hospitals in first year of large scale use of tranquilizing drugs. *American Journal of Psychiatry, 114*, 509–517.

Brill, H. R., & Patton, R. E. (1959). Analysis of population reduction in New York state mental hospitals during the first four years of large-scale therapy with psychotropic drugs. *American Journal of Psychiatry, 116*, 495–509.

Brook, B. D. (1973). Crisis hostel: An alternative to psychiatric hospitalization for emergency patients. *Hospital and Community Psychiatry, 24*, 621–624.

Brook, B. D., Cortes, M., March, R., & Sundberg-Stirling, M. (1976). Community families: An alternative to psychiatric hospital intensive care. *Hospital and Community Psychiatry, 27*, 195–197.

Broskowski, A., Marks, E., & Budman, S. H. (1981). *Linking health and mental health.* Beverly Hills, CA: Sage Publications.

Brown, P. (Ed.). (1985). *Mental health care and social policy.* Boston: Routledge & Kegan Paul.

Browning, D. H., Miller, S. I., & Tyson, R. L. (1974). The psychiatric emergency: A high risk medical patient. *Comprehensive Psychiatry, 15*, 153–159.

Buck, J. A. (1984). Effects of the Community Mental Health Centers program on the growth of mental health facilities in nonmetropolitan areas. *American Journal of Community Psychology, 12*, 609–622.

Budman, S. H. (1981). Mental health services in the health maintenance organization. In A. Broskowski, E. Marks, & S. H. Budman (Eds.), *Linking health and mental health.* Beverly Hills, CA: Sage Publications.

Budson, R. D. (1978). *The psychiatric halfway house: A handbook of theory and practice.* Pittsburgh, PA: University of Pittsburgh Press.

Buell, G. J., & Anthony, W. A. (1973). Demographic characteristics as predictors of recidivism and posthospital employment. *Journal of Counseling Psychology, 20*, 361–365.

Buell, G. J., & Anthony, W. A. (1975). The relationship between patient demographic characteristics and psychiatric rehabilitation outcome. *Community Mental Health Journal, 11*, 208–214.

Burns, B. J., Orso, C., Jacobson, A., Leet, R., & Goldner, N. (1977). Utilization of health and mental health outpatient services in organized medical care settings. (Final report for NIMH Contract No. 278–76–0027). Baltimore, MD.

Califano, J. (1979). Memorandum for the president on the basic decision in developing a national health insurance plan. In C. A. Kiesler, N. A. Cummings, & G. R. VandenBos (Eds.), *Psychology and national health insurance: A sourcebook.* Washington, DC: American Psychological Association.

Campbell, D. T., & Erlebacher, A. (1970). How regression artifacts in quasi-experimental evaluations can mistakenly make compensatory education look harmful. In J. Hellmuth (Ed.), *Compensatory education: A national debate* (vol. 3). New York: Brunner/Mazel.

Cannell, C. F. (1965). *Reporting of hospitalization in the health interview survey.* (Vital and Health Statistics, Series 2, No. 6.) Washington, DC: National Center for Health Statistics.

Cassell, W. A., Smith, C. M., Grundberg, F., Boan, J., & Thomas, R. F. (1972). Comparing costs of hospital and community care. *Hospital and Community Psychiatry, 23*, 17–20.

Caton, C.L.M. (1981). The new chronic patient and the system of community care. *Hospital and Community Psychiatry, 32*, 475–478.

Chodoff, P. (1978). Psychiatry and the fiscal third party. *American Journal of Psychiatry, 135*, 1141–1147.

Christmas, J. J. (Coordinator). (1978). *Report of the task panel on community support systems* (President's Commission on Mental Health, Vol. 2.) Washington, DC: U.S. Government Printing Office.

Cicchinelli, L. F., Bell, J. C., Dittmar, N. D., Manzanares, D. L., Sackett, K. L., & Smith, G (1981). *Factors influencing the deinstitutionalization of the mentally ill: A review and analysis.* Denver: Denver Research Institute, University of Denver.

Clinkscale, R., McCue, S., Fisher, M., & Hyatt, P. (1983). Analysis of state Medicaid program characteristics (prepared under contract No. HCFA 500–81–0040). Baltimore, MD: Health Care Financing Administration.

Code of Federal Regulations. (1984). *Title 42, Part 400 to end.* Washington, DC: U.S. Government Printing Office.

Cook, T., & Leviton, L. (1980). Reviewing the literature: A comparison of traditional methods with meta-analysis. *Journal of Personality, 48*, 449–472.

Cook, T. D., & Shadish, W. R. (1982). Meta evaluation: An assessment of the congressionally mandated evaluation system for community mental health centers. In G. Stahler & W. R. Tash (Eds.), *Innovative approaches to mental health evaluation.* New York: Academic Press.

Cooper, B.S. (1969). A study of the use of general hospitals by aged psychiatric patients, January 1965 - June 1966 and July 1966 - December 1967. Health

Insurance Statistics Series HI-13. Washington, DC: Social Security Administration.

Cummings, N. A. (1977). Prolonged (ideal) versus short-term (realistic) psychotherapy. *Professional Psychology, 8*, 491–501.

Cummings, N. A. (1979). Turning bread into stones: Our modern antimiracle. *American Psychologist, 34*, 1119–1129

Cummings, N. A., & Follette, W. T. (1968). Psychiatric services and medical utilization in a prepaid health plan setting: Part II. *Medical Care, 6*, 31–41.

Cummings, N. A., & Follette, W. T. (1976). Brief psychotherapy and medical utilization. In H. Dorken & Associates (Eds.), *The professional psychologist today.* San Francisco: Jossey-Bass.

Cummings, N. A., & VandenBos, G. R. (1979). The general practice of psychology. *Professional Psychology, 10*, 430–440.

Dain, N. (1980). *Clifford W. Beers: Advocate for the insane.* Pittsburgh, PA: University of Pittsburgh Press.

Davis, K. (1975). *National Health Insurance: Benefits, costs, and consequences.* Washington DC: Brookings Institution.

Davis, A. E., Dinitz, S., & Pasamanick, B. (1972). The prevention of hospitalization in schizophrenia: Five years after an experimental program. *American Journal of Orthopsychiatry, 42*, 375–388.

Davison, G. C., & Valins, S. (1969). Maintenance of self-attributed and drug-attributed behavior change. *Journal of Personality and Social Psychology, 11*, 25–33.

Dellario, D. J., & Anthony, W. A. (1981). On the relative effectiveness of institutional and alternative placements for the psychiactrically disabled. *Journal of Social Issues, 37*, 21–33.

Department of Health and Human Services. (1981). *Toward a national plan for the chronically mentally ill.* DHS No. (ADM) 81–1077. Washington, DC: Author.

Deutsch, A. (1949). *The mentally ill in America: A history of their care and treatment from Colonial times.* New York: Columbia University Press.

Dohrenwend, B. P., Dohrenwend, B. S., Gould, M. S., Link, B., Neugebauer, R., & Wunsch-Hitzig, R. (1980). *Mental illness in the United States: Epidemiological estimates.* New York: Praeger Publishers.

Doidge, J. R., & Rodgers, C. W. (1976). Is NIMH's dream coming true? *Community Mental Health Journal, 12*, 399–404.

Dorken, H. (1977). CHAMPUS ten-state claim experience for mental disorder: Fiscal year 1975. *American Psychologist, 32*, 697–710.

Doyle, D. N. (1966). Accuracy of selected items of Blue Cross claims information. *Inquiry, 3*, 16–27.

Dumont, M. P. (1982). Book review: E. Baxter and K. Hopper, Private Lives/Public Spaces. *American Journal of Orthopsychiatry, 52*, 367–370.

Dyck, G. (1974). The effect of a community mental health center upon state hospital utilization. *American Journal of Psychiatry, 131*, 453–456.

Eastwood, M. R. (1975). *The relation between physical and mental illness.* Toronto: University of Toronto Press.

Eaton, W. W. (1980). *The sociology of mental disorders*. New York: Praeger Publishers.

Edelman, P. B. (Coordinator). (1978). Report of the Task Panel on Community Mental Health Centers Assessment. (President's Commission on Mental Health, Vol. 2.) Washington, DC: U.S. Government Printing Office.

Endicott, J., Herz, M., & Gibbon, M. (1978). Brief versus standard hospitalization: The differential costs. *American Journal of Psychiatry, 135*, 707–712.

Estroff, S. (1981). *Making it crazy: An ethnography of psychiatric clients in an American community*. Berkeley, CA: University of California Press.

Etzioni, A. (1976). "Deinstitutionalization," a public policy fashion. *Evaluation, 3*, 9–10.

Faden, V. B., & Taube, C. A. (1977). Length of stay of discharges from nonfederal general hospital psychiatric inpatient units, United States, 1975. (Statistical Note No. 133). Rockville, MD: National Institute of Mental Health.

Falloon, I.R.H., Boyd, J. L., McGill, C. W., et al. (1982). Family management in the prevention of exacerbations of schizophrenia: A controlled study. *New England Journal of Medicine, 306*, 1437–1440.

Fenton, F. R., Tessier, L., & Struening, E. L. (1979). A comparative trial of home and hospital psychiatric care: One-year follow-up. *Archives of General Psychiatry, 36*, 1073–1079.

Fiske, S. T., & Taylor, S. E. (1984). *Social cognition*. Reading, MA: Addison-Wesley.

Flomenhaft, K., Kaplan, D. M., & Langsley, D. G. (1969). Avoiding psychiatric hospitalization. *Social Work, 14*, 38–45.

Foucault, M. (1973). *Madness and civilization: A history of insanity in the age of reason*. New York: Random House.

Frank, R. (1981). Cost-benefit analysis in mental health services: A review of the literature. *Administration in Mental Health, 8*, 161–176.

Frank, R. G. & Kamlet, M. S. (1985). Direct costs and expenditures for mental health care in the United States in 1980. *Hospital and Community Psychiatry, 36*, 165–168.

Frank, R. G. & Kamlet, M. S. (1986). Quality, quantity, and total expenditures on publicly provided goods: The case of public mental hospitals. *Journal of Public Economics, 29*, 295–316.

Franklin, J. L., Kittredge, L. D., & Thrasher, J. H. (1975). A survey of factors related to mental hospital readmissions. *Hospital and Community Psychiatry, 26*, 749–751.

Freedman, D. X. (1978). Psychiatry. *Journal of the American Medical Association, 239*, 510–512.

Freeland, M., Calat, G., & Schendler, C. E. (1980). Projections of national health expenditures, 1980, 1985, and 1990. *Health Care Financing Review, 1*, 1–27.

Friedman, L. (1985). *Caring for the mental patient in the general hospital: A comparison of hospitals with and without psychiatric units*. Unpublished doctoral dissertation, University of Pittsburgh.

Fuchs, V. R. (1974). *Who shall live? Health economics and social choice.* New York: Basic Books.

General Accounting Office. (1977). *Returning the mentally disabled to the community: Government needs to do more.* Washington, DC: U.S. Government Printing Office.

Gibson, R. M., & Waldo, D. R. (1981). National health expenditures, 1980s. *Health Care Financing Review, 3,* 1–54.

Gillis, J. S., & Moran, T. J. (1981). An analysis of drug decisions in a state psychiatric hospital. *Journal of Clinical Psychology, 37,* 32–42.

Glass, G. V., McGaw, B., & Smith, M. L. (1981). *Meta- analysis in social research.* Beverly Hills, CA: Sage Publications.

Glick, I. D., & Hargreaves, W. A. (1979). Hospitals in the 1980s: Service, training, and research. *Hospital and Community Psychiatry, 30,* 125–128.

Goffman, E. (1961). *Asylums: Essays on the social situation of mental patients and other inmates.* Garden City, NY: Doubleday.

Goldberg, I. D., & Allen, G. (1981). *Unduplicated counts of persons receiving care in psychiatric facilities in Monroe County, New York.* (Statistical Note No. 158). Rockville, MD: National Institute of Mental Health.

Goldhamer, H., & Marshall, A. W. (1953). *Psychosis and civilization: Two studies in the frequency of mental disease.* Glencoe, IL: Free Press.

Goldman, H. H. (1983). The demography of deinstitutionalization. In L. Bachrach (Ed.), *Deinstitutionalization.* San Francisco: Jossey-Bass.

Goldman, H. H., Adams, N. H., & Taube, C. A. (1983). Deinstitutionalization: The data demythologized. *Hospital and Community Psychiatry, 34,* 129–134.

Goldman, H. H., Gattozzi, A. A., & Taube, C. A. (1981). Defining and counting the chronically mentally ill. *Hospital and Community Psychiatry, 32,* 21–27.

Goldman, H. H., Taube, C. A., Regier, D. A., & Witkin, M. (1983). The multiple functions of the state mental hospital. *American Journal of Psychiatry, 140,* 296–300.

Goldstein, M. S. (1979). The sociology of mental health and illness. *Annual Review of Sociology, 5,* 381–409.

Goldstein, M. J., Rodnick, E. H., Evans, J. R., et al. (1978). Drug and family therapy in the aftercare of acute schizophrenics. *Archives of General Psychiatry, 35,* 1169–1177.

Goldstrom, I. D., & Manderscheid, R. W. (1982). The chronically mentally ill: A descriptive analysis from the Uniform Client Data Instrument. *Community Support Service Journal, 2,* 4–9.

Goodacre, R. H., Coles, E. M., MaCurdy, E. A., Coates, D. B., & Kendall, L. M. (1975). Hospitalization and hospital bed replacement. *Canadian Psychiatric Association Journal, 20,* 7–14.

Goplerud, E. N. (1981). The tangled web of clinical and epidemiological evidence. In A. Broskowski, E. Marks, & S. H. Budman (Eds.), *Linking health and mental health.* Beverly Hills, CA: Sage Publications.

Gottfredson, G. D., & Dyer, S. E. (1978). Health service providers in psychology. *American Psychologist, 33,* 314–338.

Greene, L. R., & De La Cruz, A. (1981). Psychiatric day treatment as an alternative to and transition from full-time hospitalization. *Community Mental Health Journal, 17*, 191–202.

Greenhill, M. H. (1979). Psychiatric units in general hospitals: 1979. *Hospital and Community Psychiatry, 30*, 169–182.

Grob, G. N. (1966). *The state and the mentally ill: A history of Worcester State Hospital in Massachusetts, 1830–1920*. New York: Free Press.

Grob, G. N. (1983). Mental illness and American society, 1875–1940. Princeton, NJ: Princeton University Press.

Group for the Advancement of Psychiatry. (1978). *The chronic mental patient in the community*. New York: Mental Health Materials Center.

Hansell, N. (1978). Services for schizophrenics: A lifelong approach to treatment. *Hospital and Community Psychiatry, 29*, 105–109.

Hazelton, N., Mandrill, D., & Stern, S. (1975). *Community care for the mentally ill*. Sacramento: California State Department of Health.

Health Care Financing Administration. (1983). The Medicare and Medicaid data book, 1983 (HCFA No. 03156). Office of Research and Demonstrations.

Heinrichs, D. W. (1984). Recent developments in the psychosocial treatment of chronic psychotic illnesses. In J. Talbott (Ed.), *The chronic mental patient five years later*. New York: Grune & Stratton.

Herz, M. I., Endicott, J., Spitzer, R. L., & Mesnikoff, A. (1971). Day versus inpatient hospitalization: A controlled study. *American Journal of Psychiatry, 127*, 1371–1381.

Hing, E. (1981). *Characteristics of nursing home residents, health status, and care received: National Nursing Home Survey United States, May–December 1977* (Vital and Health Statistics Series 13, No. 51.) DHHS Publication No. (PHS) 81–1712. Hyattsville, MD: National Center for Health Statistics.

Hingson, R. W., Matthews, D., & Scotch, N. A. (1979). The use and abuse of psychoactive substances. In H. E. Freeman, S. Levine, & L. G. Reeder (Eds.), *Handbook of medical sociology* (3rd edition). Englewood Cliffs, NJ: Prentice Hall.

Hoeper, E. W. (1980). Observations on the impact of psychiatric disorders upon primary medical care. In D. L. Parron and F. Solomon (Eds.), *Mental health services in primary care settings*, DHHS Publication No. (ADM) 80–995. Washington, DC: U.S. Government Printing Office.

Hogarty, G. E. (1977). Treatment and the course of schizophrenia. *Schizophrenia Bulletin, 3*, 587–599.

Intagliata, J., & Baker, F. (1984). A comparative analysis of the young adult chronic patient in New York State's community support system. *Hospital and Community Psychiatry, 35*, 45–50.

Johnson, P. J. (1983). Community support systems for deinstitutionalized patients. In L. Bachrach (Ed.), *Deinstitutionalization*. San Francisco: Jossey-Bass.

Jonas, S. (1981). *Health care delivery in the United States* (2nd ed.). New York: Springer.

Jones, K., & Vischi, T. (1980). Impact of alcohol, drug abuse, and mental health treatment on medical care utilization: Review of the research literature. *Medical Care (Supplement 17, 12)*.

Kane, J. M., & Smith, J. (1982). Tardive dyskinesia: Prevalence and risk factors 1959–1979. *Archives of General Psychiatry, 39*, 473–481.

Kane, J. M. (1984). Psychopharmacology. In J. Talbott (Ed.), *The chronic mental patient five years later*. New York: Grune & Stratton.

Karon, B. P., & VandenBos, G. R. (1981). *Psychotherapy of Schizophrenia*. New York: Aronson.

Keith, S. J., & Matthews, S. M. (1984). Research overview. In J. Talbott (Ed.), *The chronic mental patient five years later*. New York: Grune & Stratton.

Kiesler, C. A. (1973). Evaluating social change programs. In G. Zaltman (Ed.), *Processes and phenomena of social change*. New York: Wiley.

Kiesler, C. A. (1980). Mental health policy as a field of inquiry for psychology. *American Psychologist, 35*, 1066–1080.

Kiesler, C. A. (1981a). Barriers to effective knowledge use in national mental health policy. *Health Policy Quarterly, 1*, 201–215.

Kiesler, C. A. (1981b). Mental health policy: Research site for social psychology. In L. Wheeler (Ed.), *Review of Personality and Social Psychology* (Vol. 2). Beverly Hills, CA: Sage Publications.

Kiesler, C. A. (1982a). Mental hospitals and alternative care: Noninstitutionalization as potential public policy for mental patients. *American Psychologist, 37*, 349–360.

Kiesler, C. A. (1982b). Public and professional myths about mental hospitalization: An empirical reassessment of policy-related beliefs. *American Psychologist, 37*, 1323–1339.

Kiesler, C. A. (1983). Psychology and mental health policy. In M. Hersen, A. E. Kazdin, & A. S. Bellack (Eds.), *The Clinical Psychology Handbook*. New York: Pergamon Press.

Kiesler, C. A. (1984). Testimony in collaboration with the American Psychological Association and the Association for the Advancement of Psychology before the Labor-HHS-Education Appropriations Subcommittee of the Appropriations Committee, United States Senate.

Kiesler, C. A. (1985). Meta-analysis, clinical psychology, and social policy. *Clinical Psychology Review, 5*, 3–12.

Kiesler, C. A., McGuire, T., Mechanic, D., Mosher, L. R., Nelson, S. H., Newman, F. L., Rich, R., & Schulberg, H. C. (1983). Federal mental health policy making: An assessment of deinstitutionalization. *American Psychologist, 38*, 1292–1297.

Kiesler, C. A., & Sibulkin, A. E. (1983a). People, clinical episodes, and mental hospitalization: A multiple-source method of estimation. In R. F. Kidd and M. J. Saks (Eds.), *Advances in Applied Social Psychology*. Hillsdale, NJ: Erlbaum Associates.

Kiesler, C. A., & Sibulkin, A. E. (1983b). Proportion of inpatient days for mental disorders: 1969–1978. *Hospital and Community Psychiatry, 34*, 606–611.

Kiesler, C. A., & Sibulkin, A. E. (1984a). Drs. Kiesler and Sibulkin reply [Letter to the editor]. *American Journal of Psychiatry, 141,* 1497.

Kiesler, C. A., & Sibulkin, A. E. (1984b). Episodic rate of mental hospitalization: Stable or increasing? *American Journal of Psychiatry, 141,* 44–48.

Kiesler, C. A., & Sibulkin, A. E. (1984c). Episodic length of hospital stay for mental disorders. In G. M. Stephenson and J. H. Davis (Eds.), *Progress in Applied Social Psychology.* New York: Wiley.

Kirk, S. A. (1976). Effectiveness of community services for discharged mental hospital patients. *American Journal of Orthopsychiatry, 46,* 646–659.

Kirk, S. A. & Therrien, M. E. (1975). Community mental health myths and the fate of former hospitalized patients. *Psychiatry, 38,* 209–217.

Klerman, G. L. (1979a). National trends in hospitalization. *Hospital and Community Psychiatry, 30,* 110–113.

Klerman, G. L. (1979b). Patient reentry into the community: The federal viewpoint. *Journal of the National Association of Private Psychiatric Hospitals, 11,* 5–11.

Koranyi, E. K. (1972). Physical health and illness in a psychiatric outpatient department population. *Canadian Psychiatric Association Journal (Supplement), 17,* 109–116.

Koranyi, E. K. (1979). Morbidity and rate of undiagnosed physical illnesses in a psychiatric clinic population. *Archives of General Psychiatry, 36,* 414–419.

Kovacs, K. V. (1981). Telephone or letter outreach to patients who fail to keep first appointments. *Hospital and Community Psychiatry, 32,* 278–279.

Kozak, L. J., & Moien, M. (1985). *Detailed diagnoses and surgical procedures for patients discharged from short-stay hospitals United States, 1983.* (Vital and Health Statistics Series 13, No. 82). DHHS No. (PHS) 85–1743. Hyattsville, MD: National Center for Health Statistics.

Kramer, M. (1977). *Psychiatric services and the changing institutional scene, 1950–1985.* Washington, DC: U.S. Government Printing Office.

Krowinski, W. J., & Fitt, D. X. (1978). *On the clinical efficacy and cost effectiveness of psychiatric partial hospitalization versus traditional inpatient care with six month follow-up data.* Report to Capital Blue Cross, Reading Hospital and Medical Center, Day Treatment Center.

Lamb, H. R. (1979). The new asylums in the community. *Archives of General Psychiatry, 36,* 129–134.

Lamb, H. R. (1982). *Treating the long-term mentally ill.* San Francisco: Jossey-Bass.

Lamb, H. R. (1984a). Alternatives to hospitals. In J. Talbott (Ed.), *The chronic mental patient five years later.* New York: Grune & Stratton.

Lamb, H. R., (Ed.). (1984b). *The homeless mentally ill.* Washington, DC: American Psychiatric Association.

Lamb, H. R., & Goertzel, V. (1972). The demise of the state hospital: A premature obituary? *Archives of General Psychiatry, 26,* 489–495.

Lamb, H. R., & Goertzel, V. (1977). The long-term patient in the era of community treatment. *Archives of General Psychiatry, 34,* 679–682.

Landman, J. T., & Dawes, R. M. (1982). Psychotherapy outcome: Smith and Glass' conclusions stand up under scrutiny. *American Psychologist, 37*, 504–516.

Langsley, D. G., Machotka, P., & Flomenhaft, K. (1971). Avoiding mental hospital admission: A follow-up study. *American Journal of Psychiatry, 127*, 1391-1394.

Leaf, P. (1977). Patients released after Wyatt: Where did they go? *Hospital and Community Psychiatry, 28*, 366–369.

Levenson, A. I. (1982). The growth of investor-owned psychiatric hospitals. *American Journal of Psychiatry, 139*, 902–907.

Levenson, A. I. (1983). Issues surrounding the ownership of private psychiatric hospitals by investor-owned hospital chains. *Hospital and Community Psychiatry, 34*, 1127–1131.

Levenson, A. J., Lord, C. J., Sermas, C. E., Thornby, J. I., Sullender, W., & Comstock, B. S. (1977). Acute schizophrenia: An efficacious outpatient treatment approach as an alternative to full-time hospitalization. *Diseases of the Nervous System, 38*, 242–245.

Levine, D. S., & Levine, D. R. (1975). *The cost of mental illness—1971* (Mental Health Statistics, Series B, No. 7). DHEW Publication No. (ADM) 76–265. Washington, DC: U.S. Government Printing Office.

Levine, D. S., & Willner, S. G. (1976). *The cost of mental illness—1974* (Statistical Note No. 125). Rockville, MD: National Institute of Mental Health.

Levine, M. (1981). *The history and politics of community mental health.* New York: Oxford University Press.

Levine, M., & Levine, D. (1981). Report of the President's Commission on Mental health: The development of public policy. *Health Policy Quarterly, 1*, 179–192.

Lieberman, M. A., & Borman, L. D. (Eds.). (1976). A special issue on self-help groups. *The Journal of Applied Behavioral Science, 12*, 3.

Liptzin, B., Regier, D. A., & Goldberg, I. D. (1980). Utilization of health and mental health services in a large insured population. *American Journal of Psychiatry, 137*, 553–558.

Lorei, T. W., & Gurel, L. (1973). Demographic characteristics as predictors of post-hospital employment and readmission. *Journal of Consulting and Clinical Psychology, 40*, 426–430.

Love, R. E. (1984). The community support program: Strategy for reform? In J. Talbott (Ed.), *The chronic mental patient five years later.* New York: Grune & Stratton.

Manderscheid, R. W., Witkin, M. J., Bass, R. D., Bethel, H., Rosenstein, M. J., & Thompson, J. W. (1984). Care needed in counting inpatient episodes [Letter to the editor]. *American Journal of Psychiatry, 141*, 1496–1497.

Marks, J. N., Goldberg, D. P., & Hillier, V. F. (1979). Determinants of the ability of general practitioners to detect psychiatric illness. *Psychological Medicine, 9*, 337–353.

Marmor, J., Scheidemandel, P. L., & Kanno, C. K. (1975). *Psychiatrists and their patients.* Washington, DC: American Psychiatric Association.

Matthews, S. M., Roper, M. T., Mosher, L. R., & Menn, A. Z. (1979). A non-neuroleptic treatment for schizophrenia: Analysis of the two-year post-discharge risk of relapse. *Schizophrenia Bulletin, 5*, 322–333.

May, P. R. (1970). Cost-efficiency of mental health delivery systems. *American Journal of Public Health, 60*, 2060–2067.

McCaffree, K. (1969). The cost of mental health care under changing treatment methods. In C. Schulberg et al. (Eds.), *Program evaluation in the health fields*. New York: Behavioral Publications.

McEwen, C. A. (1980). Continuities in the study of total and nontotal institutions. *Annual Review of Sociology, 6*, 143–185.

McGuire, T. (1981). *Financing psychotherapy: Costs, effects, public policy.* Cambridge, MA: Ballinger.

McGuire, T. G., & Weisbrod, B. A. (Eds.) (1981) *Economics and mental health.* DHHS Publication No. (ADM) 81–1114. Washington, DC: U.S. Government Printing Office.

Mechanic, D. (Coordinator). (1978). *Report of the task panel on the nature and scope of the problem.* (President's Commission on Mental Health, Vol. 2). Washington, DC: U.S. Government Printing Office.

Mechanic, D. (1979). Physicians. In H. E. Freeman, S. Levine, & L. G. Reeder (Eds.), *Handbook of medical sociology* (3rd edition). Englewood Cliffs, NJ: Prentice Hall.

Mechanic, D. (1980). *Mental health and social policy.* Englewood Cliffs, NJ: Prentice Hall.

Mellinger, G., Balter, M., Parry, H., Manheimer, D., & Cisin, I. (1974). An overview of psychotherapeutic drug use in the United States. In E. Josephson & E. Carroll (Eds.), *Drug use: Epidemiological and sociological approaches.* Washington, DC: Hemisphere Publishing.

Melnick, G. A., Wheeler, J.R.C., & Feldstein, P. J. (1981). Effects of rate regulation on selected components of hospital expenses. *Inquiry, 18*, 240–246.

Mental Health Reports. (1985). Vol. 9, No. 16 (July 31, 1985). Arlington, VA: Capitol Publications.

Meyer, N. G. (1973). *Changes in the age, sex, and diagnostic composition of first admissions to state and county mental hospitals, United States 1962–1972.* (Statistical Note No. 97). Rockville, MD: National Institute of Mental Health.

Meyerson, A. T., & Herman, G. S. (1983). What's new in aftercare? A review of recent literature. *Hospital and Community Psychiatry, 34*, 333–342.

Minkoff, K. (1978). A map of chronic mental patients. In J. A. Talbott (Ed.), *The chronic mental patient.* Washington, DC: American Psychiatric Association.

Morrissey, J. P., Burton, N., Castellani, P., & Melnick, M. (1979). *Factors contributing to the differentials in the facility-based rate schedule for inpatient care in New York State adult psychiatric centers.* Phase II of the DMH cost-quality project. Albany: NYS Department of Mental Hygiene.

Mosher, L. R. (1982). Italy's revolutionary mental health law: An assessment. *American Journal of Psychiatry, 139*, 199–203.

Mosher, L. R. (1983). Alternatives to psychiatric hospitalization: Why has research failed to be translated into practice? *New England Journal of Medicine, 309,* 1579–1580.

Mosher, L. R., & Menn, A. Z. (1978). Community residential treatment for schizophrenia: Two year follow-up. *Hospital and Community Psychiatry, 29,* 715–723.

Mosher, L. R., Menn, A., & Matthews, S. M. (1975). Soteria: Evaluation of a home-based treatment for schizophrenia. *American Journal of Orthopsychiatry, 45,* 455–467.

Mumford, E., Schlesinger, H. J., & Glass, G. V. (1981). Reducing medical costs through mental health treatment: Research problems and recommendations. In A. Broskowski, E. Marks, & S. H. Budman (Eds.), *Linking health and mental health.* Beverly Hills, CA: Sage Publications.

Mushkin, S. J., & Dunlop, D. W. (Eds.), (1979). *Health: What is it worth?* New York: Pergamon Press.

Muszynski, S., Brady, J., & Sharfstein, S. (1983). *Coverage for mental and nervous disorders: Summaries of 300 private sector health insurance plans.* Washington, DC: American Psychiatric Press.

Myers, J. K., Weissman, M. M., Tischler, G. L., Holzer, C. E., Leaf, P. J., Orvaschel, H., Anthony, J. C., Boyd, J. H., Burke, J. D., Kramer, M., & Stoltzman, R. (1984). Six-month prevalence of psychiatric disorders in three communities. *Archives of General Psychiatry, 41,* 959–967.

National Center for Health Statistics. (1962). *International classification of diseases, adapted for indexing hospital records by disease and operations.* PHS Publication No. 719. Washington, DC: U.S. Government Printing Office.

National Center for Health Statistics. (1967–1969). *International Classification of Diseases.* Adapted for use in the United States, Eighth Revision, (PHS Publication No. 1693). Washington, DC: U.S. Government Printing Office.

National Center for Health Statistics. (1980). *International classification of diseases, Ninth Revision, Clinical Modification.* DHHS Publication No. (PHS) 80–1260. Washington, DC: U.S. Government Printing Office.

National Center for Health Statistics. (1981). *Health United States 1980.* DHHS No. (PHS) 81–1232. Hyattsville, MD: Office of Health Research, Statistics and Technology.

National Institute of Mental Health. (1976). *The financing, utilization, and quality of mental health care in the United States.* (Draft report). Rockville, MD: Author.

National Institute of Mental Health. (1980). *Provisional data on federally funded community mental health centers, 1977–1978.* Washington, DC: U.S. Government Printing Office.

Newman, H. N. (Coordinator). (1978). *Report of the task panel on cost and financing of mental health.* (President's Commission on Mental Health, Vol. 2) Washington, DC: U.S. Government Printing Office.

Nielsen, A. C., & Williams, T. A. (1980). Depression in ambulatory medical patients. *Archives of General Psychiatry, 37,* 999–1004.

O'Conner v. Donaldson, 422 U.S. 563 (1975).

Ozarin, L. D., & Sharfstein, S. S. (1978). The aftermaths of deinstitutionalization: Problems and solutions. *Psychiatric Quarterly, 50,* 128–132.

Palinkas, L. A., & Hoiberg, A. (1982). An epidemiology primer: Bridging the
gap between epidemiology and psychology. *Health Psychology, 1,* 269–287.

Pasamanick, B., Scarpitti, F. R., & Dinitz, S. (1967). *Schizophrenics in the community.* New York: Appelton-Century Crofts.

Paul, G. L., & Lentz, R. J. (1977). *Psychosocial treatment of chronic mental
patients.* Cambridge, MA: Harvard University Press.

Paul, G. L. & Licht, M. H. (1978). Resurrection of uniformity assumption myths
and the fallacy of statistical absolutes in psychotherapy research. *Journal of
Consulting and Clinical Psychology, 46,* 1531–1534.

Pepper, B., & Ryglewicz, H. (Eds.). (1982). *The young adult chronic patient.*
San Francisco: Jossey-Bass.

Pepper, B., Kirshner, M. C., & Ryglewicz, H. (1981). The young adult chronic
patient: Overview of a population. *Hospital and Community Psychiatry, 32,*
463–469.

Pepper, B., Ryglewicz, H., & Kirshner, M. C. (1982). The uninstitutionalized
generation: A new breed of psychiatric patient. In B. Pepper & H. Ryglewicz
(Eds.), *The young adult chronic patient.* San Francisco: Jossey-Bass.

Platman, S. R. (Coordinator). (1978). *Report of the task panel on
deinstitutionalization, rehabilitation, and long-term care.* (President's
Commission on Mental Health, Vol. 2.) Washington, DC: U.S. Government
Printing Office.

Polak, P. R. & Kirby, M. W. (1976). A model to replace psychiatric hospitals.
The Journal of Nervous and Mental Disease, 162, 13–22.

President's Commission on Mental Health. (1978a). *Report to the President*
(Vols. 1–4). Washington, DC: U.S. Government Printing Office.

President's Commission on Mental Health. (1978b). Vol. 2. Washington, DC:
U.S. Government Printing Office.

Rabkin, J. G. (1979). Criminal behavior of discharged mental patients: A critical
appraisal of the research. *Psychological Bulletin, 86,* 1–27.

Rabkin, J. G. (1980). Determinants of public attitudes about mental illness: Sum-
mary of the research literature. In J. G. Rabkin, L. Gelb, and J. B. Lazar
(Eds.), *Attitudes toward the mentally ill: Research perspectives.* Washington,
DC: National Institute of Mental Health.

Rabkin, J. G. (1984). Community attitudes and local psychiatric facilities. In J.
Talbott (Ed.), *The chronic mental patient five years later.* New York: Grune
& Stratton.

Ray, W. A., Federspiel, C. F., & Schaffner, W. (1980). A study of antipsychotic
drug use in nursing homes: Epidemiologic evidence suggesting misuse.
American Journal of Public Health, 70, 485–491.

Redick, R. W. (1974). *Patterns in use of nursing homes by the aged mentally ill.*
(Statistical Note No. 107). Rockville, MD: National Institute of Mental
Health.

Redick, R. W., & Witkin, M. J. (1983). *Residential treatment centers for
emotionally disturbed children, United States, 1977–78 and 1979–80.*

(Statistical Note No. 162). Rockville, MD: National Institute of Mental Health.

Redick, R. W., Manderscheid, R. W., Witkin, M. J., & Rosenstein, M. J. (1983). *A history of the U.S. national reporting program for mental health statistics, 1840–1983.* DHHS Pub. No. (ADM) 83–1296. Washington, DC: U.S. Government Printing Office.

Regier, D. A., Goldberg, I. D., & Taube, C. A. (1978). The de facto U.S. mental health services system. A public health perspective. *Archives of General Psychiatry, 35,* 685–693.

Regier, D. A., & Taube, C. A. (1981). The delivery of mental health services. In S. Arietti & H.K.H. Brodie (Eds.), *American Handbook of Psychiatry.* New York: Basic Books.

Rich, R. F. (1979). The pursuit of knowledge. *Knowledge: Creation, Diffusion, Utilization, 1,* 6–28.

Rich, R. F. (1981). *Social science information and public policy making: The interaction between bureaucratic politics and the use of survey data.* San Francisco: Jossey-Bass.

Rittenhouse, J. D. (1970). Endurance of effect: Family unit treatment compared to identified patient treatment. *Proceedings of the Annual Convention of the American Psychological Association, 2,* 535–536.

Rose, S. M. (1979). Deciphering deinstitutionalization: Complexities in policy and program analysis. *Milbank Memorial Fund Quarterly/Health and Society, 57,* 429–460.

Rosenblatt, A., & Mayer, J. E. (1974). The recidivism of mental patients: A review of past studies. *American Journal of Orthopsychiatry, 44,* 697–705.

Rosenhan, D. L. (1973). On being sane in insane places. *Science, 179,* 250–258.

Rosenstein, M. J., & Millazzo-Sayre, L. (1981). *Characteristics of admissions to selected mental health facilities, 1975: An annotated book of charts and tables.* (Mental Health National Statistics Series CN, No. 2). DHEW No. (ADM) 81–1005. Washington, DC: U.S. Government Printing Office.

Rubin, J. (1978). *Economics, mental health, and the law.* Lexington, MA: D.C. Heath.

Rubin, J. (1982). Cost measurement and cost data in mental health settings. *Hospital and Community Psychiatry, 33,* 750–754.

Sainer, J. S. (1976). The community cares: Older volunteers. *Social Policy, 7,* 73–75.

Saltman, R. B., & Young, D. W. (1981). The hospital power equilibrium: An alternative view of the cost containment dilemma. *Journal of Health Politics, Policy and Law, 6,* 391–418.

Saxe, L. (1980). *The efficacy and cost-effectiveness of psychotherapy.* Office of Technology Assessment, Congress of the U.S. Washington, DC: U.S. Government Printing Office.

• Schlesinger, H. J., Mumford, E., Glass, G. V., Patrick, C., & Sharfstein, S. (1983). Mental health treatment and medical care utilization in a fee-for-service system: Outpatient mental health treatment following the onset of a chronic disease. *American Journal of Public Health, 73,* 422–429.

Schulberg, H. C. (1979). Community support programs: Program evaluation and public policy. *American Journal of Psychiatry, 136*, 1433–1437.

Schur, E. M. (1971). *Labeling deviant behavior.* New York: Harper & Row.

Schwab, J. J., Bell, R. A., Warheit, G., & Schwab, R. B. (1979). *Social order and mental health.* New York: Brunner/Mazel.

Schwartz, W. B. (1981). The regulation strategy for controlling hospital costs. *New England Journal of Medicine, 305*, 1249–1255.

Schwartz, S. R., & Goldfinger, S. M. (1981). The new chronic patient: Clinical characteristics of an emerging subgroup. *Hospital and Community Psychiatry, 32*, 470–474.

Schwartz, A. H., Perlman, B. B., Paris, M., Schmidt, K., & Thornton, J. C. (1980). Psychiatric diagnoses as reported to Medicaid and as recorded in patient charts. *American Journal of Public Health, 70*, 406–408.

Scull, A. (1977). *Decarceration: Community treatment and the deviant: A radical view.* Englewood Cliffs, NJ: Prentice-Hall.

Shadish, W. R., Silber, B. G., & Bootzin, R. R. (1984). Mental patients in nursing homes: Their characteristics and treatment. *International Journal of Partial Hospitalization, 2*, 153–163.

Shadish, W. R., Straw, R. B., McSweeny, A. J., Koller, D. L., & Bootzin, R. R. (1981). Nursing home care for mental patients: Descriptive data and some propositions. *American Journal of Community Psychology, 9*, 617–633.

Shaeffer, D. E., Schulberg, H. C., & Board, G. (1978). Effects of community mental health services on state hospital admissions: A clinical-demographic study. *Hospital and Community Psychiatry, 29*, 578–583.

Shapiro, S., Skinner, E. A., Kessler, L. G., Von Korff, M., German, P. S., Tischler, G. L., Leaf, P. J., Benham, L., Cottler, L., & Regier, D. A. (1984). Utilization of health and mental health services. *Archives of General Psychiatry, 41*, 971–978.

Sharfstein, S. S., Towery, O. B., & Milowe, I. D. (1980). Accuracy of diagnostic information submitted to an insurance company. *American Journal of Psychiatry, 137*, 70–73.

Sheehan, D. M., & Atkinson, J. A. (1974). Comparative costs of state hospital and community-based inpatient care in Texas: Who benefits most? *Hospital and Community Psychiatry, 25*, 242–244.

Sibulkin, A. E., & Kiesler, C. A. (1982). Guide to national data on inpatient care for mental disorders. *JSAS Catalog of Selected Documents in Psychology, 12*, 47, Ms. 2508.

Silverman, P. R. (1978). *Mutual help groups: A guide for mental health workers.* Rockville, MD: National Institute of Mental Health.

Silverman, I., & Saunders, D. (1980). Creating the mental illness culture: Demographic studies of mental institutionalization in Ontario. *Canadian Psychology, 21*, 121–128.

Sirrocco, A. (1974). *Inpatient health facilities as reported from the 1971 MFI survey.* (Vital and Health Statistics Series 14, No. 12). DHEW No. (HRA) 74–1807. Rockville, MD: National Center for Health Statistics.

Sirrocco, A. (1976). *Inpatient health facilities as reported from the 1973 MFI survey.* (Vital and Health Statistics Series 14, No. 16) DHEW No. (HRA) 76–1811. Rockville, MD: National Center for Health Statistics.

Smith, M. L., & Glass, G. V. (1977). Meta-analysis of psychotherapy outcome studies. *American Psychologist, 32,* 752–760.

Smith, M. L., Glass, G. V., & Miller, T. I. (1980). *The benefits of psychotherapy.* Baltimore, MD: Johns Hopkins University Press.

Social Security Administration. (1984a). *Annual statistical supplement, 1983.* (SSA No. 13–11700). Washington, DC: U.S. Government Printing Office.

Social Security Administration. (1984b) *Social security handbook* (8th edition). SSA No. (05–10135). Social Security Administration.

Solomon, P., Davis, J., & Gordon, B. (1984). Discharged state hospital patients' characteristics and use of aftercare: Effect on community tenure. *American Journal of Psychiatry, 141,* 1566–1570.

Solomon, P., Davis., J. M., Gordon, B., Fishbein, P., & Mason, A. (1983). *The aftercare mosaic.* Cleveland, OH: Federation for Community Planning.

Spearly, J. L. (1980). Evaluating the impact of community mental health centers on hospital admissions: An interrupted time-series analysis. *American Journal of Community Psychology, 8,* 229–241.

Stein, L. I., & Test, M. A. (1980). Alternative to mental hospital treatment: I. Conceptual model, treatment program, and clinical evaluation. *Archives of General Psychiatry, 37,* 392–397.

Stein, L. I., & Test, M. A. (1982). Community treatment of the young adult patient. In B. Pepper & H. Ryglewicz (Eds.), *The young adult chronic patient.* San Francisco: Jossey-Bass.

Stein, L. I., Test, M. A., & Marx, A. J. (1975). Alternative to the hospital: A controlled study. *American Journal of Psychiatry, 132,* 517–522.

Stickney, S. K., Hall, R.C.W., & Gardner, E. R. (1980). The effect of referral procedures on aftercare compliance. *Hospital and Community Psychiatry, 31,* 567–569.

Strahan, G. W. (1981). *Inpatient health facilities statistics United States, 1978.* (Vital and Health Statistics Series 14, No. 24). DHHS No. (PHS) 81–1819. Hyattsville, MD: National Center for Health Statistics.

Strauss, J. S., Carpenter, W. T., & Nasrallah, A. T. (1978). How reliable is the psychiatric history? *Comprehensive Psychiatry, 19,* 213–219.

Straw, R. B. (1982). *Meta-analysis of deinstitutionalization in mental health.* Unpublished doctoral dissertation, Northwestern University.

Strayer, R. G., & Keith, R. A. (1979). An ecological study of the recently discharged chronic psychiatric patient. *Journal of Community Psychology, 7,* 313–317.

Sutton, J. F., & Sirrocco, A. (1980). *Inpatient health facilities as reported from the 1976 MFI survey.* (Vital and Health Statistics Series 14, No. 23). DHEW No. (PHS) 80–1818. Hyattsville, MD: National Center for Health Statistics.

Szasz, T. S. (1963). *Law, liberty, and psychiatry: An inquiry into the social uses of mental health practices.* New York: Macmillan.

Taber, M. A. (1980). *The social context of helping: A review of the literature on alternative care for the physically and mentally handicapped.* Washington, DC: National Institute of Mental Health.

Talbott, J. A. (1978). *The chronic mental patient.* Washington, DC: American Psychiatric Association.

Talbott, J. A. (Ed.). (1984). *The chronic mental patient five years later.* New York: Grune & Stratton.

Taube, C. A. (1973a). *Admissions to private mental hospitals, 1970.* (Statistical Note No. 75). Rockville, MD: National Institute of Mental Health.

Taube, C. A. (1973b). *Utilization of mental health facilities, 1971.* (Mental Health Statistics Series B, No. 5). DHEW No. NIH-74-657. Washington, DC: U.S. Government Printing Office.

Taube, C. A. (1974). *Readmissions to inpatient services of state and county mental hospitals, 1972.* (Statistical Note No. 110). Rockville, MD: National Institute of Mental Health.

Taube, C. A., & Barrett, S. A. (Eds.). (1983). *Mental Health United States 1983.* DHHS No. (ADM) 83–1275. Rockville, MD: National Institute of Mental Health.

Taube, C. A., & Barrett, S. A. (Eds.). (1985). *Mental Health United States 1985.* DHHS No. (ADM) 85–1378. Washington, DC: U.S. Government Printing Office.

Taube, C. A., Thompson, J. W., Rosenstein, M. J., Rosen, B. M., & Goldman, H. H. (1983). The chronic mental hospital patient. *Hospital and Community Psychiatry, 34,* 611–615.

Tenney, J. B. (1968). Diagnostic precision for insurance records: A physicians' survey. *Inquiry, 5,* 14–19.

Tessler, R., & Mason, J. H. (1979). Continuity of care in the delivery of mental health services. *American Journal of Psychiatry, 136,* 1297–1301.

Tessler, R. C., Bernstein, A. G., Rosen, B. M., & Goldman, H. H. (1982). The chronically mentally ill in community support systems. *Hospital and Community Psychiatry, 33,* 208–211.

Tessler, R., Mechanic, D., & Dimond, M. (1976). The effect of psychological distress on physician utilization: A prospective study. *Journal of Health and Social Behavior, 17,* 353–364.

Test, M. A. (1981). Effective treatment of the chronically mentally ill: What is necessary? *Journal of Social Issues, 37,* 71–86.

Test, M. A., & Stein, L. I. (1978). Training in community living: Research design and results. In L. Stein & M. Test (Eds.), *Alternatives to mental hospital treatment.* New York: Plenum Press.

Thompson, J. W., Bass, R. D., & Witkin, M. J. (1982). Fifty years of psychiatric services: 1940–1990. *Hospital and Community Psychiatry, 33,* 711–717.

Toff, G. (1984). *Mental health benefits under Medicaid: A survey of the states.* Washington, DC: Intergovernmental Health Policy Project.

Tringo, J. (1970). The hierarchy of preference toward disability groups. *The Journal of Special Education, 4,* 295–306.

U.S. Bureau of the Census. (1984). *Statistical abstract of the United States: 1985.* Washington, DC: U.S. Bureau of the Census.

U.S. Senate. (1976). *Nursing home care in the United States: Failure in public policy.* Prepared by the subcommittee on long-term care of the Special Committee on Aging. Washington, DC: Government Printing Office.

Uyeda, M. K., & Moldawsky, S. (1986). Prospective payment and psychological services. *American Psychologist, 41*, 60–63.

Van Nostrand, J. F., Zappolo, A., Hing, E., Bloom, B., Hirsch, B., & Foley, D. J. (1979). *The national nursing home survey—1977: Summary for the United States.* (Vital and Health Statistics Series 13, No. 43). DHEW No. (PHS) 79–1794. Hyattsville, MD: National Center for Health Statistics.

Vischi, T. R., Jones, K. R., Shank, E. L., & Lima, L. H. (1980). *The alcohol, drug abuse, and mental health national data book.* DHHS No. (ADM) 80–938. Washington, DC: U.S. Department of Health, Education and Welfare.

Wallen, J. (1985). *Use of short-term general hospitals by patients with psychiatric diagnoses.* Hospital Cost and Utilization Project Research Note 8, Hospital Studies Program. DHHS Publication No. (PHS) 86–3395. National Center for Health Services Research and Health Care Technology Assessment.

Washburn, S., Vannicelli, M., Longabaugh, R., & Scheff, B. H. (1976). A controlled comparison of psychiatric day treatment and inpatient hospitalization. *Journal of Consulting and Clinical Psychology, 44*, 665–675.

Weinstein, A. S. (1983). The mythical readmissions explosion. *American Journal of Psychiatry, 140*, 332–335.

Weisbrod, B. (1983). A guide to benefit-cost analysis, as seen through a controlled experiment in treating the mentally ill. *Journal of Health Politics, Policy and Law, 7*, 805–845.

Weisbrod, B. A., Test, M. A., & Stein, L. I. (1980). Alternative to mental hospital treatment: II. Economic benefit-cost analysis. *Archives of General Psychiatry, 37*, 400–405.

Weiss, C. H. (1977). Research for policy's sake: The enlightenment function of social research. *Policy Analysis, 3*, 531–545.

Wilder, J. F., Levin, G., & Zwerling, I. (1966). A two-year follow-up evaluation of acute psychotic patients treated in a day hospital. *American Journal of Psychiatry, 122*, 1095–1101.

Wilson, F. A., & Neuhauser, D. (1982). *Health services in the United States* (2nd edition). Cambridge, MA: Ballinger

Windle, C., & Scully, D. (1976). Community mental health centers and the decreasing use of state mental hospitals. *Community Mental Health Journal, 12*, 239–243.

Witkin, M. J. (1980). *Trends in patient care episodes in mental health facilities, 1955–1977.* (Statistical Note No. 154). Rockville, MD: National Institute of Mental Health.

Wolford, J. A., Hitchcock, J., Ellison, D. L., Sonis, A. C., & Smith, F. (1972). The effect on state hospitalization of a community mental health/mental retardation center. *American Journal of Psychiatry, 129*, 202–206.

Wolpert, J., & Wolpert, E. R. (1976). The relocation of released mental hospital patients into residential communities. *Policy Sciences, 7*, 31–51.

World Health Organization. (1973). *Psychiatry and primary medical care.* Report on a working group convened by the regional office for Europe of the World Health Organization, Lysebu, Oslo, April 10–13, 1973.

Wyatt v. Stickney, 344 F. Supp. 373, 344 F. Supp. 387 (M.D. Ala. 1972), enforcing 325 F. Supp. 781, 334 F. Supp. 1341 (M.D. Ala. 1971), aff'd in part, remanded in part, decision reserved in part sub nom. Wyatt v. Aderholt, 503 F. 2d 1305 (5th Cir. 1974).

Yates, B. T., & Newman, F. L. (1980). Findings of cost-effectiveness and cost-benefit analyses of psychotherapy. In G. R. VandenBos (Ed.), *Psychotherapy: From practice to research to policy.* Beverly Hills, CA: Sage Publications.

Zeldow, P. B., & Taub, H. A. (1981). Evaluating psychiatric discharge and after-care in a VA medical center. *Hospital and Community Psychiatry, 32*, 57–58.

Zimmer, J. G., Watson, N., & Treat, A. (1984). Behavioral problems among patients in skilled nursing facilities. *American Journal of Public Health, 74*, 1118–1121.

Zook, C. J., & Moore, F. D. (1980). High-cost users of medical care. *New England Journal of Medicine, 302*, 996–1002.

Zook, C. J., Moore, F. D., & Zeckhauser, R. J. (1981). "Catastrophic" health insurance—a misguided prescription? *The Public Interest, 62*, 66–81.

Zusman, J. (1967). Some explanations of the changing appearance of psychotic patients. *International Journal of Psychiatry, 3*, 216–237.

Zwerling, I., & Wilder, J. F. (1964). An evaluation of the applicability of the day hospital in treatment of acutely disturbed patients. *The Israel Annals of Psychiatry and Related Disciplines, 2*, 162–185.

AUTHOR INDEX

Action for Mental Health, 29, 33, 182, 252
Adams, N. H., 47, 62, 65, 69
Adams, R. L., 140
Albee, G. W., 241, 254
Alcohol, Drug Abuse, and Mental Health Administration, 218
Allen, G., 133, 134
Althoff, M. E., 135
Altman, H., 130
American Hospital Association (AHA), 26, 103, 213, 226
American Psychiatric Association, 13, 32, 244
Anthony, W. A., 15, 135, 136, 137, 138, 171, 190
Arce, A., 196
Atkinson, J. A., 205

Babigian, H. M., 140, 141
Bachrach, L. L., 19, 177, 179, 182, 183, 188, 194, 196, 239, 240
Bahn, A. K., 132, 133, 134
Baker, F., 187, 189
Balter, M., 241
Bandura, A., 145, 177, 181, 255, 258, 261
Barnes, R. H., 140
Barrett, S. A., 42, 43, 85, 91, 206, 207, 256
Bass, R. D., 57, 65, 139
Bassuk, E. L., 69, 130, 189, 196, 197
Baxter, E., 197
Beard, J. H., 138, 139
Beers, C. W., 35, 272
Bell, J. C., 110
Benham, L., 15
Berger, P. A., 244
Bernstein, A. G., 186
Bethel, H. E., 65
Billings, A., 142
Binner, P. R., 205, 206

Bloom, B., 121
Boan, J., 206
Board, G., 141
Bockoven, J., 30, 34, 39, 40
Bond, E. D., 34
Bootzin, R. R., 125
Borman, L. D., 236
Boyd, J. L., 15, 195
Brady, J., 14
Braff, J., 136, 137
Braun, P., 152, 168, 169
Brenner, M. H., 34
Brill, H. R., 38, 39
Brook, B. D., 158, 164
Broskowski, A., 249
Brown, P., 268
Browning, D. H., 245
Buck, J. A., 252
Budman, S. H., 241, 249
Budson, R. D., 235, 236
Buell, G. J., 135, 136, 137
Burke, J. D., 15
Burns, B. J., 245
Burton, N., 206

Calat, G., 102
Califano, J., 247
Campbell, D. T., 151
Cannel, C. F., 128
Carpenter, W. T., 128
Cassell, W. A., 206
Castellani, P., 206
Caton, C. L., 188, 191
Chodoff, P., 26
Christmas, J. J., 235, 236
Cicchinelli, L. F., 110, 115, 120, 121, 123, 124, 125, 126
Cisin, I., 241
Clinkscale, R., 230
Coates, D. B., 166
Code of Federal Regulations, 232
Cohen, M. R., 135

Coles, E. M., 166
Cook, T. D., 252, 255
Cooper, B. S., 232
Cortes, M., 164
Cottler, L., 15
Cummings, N. A., 202, 241, 246, 262

Dain, N., 33, 40, 272
Davis, A. E., 161
Davis, J., 186
Davis, K., 247
Davison, G. C., 263
Dawes, R. M., 241
De La Cruz, A., 152, 168
Dellario, D. J., 171
Department of Health and Human
    Services, 183
Deutsch, A., 29, 36, 40
Dimond, M., 247
Dinitz, S., 161
Dittmar, N. D., 110
Dix, D., 30, 31
Dohrenwend, B. P., 15, 16, 203
Dohrenwend, B. S., 15
Doidge, J. R., 140
Dorken, H., 248
Doyle, D. N., 14
Dumont, M. P., 178
Dunlop, D. W., 203
Dyck, G., 140
Dyer, S. E., 254

Earle, P., 34
Eastwood, M. R., 13, 245
Eaton, W. W., 28, 30, 40
Edelman, P. B., 18, 19
Ellison, D. L., 140
Endicott, J., 143
Erlebacher, A., 151
Estroff, S., 144
Etzioni, A., 178
Evans, J. R., 195

Faden, V. B., 91
Falloon, I. R. H., 195
Federspiel, C. F., 242

Feldstein, P. J., 102
Fenton, F. R., 166, 167, 174
Fishbein, P., 186
Fisher, M., 230
Fiske, S. T., 250
Fitt, D. X., 163, 164, 178, 198
Flomenhaft, K., 159, 160, 176
Foley, D. J., 121
Follette, W. T., 246
Foucault, M., 28, 146
Frank, R. G., 206, 219, 223
Franklin, J. L., 139
Freedman, D. X., 204
Freeland, M., 102
Friedman, L., 77, 78, 268
Fuchs, V. R., 258, 261
Fuller, R., 35
Fuller, R., G., 36

Gardner, E. R., 138
Gattozzi, A. A., 63, 183, 187
General Accounting Office (GAO),
    140, 146
German, P. S., 15
Gerson, S., 69, 130, 189
Gibbon, M., 144
Gibson, R. M., 102
Gillis, J. S., 242
Glass, G. V., 172, 240, 241, 247
Glick, G. V., 78
Goertzel, V., 187, 189, 190
Goffman, E., 144
Goldberg, D. P., 13
Goldberg, I. D., 15, 133, 134, 245,
    248
Goldfinger, S. M., 189, 190, 192
Goldhamer, H., 34
Goldman, H. H., 47, 62, 63, 65, 66,
    69, 110, 183, 186, 187, 197
Goldner, N., 245
Goldstein, M. J., 195
Goldstein, M. S., 144
Goldstrom, I. D., 186, 191
Goodacre, R. H., 166, 174
Goplerud, E. N., 244, 246
Gordon, B., 186

Gorwitz, K., 132
Gottfredson, G. D., 254
Gould, M. S., 15
Gray, J., 32
Greenberg, S., 152
Greene, L. R., 152, 168
Greenhill, M. H., 108
Grob, G. N., 31, 32, 33, 36, 40, 109, 131, 146, 179
Group for the Advancement of Psychiatry (GAP), 183, 184, 185
Grundberg, F., 206
Gudeman, J. E., 152
Gurel, L., 148

Hall, R. C. W., 138
Hanbery, G. W., 213
Hansell, N., 180
Hargreaves, W. A., 78
Hazelton, N., 264
Health Care Financing Administration (HCFA), 21, 26, 225, 232
Heinrichs, D. W., 195
Herman, G. S., 138, 139
Herz, M. I., 143, 160
Hillier, V. F., 13
Hing, E., 63, 117, 121
Hingson, R. W., 241
Hirsch, B., 121
Hitchcock, J., 140
Hoeper, E. W., 13
Hogarty, G. E., 171
Hoiberg, A., 45
Holzer, C., 15
Hopper, K., 197
Hyatt, P., 230

Intagliata, J., 187, 189

Jacobson, A., 245
Joffe, J. M., 241
Johnson, P. J., 234
Johnson, S., 152
Johnston, M., 36
Jonas, S., 102

Jones, K., 93, 241, 246

Kamlet, M. S., 219, 223
Kane, J. M., 263
Kaplan, D. M., 159
Karon, B. P., 128
Keith, S. J., 186, 188, 263
Kendall, L. M., 166
Kessler, L. G., 15
Kessler, M., 241
Kiesler, C. A., 14, 16, 18, 45, 65, 66, 77, 79, 80, 99, 100, 109, 152, 153, 167, 170, 174, 176, 180, 198, 235, 241, 247, 253, 254, 261, 266, 267, 273
Kirby, M. W., 164, 165, 166, 172, 176
Kirk, S. A., 136, 138, 184
Kirshner, M. C., 183
Kittredge, L. D., 139
Klee, G. D., 132
Klerman, G. L., 65, 131
Kochansky, G., 152
Koller, D. L., 125
Koranyi, E. K., 244, 245
Kovacs, K. V., 138
Kozak, L. J., 79
Kramer, M., 15, 133, 204
Krowinski, W. J., 163, 164, 178, 198

Lamb, H. R., 180, 183, 187, 189, 190, 194, 195, 197
Landman, J. T., 241
Langsley, D. G., 159, 160
Lauriat, A. S., 196, 197
Leaf, P., 15, 186, 188
Leet, R., 245
Lefkowitz, M. M., 136, 137
Lentz, R. J., 172, 180, 238
Levenson, A. I., 55
Levenson, A. J., 161
Levin, G., 163
Levine, D., 262
Levine, D. R., 24, 204
Levine, D. S., 24, 204
Levine, M., 40, 262

Leviton, L., 255
Licht, M. H., 255
Lieberman, M. A., 236
Lima, L. H., 93
Link, B., 15
Liptzin, B., 248, 254
Longabaugh, R., 162
Lorei, T. W., 148
Love, R. E., 180, 235

Machotka, P., 160
MaCurdy, E. A., 166
Malamud, T. J., 138, 139
Manderscheid, R. W., 41, 65, 186, 191
Mandrill, D., 264
Manheimer, D., 241
Mann, H., 30
Manzanares, D. L., 110
March, R., 164
Marks, E., 249
Marks, J. N., 13
Marmor, J., 254
Marshall, A. W., 34
Marx, A. J., 153
Mason, A., 186
Mason, J. H., 138, 139
Matthews, D., 241
Matthews, S. M., 158, 263
May, P. R., 205
Mayer, J. E., 136
McCaffree, K., 206
McCue, S., 230
McEwen, C. A., 144
McGaw, B., 240
McGill, C. W., 195
McGuire, T. G., 18, 241, 247, 248, 249, 254
McSweeny, A. J., 125
Mechanic, D., 15, 18, 31, 39, 201, 220, 247, 254, 261, 272
Mellinger, G., 241
Melnick, G. A., 102
Melnick, M., 206
Menn, A. Z., 158
Mental Health Reports, 228, 239

Mesnikoff, A., 143
Meyer, N. G., 131
Meyerson, A. T., 138, 139
Millazzo-Sayre, L., 85, 91
Miller, S. I., 245
Miller, T. I., 172
Milowe, I. D., 25
Minkoff, K., 183, 185, 204
Moien, M., 79
Moldawsky, S., 227
Moore, F. D., 222
Moran, T. J., 242
Morrissey, J. P., 206
Mosher, L. R., 18, 158, 169, 177, 178, 179
Mumford, E., 247
Mushkin, S. J., 203
Muszynski, S., 14, 21, 24
Myers, J. K., 15

Nasrallah, A. T., 128
Nassimbene, R., 205, 206
National Center for Health Statistics, 13, 67, 78
National Institute of Mental Health (NIMH), 22, 36, 42-43, 134, 213, 235, 248,   257, 258-259
Nebel, M. E., 130
Nelson, S. H., 18
Neugebauer, R., 15
Neuhauser, D., 232
Newman, F. L., 18, 240
Newman, H. N., 21, 24, 26
Nielson, A. C., 13

Orso, C., 245
Orvaschel, H., 15
Ozarin, L. D., 130

Packard, E. P. W., 35
Palinkas, L. A., 45
Paris, M., 25
Parry, H., 241
Pasamanick, B., 161
Patrick, C., 247
Patton, R. E., 38, 39

Paul, G. L., 172, 180, 181, 182, 185, 238, 255, 270
Pepper, B., 182, 183, 187, 188, 189, 190
Perlman, B., 25
Pinel, P., 30, 33
Platman, S. R., 184
Polak, P. R., 164, 165, 166, 172, 176
President's Commission on Mental Health, 15, 39, 182, 183, 184, 236, 262

Rabkin, J. G., 190, 264, 265
Ray, W. A., 242, 262
Redick, R. W., 41, 59, 62, 98
Regier, D. A., 15, 57, 58, 65, 242, 245, 248
Rich, R. F., 18, 257
Rittenhouse, J. D., 165
Rodgers, C. W., 140
Rodnick, E. H., 195
Roper, M. T., 158
Rose, S. M., 236
Rosen, B. M., 66, 186
Rosenblatt, A., 136
Rosenhan, D. L., 144, 175
Rosenstein, M. J., 41, 65, 66, 85, 91
Rossman, E., 138, 139
Rothman, D. J., 146
Rubin, J., 39, 108, 204, 205, 206, 213, 264, 272
Rush, B., 29
Ryglewicz, H., 182, 183

Sackett, K. L., 110
Sainer, J. S., 238
Saltman, R. B., 102
Saunders, C. A., 129
Saxe, L., 240
Scarpitti, F. R., 161
Schaffner, W., 242
Scheff, B. H., 162
Schendler, C. E., 102
Schlesinger, H. J., 247, 254
Schmidt, K., 25
Schulberg, H. C., 18, 141, 236

Schur, E. M., 145
Schwab, J. J., 244
Schwartz, A. H., 25
Schwartz, S. R., 189, 190, 192
Schwartz, W. B., 102
Scotch, N. A., 241
Scull, A. T., 39, 146
Scully, D., 140
Shadish, W. R., 125, 126, 252
Shaeffer, D. E., 141
Shank, E. L., 93
Shapiro, R., 152
Shapiro, S., 15
Sharfstein, S. S., 14, 25, 130, 247
Sharratt, S., 135
Sheehan, D. M., 205
Shore, M. F., 152
Sibulkin, A. E., 45, 65, 66, 79, 80, 99, 100, 109
Silber, B. G., 125
Silverman, I., 129
Silverman, P. R., 236
Sirrocco, A., 89
Skinner, E. A., 15
Sletten, I. W., 130
Smith, C. M., 206
Smith, F., 140
Smith, G., 110
Smith, J., 263
Smith, M. L., 172, 240, 241, 242, 243, 244
Social Security Administration, 21, 232, 233
Solomon, P., 186, 190, 193, 194
Sonis, A. C., 140
Sorenson, J. E., 213
Spearly, J. L., 142
Spitzer, R. L., 143
Stein, L. I., 145, 153, 156, 171, 173, 178, 180, 195, 238, 272, 273
Stern, S., 264
Stickney, S. K., 138
Stoltzman, R., 15
Strahan, G. W., 89
Strauss, J. S., 128
Straw, R. B., 125, 152, 176

Strayer, R. G., 186, 188
Struening, E. L., 166
Sundberg-Stirling, M., 164
Sutton, J. F., 89
Szasz, T., 144

Taber, M. A., 236
Talbott, J. A., 183
Taub, H. A., 138
Taube, C. A., 15, 42, 43, 47, 57, 62, 63, 65, 66, 69, 85, 91, 131, 183, 187, 188, 206, 207, 245, 256
Taylor, S. E., 250
Tenney, J. B., 14
Tessier, L., 166
Tessler, R., 138, 139, 186, 247
Test, M. A., 145, 152, 153, 156, 168, 171, 178, 180, 195, 238, 272, 273
Therrien, M. E., 184
Thomas, R. F., 206
Thompson, J. W., 57, 65, 66, 139, 206
Thornton, J. C., 25
Thrasher, J. H., 139
Tischler, G. L., 15
Toff, G., 230, 232
Towery, O. B., 25
Treat, A., 120
Tringo, J., 264
Tuerk, I., 133
Tuke, W., 30, 33
Tyson, R. L., 245

Urban Institute, 183
U.S. Bureau of the Census, 42, 208
U.S. Senate, 62, 112
Uyeda, M. K., 227, 232

Valins, S., 263

Van Nostrand, J. F., 121
VandenBos, G. R., 128, 241
Vannicelli, M., 162
Vergare, M., 196
Vischi, T. R., 93, 213, 220, 241, 246
Vitalo, R., 135
Von Korff, M., 15

Waldo, D. R., 102
Wallen, J., 77, 78
Washburn, S., 162
Watson, N., 120
Weinstein, A. S., 131, 132, 135
Weisbrod, B. A., 156, 157, 158, 173, 247
Weiss, C. H., 257
Weissman, M. M., 15
Wheeler, J. R. C., 102
Wilder, J. F., 162, 163, 170
Williams, T. A., 13
Willner, S. G., 204
Wilson, F. A., 232
Windle, C., 140
Witkin, M. J., 19, 27, 41, 57, 59, 65, 139, 213
Wolford, J. A., 140
Wolpert, E. R., 184
Wolpert, J., 184
World Health Organization, 245
Wunsch-Hitzig, R., 15

Yates, E. T., 240
Young, D. W., 102

Zappolo, A., 121
Zeckhauser, R. J., 222
Zeldow, P. B., 138
Zimmer, J. G., 120
Zook, C. J., 222, 250
Zusman, J., 39
Zwerling, I., 162, 169

INDEX

Admissions
  definition, 44
  private mental hospitals, 55
  state mental hosptals, 46-47
  VA medical centers, 50-55
Alternative care, 148-175, 234-240
  alternative explanations for effects,
    169-170
  alternative services, 236, 271
  community living approach,
    153-158
  comparison with mental
    hospitalization, 270
  complexities of treatment, 171-172
  components of successful programs,
    239
  cost-benefit analysis, 157-158
  covariance techniques, 150-151
  day care treatment, 160-161,
    162-163, 163-164
  developing concensus, 167-169
  family crisis therapy, 159-160
  family unit therapy, 165-166
  home treatment, 166-167
  hostel, 158-159
  incentives, 180, 273
  interaction of diagnosis and
    efficacy, 173
  issues, 238-240
  length of assessment period, 171
  matched pairs technique, 151
  power of the effect, 171
  problems in measurement, 170
  public health nurse visits, 161
  random assignment, 150-151
  readmissions, 174
  research design requirements,
    148-151
  Soteria, 158
  summary, 174-175
  true experiments, 152-167

  types of alternative treatment,
    173-174
  use of drugs, 172
  volunteer groups, 236
Antipsychotic medication
  see Drugs
Attitudes
  and public policy, 265
  group homes, 264
  quality of care, 264
  stigma, 264
  toward mental illness, 264-265

Beers, Clifford, 35, 272

Chronic mental patient, 182-195
  characteristics of, 188-192
  Community Support Program, 186,
    190, 191, 192-195, 235
  crime, 190-192
  definition, 183-185, 270
  estimated number of, 183
  living arrangements, 185-188
  use of services, 192-195
Community mental health centers,
    18-19, 27
  deinstitutionalization, 266
  effect on reducing state hospital
    admissions, 140-142
  episodes, 55
  inpatient days, 55, 104, 105
  length of stay, 93-94
  mental health service delivery,
    252-253
  national expenditures, 213
  rate of episodes, 71
  shift in locus of inpatient care,
    139-142
  Systems Act, 18, 36, 37
Community support system, 234-236,
    271

Community Support Program, 186, 190. 191, 192-195, 235
Costs
  see National Expenditures

Decision to hospitalize, 177-180, 250-252, 270, 271
  assumptions, 250-251
  systematic error, 250
Deinstitutionalization, 19-20, 38
  alternative services, 236
  characteristics of the deinstitutionalized, 188-192
  chronicity, 177-198, 184
  community mental health centers, 266
  controversy, 11, 145-147
  crime, 190-192
  drugs, 38-39, 262, 263
  forms of hospital treatment, 143
  homeless, 195-198
  ideological clash, 178-179
  length of stay, 97-99
  living arrangements, 185-188
  nursing homes, 269
  open hospital system, 38
  O'Connor v. Donaldson, 39
  subsequent treatment, 177-198
  themes, 11
  use of services, 192-195
  Wyatt v. Stickney, 39
Diagnosis of mental disorder
  mislabeling, 13
  recognition and detection of, 13, 120, 219, 245
Diagnostic and Statistical Manual, 13
Discharges
  general hospitals, 58-59
  Indian Health Services, 63
  military hospitals, 64
  VA medical centers, 51-55
Dix, Dorothea, 30-31
Drugs
  alternative care, 172
  and mental health policy, 241-244, 262-264

and psychotherapy, 242-244
attribution for changes in behavior, 263
deinstitutionalization, 38-39, 262, 263
effectiveness, 241-244, 263-264, 271
in nursing homes, 262-263
types of, 243

Earle, Pliny, 34
Epidemiologic Catchment Area (ECA) study, 5-16
Epidemiology of mental disorders, 15
Episodes
  community mental health centers, 55
  definition, 44
  duplication in reporting, 73-75
  general hospitals, 58-59, 256
  general hospitals without units, 58-59, 268
  Indian Health Service, 63
  military hospitals, 64
  national total, 65
  private mental hospitals, 55
  residential treatment centers, 59
  state mental hospitals, 47
  VA medical centers, 50-55

Fuller, Robert, 35

General hospitals
  characteristics of discharges, 76-77
  discharges, 58-59
  episodes, 58-59, 256
  inpatient days, 105
  length of stay, 91-93, 268, 270
  national expenditures, 213, 270
  rate of episodes, 71, 75, 268
  referral to other facilities, 78
  without psychiatric units, 27, 58-59, 75, 76-77, 268
Gray, John, 32

Homeless, 11, 195-198, 270, 273

Indian Health Service
  discharges, 63
  episodes, 63
  length of stay, 94
Inpatient days for mental disorders,
      273
  community mental health centers,
      55, 104, 105
  definition, 81-83, 101
  general hospitals, 105
  hospital cost containment, 102-103,
      108, 109, 256
  private mental hospitals, 105
  proportion of all hospital days,
      101-109, 256, 268-269
  residential treatment centers, 104,
      105
  sources of data, 103-104
  state mental hospitals, 105
  VA medical centers, 105
Insurance, 247-250
  adverse selection, 248-249
  alternative care, 179
  community care programs, 178
  effects on hospitalization rates, 28,
      220-222
  moral hazard, 247
  price elasticity, 247-248
  reimbursement, 13
    see also Medicaid, Medicare
Intermediate care facilities, 229-233
International Classification of
      Diseases, 13

Joint Commission on Mental Illness
      and Health, 29, 31, 32, 36, 37, 38,
      182

Knowledge acquisition
  see Knowledge use
Knowledge use, 256-266
  barriers to, 256-266
  for public policy, 257
  resistance to change, 265-266, 271,
      272

Length of stay
  community mental health centers,
      93-94
  definitions, 81-83
  deinstitutionalization, 97-99
  general hospitals, 91-93, 268, 270
  general hospitals without psychiatric
      units, 93, 268
  Indian Health Service, 94
  military hospitals, 94-95
  private mental hospitals, 89-90
  sources of data, 83-84
  state mental hospitals, 84-85, 256,
      268
  summary of trends, 95-99
  VA medical centers, 85-89, 268

Mann, Horace, 30
Medicaid, 21-22, 224-233, 262
  coverage and limitations, 228-230
  Social Security Act, 224-225
  state variation in mental health
      coverage, 230-233
Medical offset
  see Medical Utilization
Medical utilization, 246-247
  effect of mental health services on,
      246-247
Medicare, 21, 224-233, 259
  coverage and limitations, 225-228
  Social Security Act, 224-225
Mental and physical health, 244-246,
      258, 271
Mental health policy
  and primary care, 260
  cooperation between public and
      private sectors, 273
  coordination of state and federal
      programs, 266, 271
  cost-effectiveness, 218
  court decisions, 257, 272
  de facto policy, 17, 20-24, 199, 220,
      234, 265, 268
  de jure policy, 17-20, 41, 81, 265,
      268

Mental health policy (*continued*)
  definition, 16
  drugs, 241-244, 262-264
  health policy domination of,
      258-262, 271
  national data base, 12, 14, 273
  national health insurance, 250
  resistance to change, 265-266, 271,
      272
  service delivery sites, 271, 273
  sickness ideology, 261
Mental health service delivery,
      252-255, 271, 273
  community mental health centers,
      252-253, 254
  health maintenance organizations,
      252-254
  private practice, 254
Mental Health Systems Act, 39-40
Mental hospitalization,
  19th century, 30-35
  20th century, 35-40
  active treatment, 144-145
  appropriate training of personnel,
      238, 271
  barriers to, 249
  colonial United States, 29-30
  dangerous behavior, 272
  decision to hospitalize, 270, 271
  definition, 17, 43
  drugs, 32, 38
  early history, 28
  effectiveness of, 12, 27, 33-34,
      143-147, 180-182, 268
  history, 27-40
  moral treatment, 30, 31, 32, 33, 34
  myths, 256, 267
  quality of care, 145, 271
  relearning, 145
  research needs, 234-255, 271
  self-labeling, 145
  social learning approach, 180-182
  state hospital system, 27
  stigma, 78
  total institutions, 144-145

  see also Alternative care,
      Episodes, Inpatient days for
      mental disorders, Length of
      stay, Rate of mental
      hospitalization, Residents,
      Trends in mental hospitalization
Military hospitals
  discharges, 64
  episodes, 64
  length of stay, 94-95

National expenditures, 201-222, 270
  community mental health centers,
      213
  cost-effectiveness, 218
  cost per inpatient day, 205-206, 270
  cost per stay, 205-206, 215, 270
  costs of inappropriate treatment, 220
  direct costs, 203-205, 270
  effects of insurance practices on
      hospitalization rates, 220-222
  general hospitals, 213, 270
  indirect costs, 203-205, 220
  issues in calculating cost, 203-205
  personal distress, 203
  policy condiderations, 201-203
  private psychiatric hospitals, 208
  proportion for inpatient care,
      218-220
  residential treatment centers, 213
  sources of data, 207-208
  state mental hospitals, 208
  summary, 222
  total costs, 216
  transfer payments, 204-205
  VA medical centers, 211
National Institute of Mental Health,
      22, 36, 42-43, 134, 213, 235,
      248, 257, 258-259
National Institutes of Health, 258-259
National Plan for the Chronically
      Mentally Ill, 182, 185
Nursing homes, 110-126, 273
  beds, 110-112
  chronically mentally ill, 120

comparison of nursing home and
   state mental hospital trends,
   117-126
deaths, 112
deinstitutionalization, 110-126, 269
drugs, 262-263
rate of residents with mental
   disorders, 117, 123
residents, 62-63, 110-112
residents with mental disorders,
   114-117, 269
senility, 63, 115
state mental hospitals, 110-126
transfer to state hospitals, 121-126

O'Connor v. Donaldson, 39
Omnibus Budget Reconciliation Act,
   40, 232

Packard, E.P.W.,, 35
Physical and mental health, 244-246,
   258, 271
Pinel, Phillipe, 30, 33
President's Commission on Mental
   Health, 15, 39, 182, 183, 184,
   236, 262
Private mental hospitals
   admissions, 55
   episodes, 55
   inpatient days, 105
   length of stay, 89-90
   national expenditures, 208
   rate of episodes, 71
   residents, 55
Psychoactive Drugs
   see Drugs
Psychotherapy
   and drugs, 242-244
   effectiveness, 240-241, 271
   meta-analysis, 240
Psychotropic Drugs
   see Drugs

Rate of mental hospitalization, 69-80,
   268, 273

community mental health centers,
   71
duplication in reporting of episodes,
   73-75, 78
general hospitals, 71, 75, 268
national total, 73
NIMH data, 69, 71
population at risk, 270
private mental hospitals, 71
sources of data, 70-73
state mental hospitals, 71
VA medical centers, 71
Readmissions, 127-142
   alternative care, 174
   characteristics of person related to,
      136-137
   characteristics of treatment related
      to, 137
   deinstitutionalization, 127, 129
   insufficient time span, 128
   methodological problems, 128-129
   national needs, 129-130
   net live releases, 131, 132
   New York State, 131-132
   NIMH data, 130-131
   percentage rehospitalized, 135-136
   readmission index, 132
   relation of aftercare to, 137-139
   reliability of data, 128
   research design flaws, 128-129
   revolving door, 79, 127, 129-135,
      269
   state and county registers, 132-135
   summary of revolving door data,
      142
   treatment effectiveness and, 130
Research needs, 234-255, 271
Residential treatment centers
   definition, 59
   episodes, 59
   inpatient days, 104, 105
   national expenditures, 213
Residents
   definition, 44
   nursing homes, 62-63, 110-112

Residents (*continued*)
  private mental hospitals, 55
  state mental hospitals, 27, 46
  VA medical centers, 50-55
Revolving door, 79, 127, 129-135,
    269
  summary of data, 142
    See also Readmissions
Rush, Benjamin, 29

Skilled nursing facilities, 229-233
State mental hospitals
  admissions, 46-47
  comparison of nursing home and
      state mental hospital trends,
      117-126
  deaths, 112
  episodes, 47
  inpatient days, 105
  length of stay, 84-85, 256, 268
  national expenditures, 208
  net releases by age, 114, 269
  nursing homes, 110-126
  rate of episodes, 71
  residents, 27, 46
  residents with organic brain
      disorder, 112-114
  transfer from nursing homes,
      121-126
  trends in residents by age, 112-114,
      269

Trends in mental hospitalization
  commmunity mental health centers,
      55

general hositals without psychiatric
    units, 58-59
general hospitals, 58-59
history of surveys, 41-43
Indian Health Service, 63
military hospitals, 64
nursing homes, 62-63, 269
private mental hospitals, 55
rate of mental hospitalization, 69-80
residential treatment centers, 59
sources of data, 44-45
state mental hospitals, 46-47
summary, 64-65
VA medical centers, 50-55
Tuke, William, 30, 33

VA medical centers
  admissions, 50-55
  discharges, 51-55
  episodes, 50-55
  inpatient days, 105
  length of stay, 85-89, 268
  national expenditures, 211
  rate of episodes, 71
  residents, 50-55
Volunteer groups, 234, 236-238
  self-help groups, 236-237
  self-selection, 237

Wyatt v. Stickney, 39

About the Authors

Charles A. Kiesler is Provost of Vanderbilt University. He received a Ph.D. in social psychology from Stanford University in 1963 and has published extensively in the area of attitude change. Dr. Kiesler was formerly Bingham Professor of Psychology and Dean of Humanities and Social Sciences at Carnegie-Mellon University. He previously held positions as Executive Director of the American Psychological Association, Chairman of the Psychology Department at the University of Kansas, and Associate Professor of Psychology at Yale University. His research interests are in public policy, particularly mental health policy. A current federally funded project supports a reanalysis of the national data base regarding the treatment of mental disorders in general hospitals.

Amy E. Sibulkin is Research Associate at the Vanderbilt Institute for Public Policy Studies, where she is studying the characteristics of people treated for mental disorders in general hospitals. After receiving a Ph.D. in human development and family studies at Cornell University in 1981, she was Research Associate in the Department of Psychology at Carnegie-Mellon University. Dr. Sibulkin has published a series of articles on national trends in mental hospitalization with Dr. Charles Kiesler.